CANCER ETIOLOGY, DIAGNOSIS AND TREATMENTS

FIGHTING LUNG CANCER THROUGH THE HER FAMILY OF SURFACE RECEPTORS

CANCER ETIOLOGY, DIAGNOSIS AND TREATMENTS

Additional books in this series can be found on Nova's website
under the Series tab.

Additional e-books in this series can be found on Nova's website
under the e-book tab.

CANCER ETIOLOGY, DIAGNOSIS AND TREATMENTS

FIGHTING LUNG CANCER THROUGH THE HER FAMILY OF SURFACE RECEPTORS

DIEGO MÁRQUEZ-MEDINA, M.D., PH.D.
EDITOR

NOVA BIOMEDICAL

New York

Library of Congress Cataloging-in-Publication Data

ISBN: 978-1-63321-092-9

Library of Congress Control Number: 2014939923

Published by Nova Science Publishers, Inc. † New York

To all those who think that no place is small,
Or that no one is trifling.
Eventual help can arrive from the littlest being.
So, if you look around,
The hardest condition can be mitigated.
Encourage, believe, fight, live.
Reward is the own way.

Contents

Foreword

Rafael Rosell, M.D.
Medical Oncology Service, Catalan Institute of Oncology,
Germans Trias i Pujol University Hospital of Badalona (Spain),
President of the Spanish Lung Cancer Group

This book tackles the challenges posed by lung cancer, which remains one of the diseases with most dismal prognosis. To this end, Diego Marquez has gathered together a group of knowledgeable clinical investigators and researchers to provide their views and experience on this difficult and complex disease. New evidence in the genetic landscape of lung cancer clearly indicates that even the subgroup of adenocarcinomas could represent different types of diseases. Epidermal growth factor receptor (EGFR) signaling is an essential aspect of lung cancer biology and one of the major aims of this book is to decipher the clinical relevance of this pathway, especially with regard to management of non-small-cell lung cancer (NSCLC) patients.

Chemotherapy in NSCLC is not curative and has limited benefit, which can be measured in weeks or months. Cytotoxic therapy removes the incumbent clones, like a "mass extinction" event and shifts the evolutionary landscape in favor of more aggressive clones with increased levels of human epidermal growth factor receptor (HER) signaling, due in part to the enrichment of a preexisting neuregulin 1 subpopulation. Neuroregulin signaling can be mediated in these models either by the HER3 or HER4 receptor, resulting in the differential activation of downstream effectors [1]. EGFR-driven resistance in lung cancer with BRAF mutations has recently been reported. Autocrine EGFR signaling is led by c-Jun ligand expression and EGFR activation. This is one of the first examples of BRAF-EGFR signaling crosstalk in NSCLC [2].

EGFR mutations occur in 17% of NSCLC patients, who have remarkable response to EGFR-TKI but very low complete remission rates. Despite clinical response in these patients, disease progresses, as was observed in the first large-scale study in NSCLC patients with *EGFR* mutations [3]. Since then, EGFR mutation screening has been incorporated into routine clinical practice and many clinical trials have been performed, including the EURTAC study [4]. One mechanism of acquired resistance described was the presence of the T790M mutation; we and others observed have the initial presence of T790M in a significant proportion of patients [5]. We were able to validate the initial findings: more than 50% of patients included in the EURTAC study harbored the T790M before treatment and T790M significantly influenced progression-free survival (PFS) in the erlotinib arm [6]. Moreover, we were able to show the independent prognostic value of BIM mRNA expression on response, PFS and overall survival. For patients with high expression of BIM mRNA response rate was 89%, while for patients with low or intermediate expression response rate was only 22% [6]. These observations, attained through the opportunity of the EURTAC study, are of paramount relevance for new therapeutic approaches based on synthetic lethal combinations [7].

With the discovery of *EGFR* mutations in NSCLC in 2004, it was hypothesized that NSCLC cell lines with *EGFR* mutations undergo extensive apoptosis following treatment with AKT and STAT3 inhibitors and are relatively resistant to apoptosis induced by chemotherapy. This first evidence showed that mutant *EGFR* cells selectively activate AKT and signal transduction and activator of transcription (STAT) signaling pathways, which promote cell survival [8]. Surprisingly, *EGFR* mutant cells result in transient prodeath imbalance of survival and apoptotic signaling in response to EGFR inhibition. This is explained in part since expression of SHP2 is essential to the balance between ERK and PI3K/AKT and STAT activity [9]. Gefitinib never inhibits STAT3 phosphorylation in *EGFR* mutant cell lines [10], indicating that treatment with single EGFR-TKIs in *EGFR* mutant NSCLC can be incomplete and requires synthetic lethal approaches. This has been demonstrated in cell lines harboring T790M, in which afatinib is not able to abrogate phosphorylation of STAT3 or could even be more activated. For example, in the H1975 and PC9-GR, respectively [11]. The addition of IL-6 antibodies or JAK1 or STAT3 blockers to afatinib achieves inhibition of STAT3 in these afatinib-resistant cell lines, providing strong evidence that synthetic lethal approaches are warranted for optimizing therapy of *EGFR* mutant lung cancer [7].

Also, experimental evidence shows that in a subgroup of patients early adaptive drug escape to erlotinib could occur with activation of STAT3, Bcl2 and BCLXL, which is associated with a proliferative quiescence state [12]. Further clinical research is warranted since this subgroup of patients could be identified from the beginning and offered the opportunity to further improve clinical outcomes. However, in the majority of *EGFR* mutant NSCLC patients, response is meager, as we have demonstrated based on BIM mRNA expression [6, 7]. This raises the hypothesis that in the majority of patients, intrinsic mechanisms of resistance could be led by activation of other receptor tyrosine kinases, independent of EGFR signaling. One potential mechanism could be activation of these receptors and crosstalk between them through production of hepatic growth factor (HGF) from stromal cells [13]. In the near future, synthetic lethal approaches could be tested for a large group of patients in which BIM mRNA expression is low, something which can be associated with overexpression of other receptor tyrosine kinases [7]. Therefore, this inspiring book is very welcome and permits a review of several perspectives and views in the field of EGFR signaling and *EGFR* mutations in lung cancer. It can pave the way for further exploration of the multifaceted molecular mechanisms, which make NSCLC still an incurable disease. The reader will find much useful information, of great interest and applicability for clinical practice. This can also serve as stimuli for further translational research endeavors and as motivation to participate in clinical trials devoted to identification of useful biomarkers and signaling pathway crosstalk. These can be definitively treated with EGFR-TKIs partnered with drugs targeting identified components of the signaling pathways responsible for resistance to single EGFR-TKIs [7].

References

[1] Hegde GV, De La Cruz CC, Chiu C, et al. Blocking NRG1 and other ligand-mediated Her4 signaling enhances the magnitude and duration of the chemotherapeutic response of non-small cell lung cancer. *Sci Transl Med.* 2013; 5 (171): 171-118.

[2] Lin L, Asthana S, Chan E, et al. Mapping the molecular determinants of BRAF oncogene dependence in human lung cancer. *Proc Natl Acad Sci U S A.* 2014; 111 (7): E748-57.

[3] Rosell R, Moran T, Queralt C, et al. Screening for epidermal growth factor receptor mutations in lung cancer. *N Engl J Med.* 2009; 361 (10): 958-67.

[4] Rosell R, Carcereny E, Gervais R, et al. Erlotinib versus standard chemotherapy as first-line treatment for European patients with advanced EGFR mutation-positive non-small-cell lung cancer (EURTAC): a multicentre, open-label, randomised phase 3 trial. *Lancet Oncol.* 2012; 13 (3): 239-46.

[5] Rosell R, Molina MA, Costa C, et al. Pretreatment EGFR T790M Mutation and BRCA1 mRNA Expression in Erlotinib-Treated Advanced Non-Small-Cell Lung Cancer Patients with EGFR Mutations. *Clin Cancer Res.* 2011; 17 (5): 1160-8.

[6] Costa C, Molina MA, Drozdowskyj A, et al. The impact of EGFR T790M mutations and BIM mRNA expression on outcome in patients with EGFR-mutant NSCLC treated with erlotinib or chemotherapy in the randomized phase III EURTAC trial *Clinical Cancer Research.* (2014) [Epub ahead of print].

[7] Rosell R, Bivona TG, Karachaliou N. Genetics and biomarkers in personalisation of lung cancer treatment. *Lancet.* 2013; 382 (9893): 720-31.

[8] Sordella R, Bell DW, Haber DA, Settleman J. Gefitinib-sensitizing EGFR mutations in lung cancer activate anti-apoptotic pathways. *Science.* 2004; 305 (5687): 1163-7.

[9] Lazzara MJ, Lane K, Chan R, et al. Impaired SHP2-mediated extracellular signal-regulated kinase activation contributes to gefitinib sensitivity of lung cancer cells with epidermal growth factor receptor-activating mutations. *Cancer Res.* 2010; 70 (9): 3843-50.

[10] Gao SP, Mark KG, Leslie K, et al. Mutations in the EGFR kinase domain mediate STAT3 activation via IL-6 production in human lung adenocarcinomas. *J Clin Invest.* 2007; 117 (12): 3846-56.

[11] Kim Y, Ko J, Cui Z, et al. The EGFR T790M mutation in acquired resistance to an irreversible second-generation EGFR inhibitor. *Mol Cancer Ther.* 2012; 11 (3): 784-91.

[12] Fan W, Tang Z, Yin L, et al. MET-independent lung cancer cells evading EGFR kinase inhibitors are therapeutically susceptible to BH3 mimetic agents. *Cancer Res.* 2011; 71 (13): 4494-505.

[13] Gusenbauer S, Vlaicu P, Ullrich A. HGF induces novel EGFR functions involved in resistance formation to tyrosine kinase inhibitors. *Oncogene.* 2013; 32 (33): 3846-56.

About the Editor

Diego Márquez-Medina, M.D., Ph.D.

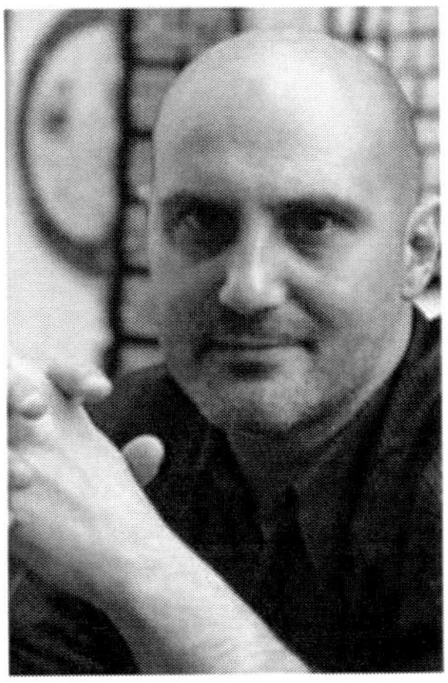

Dr. Márquez-Medina obtained his Practitioner Accreditation for the Public Health Systems of the European Community States and Medical and Surgical Degree at the Spanish University of Córdoba in 1994. From 1995 to 1998, he was awarded with a University Scholarship and trained as a basic researcher in the Experimental Unit of the University Hospital Reina Sofia of Córdoba that culminated obtaining his Doctor of Philosophy Degree in Medicine and Surgery in 1998.

In 1995, he won a position as a Medical Oncology Resident and was trained in the Integral Oncology Department of the University Hospital San Cecilio of Granada from 1998 to 2002, alternating with stages in Pediatric Oncology, and Hematology and Bone Marrow Transplant Divisions in the Italian Istituto Nazionale per lo Studio e la Cura dei Tumori of Milano.

Currently, he is a Staff Physician in the Medical Oncology Department of the University Hospital Arnau de Vilanova of Lleida (Spain) on charge of patients with thoracic malignancies, and he has focused on medical practice and research in this area.

Tel: 00346 292 85969
Email: dmarmed@hotmail.com

Introduction

1. Why Lung Cancer?

Lung cancer remains one of the biggest challenges for modern oncology. It is the most common and most lethal malignancy worldwide, with the same incidence as breast or colorectal cancer, but causing 1.4 million diseases every year; almost as many as breast and colorectal cancers combined. As a disease, lung cancer demands our maximum abilities as researchers, physicians, and care-givers; Moreover, it warrants a multidisciplinary approach. Geneticists, biologists and pharmaceutics form the basis of molecular investigation and knowledge. Pneumology, internal medicine, radiology, pathology, thoracic surgery, radiation, and medical oncology departments are essential members of thoracic tumor boards. Palliative care physicians, specialized nurses, psycho-oncologists, general practitioners, and trained volunteers are indispensable for the healing and management of lung cancer patients.

Nevertheless, 5-year overall survival rates are less than 20% for lung cancer patients. Half these patients are diagnosed at such an advanced stage that cure cannot be considered a realistic aim, and over 75% of cases selected for a curative treatment eventually relapse within five years. Moreover, recent advances in treatment have been limited to the metastatic setting and do not provide a great long-term benefit in terms of survival.

2. Why the Epidermal Growth Factor Receptor?

The epidermal growth factor receptor (EGFR) is overexpressed in over 80% of lung cancer. The identification of some conformational mutations in the *EGFR* that increases the efficacy of tyrosine kinase inhibitors against the receptor unlocks a new era in understanding and treatment of lung cancer. EGFR tyrosine kinase inhibitors (EGFR-TKI) greatly prolong disease-free survival of those patients harboring sensitizing *EGFR* mutations, and have been suggested as an essential tool in the therapeutic repertoire.

This volume has been put together with the aim of serving as an updated compendium of biology and applications and a look at the future of anti-human epidermal growth factor family of surface receptors therapy in lung cancer. It pretends to be the first of a series of monographs covering different strategies for lung cancer treatment. Each one of these monographs are expected to be written by members of different internationally recognized collaborative groups; the Spanish Lung Cancer Group (SLCG) has been chosen to write the first volume.

Headed by Rafael Rosell, the SLCG is a multicentre and multidisciplinary group of over 300 oncologists, surgeons, and researchers from more than 150 hospitals. It was created in 1991 with the purpose of improving the treatment of lung cancer through investigation and prevention. The SLCG has taken part in more than 70 protocols and clinical trials involving at least 10,000 lung cancer patients, and has made great contributions to many therapeutic arenas. The NATCH trial in the neoadjuvant setting, the SCAT and the BREC trials of customized treatment, and the RENO trial of chemoradiation stand out among their recent contributions. The performance and publication of a large-scale screening for *EGFR*-mutations in 2105 NSCLC patients from 129 Spanish institutions, as well as the TARGET trial, were early efforts to study anti-EGFR treatments. This culminated in the publication of the EURTAC trial, the first study to confirmed the improvement in tolerability, response rate and progression-free survival of erlotinib over conventional chemotherapy as first line therapy for Caucasian patients.

3. Summary of the Book

"Fighting lung cancer through the HER family of surface receptors" aims to exhaustively review the molecular basis and applications of any therapy targeted against HER receptors in lung cancer; each chapter in the book has been overseen by a recognized member of the SLCG. Nevertheless, this handbook is not an official SLCG publication. Authors have contributed their respective chapters independently of their membership in the SLCG, and chapters reflect authors' own opinions. Neither the SLCG, the Editor, nor the Publisher of the book are responsible for authors' viewpoints.

The *foreword* of this edition was kindly and perspicaciously written by Dr. Rafael Rosell, president of the SLCG and one of the most important lung cancer investigators and practitioners in the world. I would like to thank him publically for his continuous support of all my humble initiatives.

To begin with, Amaia Ojanguren et al. explore the lung cancer predicament in the chapter *Lung cancer I. Epidemiology, pathology, and diagnosis.* They exhaustively review the epidemiology of lung cancer, and discuss the main risk factors for the disease. New histological classifications and techniques to provide an accurate diagnosis and work up are described, linked to future challenges in molecular diagnostics.

Next, Oscar Juan reviews the role of conventional chemotherapy as systemic treatment for lung cancer in contrast to target therapies. *Lung cancer II. Conventional treatment for advanced non-small cell lung cancer* describes the history of chemotherapy from the introduction of platinum-based doublets to the development of customized therapies according to histology or molecular findings, the combination with anti-angiogenic drugs, the indications and benefits of second and third line therapies, and the maintenance chemotherapy.

Angeles Montero describes several advances in the understanding of molecular alterations in lung cancer that have improved survival and patients' quality of life. The nature and significance of activating mutations in *EGFR* are explained in *Biology I. Human*

Epidermal Growth Factor Receptors in health and tumor cells. Following directly on from this, *Biology II. Etiology and histology of lung cancer according to the presence of alterations in the human epidermal growth factor family of receptors* explores those clinical and pathological phenomena related to HER alterations, and the ability to predict response to EGFR-TKI.

In addition, Beatriz Bellosillo et al. explain the most common methodologies to analyze HER in *Laboratory I. Analysis of Human Epidermal Growth Factor Receptors: Conventional analysis,* while Javier Hernández anticipates the future of HER analysis in *Laboratory II. Experimental analysis of Human Epidermal Growth Factor Receptors*.

Evolutionary changes in the HER expression are discussed by Santiago Viteri in *Timing I. Dynamic analysis of Human Epidermal Growth Factor Receptors. Role of rebiopsy.* Teresa Moran et al. analyze the right time to analyze EGFR mutations and begin anti-EGFR treatment in *Timing II. Appropriate time to determine the presence of EGFR mutation and sequence of treatment*.

Results of EGFR-TKI application in unselected patients with lung cancer are described by Edurne Arriola et al. in *Treatment I. Treatment of unselected patients with Epidermal Growth Factor Tyrosine Kinase Inhibitors.* Ramón Palmero reviews the efficacy of those EGFR-TKIs over molecularly selected patients in *Treatment II. Treatment of selected NSCLC patients*.

Upcoming anti-HER therapies are advanced by García-Campelo et al. in *Future I. Still un-approved drugs.* Elsa Dalmau et al. explore the eventual role of anti-HER therapies in early lung cancer in the chapter *Future II. Targeted therapies in early-stage non-small cell lung cancer*.

Jordi Remón et al. describe mechanisms which permit acquired resistance to anti-HER therapies and the experimental strategies to bypass them in *Resistance I. Acquired resistance to Epidermal Growth Factor Receptor Tyrosine Kinase Inhibitors in EGFR-mutant Non-Small Cell Lung Cancer,* whilst I review conventional salvage therapies for anti-HER resistance in *Resistance II. Conventional salvage therapies for the resistance to anti-human epidermal growth factor receptor treatments*.

Finally, the application of anti-HER therapies in other malignancies is examined by Elena Aguirre, Yolanda García and Teresa Taberner in *Other malignancies. Breast, gynecological, head and neck, and Digestive cancers,* accompanied by a *self-correcting test* for readers.

I sincerely hope you enjoy the book and learn from it as much as we have learned and enjoyed writing it.

Diego Márquez-Medina, M.D., Ph.D.
February, the 26th, 2014

In: Fighting Lung Cancer through the HER Family ...
Editor: Diego Márquez-Medina
ISBN: 978-1-63321-092-9

Chapter 1

Lung Cancer I. Epidemiology, Pathology and Diagnosis. Tissue Sampling

***Amaia Ojanguren, M.D., Ph.D.*[1]*, Miriam Barrecheguren, M.D.*[2] *and Iñigo Ojanguren, M.D.*[2]**

[1]General Surgery Department, Thoracic Surgery Division,
Arnau de Vilanova University Hospital of Lleida, Spain
[2]Respiratory Department,
Vall d'Hebron University Hospital of Barcelona, Spain

Abstract

Lung cancer is the leading cause of cancer and cancer death since 1985. The 5-year survival rate in the United States and Europe is 15.6% and 10%, respectively. Lung cancer is the consequence of combining the exposure to etiologic agents with the individual susceptibility. Smoke is the main risk factor for the lung cancer development. There are over 1.1 billion smokers worldwide and, if the smoke patterns do not change, this number will increase to 1.9 billion by 2025. Over 70% of lung cancer debuts in an advanced, un-resectable stage, which warrants an accurate histological diagnosis based on cytology and small biopsies to define the better treatment for each lung cancer subtype. The International Association for the Study of Lung Cancer/American Thoracic Society/European Respiratory Society has recently introduced modifications in the lung adenocarcinoma classification, and modified the previous Word Health Organization carcinoma classification. Immunohistochemistry based on the antibody identification of specific antigens plays a main role in the histological diagnosis of lung cancer. The development of techniques to detect eventual targets for molecular treatments in lung cancer specimens is necessary for modern treatment algorithms.

1. Epidemiology

Since 1985, lung cancer is considered the most common and lethal malignancy worldwide. In 2010, the American Cancer Society estimated a total of 239,320 new cases and 161,250 lung cancer related deaths in the United States. In 2008, more than 1.6 million people were diagnosed with lung cancer and 1.4 million died as a consequence of the disease around the World; it represents 18% of cancer deaths [1, 2].

Smoke is the main risk factor for the development of lung cancer. Almost 80-90% of bronchopulmonary carcinomas are related to tobacco smoking [3, 4], there are over 1.1 billion smokers worldwide and, if the smoke patterns do not change, this number will increase to 1.9 billion by 2025 [5].

1.1. Survival

The 5-year overall survival rate for lung cancer in the United States and Europe is 15.6% and 10%, respectively, although it widely varies according to the baseline stage from 52% in early, to 24% in locally advanced, and to 4% in advanced lung cancer [6].

1.2. Temporal Trends

1. 3. Age

According to the Surveillance, Epidemiology and End Results (SEER) data from 2004-2008, the median age for lung cancer diagnosis was 71 years-old. The incidence of lung cancer varies depending on the age stratum [5]: 0% from 0 to 20 years; 0.2% from 21-34 years; 1.5% from 35-44 years; 8.8% from 45-54 years; 20.9% from 55-64 years; 31.1% from 65-74 years; 29% from 75-84 years; and 8.3% beyond 85 years of age [5].

1.4. Gender

In 2008, lung cancer was the leading cause of cancer death and the most common malignancy among men worldwide. It was the second leading cause of cancer death and the fourth most common cancer among women. From 1995 to 2006, the lung cancer mortality decreased by 2% per year in men [2] meanwhile it maintained a rising incidence by 0.3% per year in women, due to the genetic predisposition and the later introduction of smoke in the female gender [7].

1.5. Geographic Patterns

The Word Health Organization (WHO) estimates that lung cancer deaths will continue increasing worldwide as a consequence of cigarette smoking. The international lung cancer rates vary depending on the smoking prevalence. Central and Eastern Europe and North America present the highest incidence of lung cancer in men (65.7 and 61.2 per 100,000 respectively), Northern Europe and North America have the highest incidence in women (35.6 and 21.3 per 100,000 respectively), and Africa has the lowest incidence of lung cancer for both gender [8].

1.6. Socioeconomic Status

The lower socioeconomic and educational status is considered and unfavorable epidemiological factor for a higher incidence of lung cancer, and a more advanced stage at diagnosis [9, 10].

2. Etiology of Lung Cancer

Lung cancer is the consequence of an exposure to different etiologic agents combined with the individual susceptibility to develop the malignancy. In 1938, Pear et al. [11] first time reported an association between the cigarette smoking and the higher risk of premature death. In 1950, two large landmark epidemiologic studies [12, 13] demonstrated that tobacco smoking was a causal factor in the development of bronchogenic carcinoma. In 1964, a case-control study by Wynder and Graham [13, 14] including 605-patients determined that, 1) the disproportionate and prolonged tobacco smoking was very important to induce bronchogenic carcinomas, 2) lung cancer in non-smoker was uncommon, and 3) a gap of 10 years or more between the smoking cessation and the lung cancer development was possible.

2.1. Tobacco

Cigarette smoking is the leading cause of lung cancer, and accounts for 80-90% of cases in the United States [15]. One in nine smokers will develop lung cancer. Long-term and heavy smokers have a 10-30-fold relative risk to develop lung cancer in comparison to never smokers (30% versus <1%) [16], and a direct relationship between this risk and the amount of smoked cigarettes (packs per day, smoking onset age, inhalation degree, nicotine and tar content, and consume of unfiltered cigarettes) have been established [17, 18].

More than 80% of lung cancer patients are tobacco smokers, and approximately 20% of cancer deaths worldwide could be prevented if tobacco smoking was eliminated. However, fewer than 20% of smokers develop a lung carcinoma [19]. The genetic susceptibility to tobacco and the exposure to environmental agents explain this variability in the lung cancer development.

The cigarette smoke contains more than 4000 chemical agents composing a complex aerosol of gas and particles in which nicotine, water, and tar are the main components. Nicotine is the most addictive factor, and tar and N-nitrosamines (TSNAs) are the main carcinogenic agents in the tobacco smoke. The International Agency for Research on Cancer has identified over 50 carcinogens in the tobacco smoke [20, 21]. TSNAs are the consequence of the nicotine nitrosation during smoking and have been related to the development of lung, oral cavity, larynx, esophagus, pancreas, and bladder carcinomas. The four-(methylnitrosamino)-1(3-pyridil)-1-butanone (NNK) interferes with oncogenic and tumor suppressor genes such as the activated K-ras oncogenes reported in 24% of lung adenocarcinomas [22, 23, 24].

2.2. Never Smokers

Up to 53% of lung cancer in women, and 15% in men occur in never smokers, including all those patients that did not smoke or smoked less than 100 cigarettes during the lifetime. This incidence widely varies according to geography and for instance, up to 80% of South Asian women with lung cancer are never smokers. Adenocarcinoma is the most common histology among them. Environmental exposure, genetic factors, prior lung diseases, and infections have been proposed as risk factors for the development of lung cancer in never smokers [25].

2.3. Environmental Exposures

Lung cancer is the most common cancer associated to occupational exposures. Over 10% of lung cancer mortality could be attributable to occupational carcinogens such as asbestos, arsenic, beryllium, cadmium, chromium, nickel, silica, and diesel fumes [26, 27].

a) Asbestos:

Asbestos is the most common cause of occupational lung cancer and has a synergic effect with cigarette smoke. Those fibrous silicate minerals with fire-retardant properties and structural strength have been widely used in construction since 1800 [28]. The carcinogenic action of asbestos is known since 1940, and widely recognized as a lung carcinogen since 1950s. Those patients then have been exposed to asbestos exposure and has a fivefold excess of risk for the development of lung cancer [29].

b) Radon:

Radon is an inert gas, a decay product of radium 226 and uranium 238, which are omnipresent in soil and rock [30, 31]. Two decay products of radon emit highly damaging alpha particles that modify the DNA of the respiratory epithelium. Epidemiologic studies have demonstrated a linear relationship between radon exposure and lung cancer risk [32, 33].

2.4. Host Factors

a. Family history of lung disease:

In the meta-analyses by Lissowska et al. [34], patients with a positive family history of lung cancer present a 1.7 fold increased risk to develop a bronchogenic carcinoma.

b. Acquired lung disease:

The acquired lung diseases can be divided in two main groups, 1) the respiratory obstructive disease and, 2) the pulmonary fibrotic disease.

Table 1. Modified from the 2004 WHO Classification and the 2011 IASLC/ATS/ERS Classification of Lung Adenocarcinoma

HISTOLOGIC CLASSIFICATION OF LUNG CANCER
PREINVASIVE LESIONS • Squamous dysplasia/ carcinoma in situ (CIS) • Atypical adenomatous hyperplasia (AAH) • Adenocarcinoma in situ (AIS) (nonmucinous, mucinous, or mixed nonmucinous/mucinous) • Diffuse idiopathic pulmonary neuroendocrine cell hyperplasia (DIPNECH)
SQUAMOUS CELL CARCINOMA • Papillary • Clear cell • Small cell • Basaloid
SMALL CELL CARCINOMA • Combined small cell carcinoma
ADENOCARCINOMA • Minimally invasive adenocarcinoma (MIA) ($\leq$3 cm lepidic predominant tumour with $\leq$5 mm invasion): nonmucinous, mucinous, mixed mucinous/nonmucinous) • Invasive adenocarcinoma: lepidic predominant (formerly nonmucinous bronchioloalveolar carcinoma (BAC) pattern, with >5 mm invasion), acinar predominant, papillary predominant, micropapillary predominant, solid predominant with mucin • Variants of invasive adenocarcinoma: invasive mucinous adenocarcinoma (formerly mucinous BAC), colloid, fetal, enteric.
LARGE CELL CARCINOMA • Large cell neuroendocrine carcinoma (LCNEC) • Basaloid carcinoma • Lymphoepithelioma-like carcinoma • Clear cell carcinoma • Large cell carcinoma with rhabdoid phenotype
ADENOSQUAMOUS CARCINOMA
SARCOMATOID CARCINOMAS • Pleomorphic carcinoma • Spindle cell carcinoma • Giant cell carcinoma • Carcinosarcoma • Pulmonary blastoma • Other
CARCINOID TUMOR • Typical carcinoid (TC) • Atypical carcinoid (AC)
CARCINOMAS OF SALIVARY GLAND TYPE • Mucoepidermoid carcinoma • Adenoid cystic carcinoma • Epimyoepithelial carcinoma

Chronic obstructive pulmonary disease (COPD) is defined as an obstructive disorder of the main airflow. Tobacco smoking is the first cause of both COPD and lung cancer, and the presence of COPD is a clinically useful marker for lung cancer risk [35, 36].

The pulmonary fibrotic disease has been associated with an increased risk of lung cancer [37]. Hypothetical mechanisms for the lung carcinogenesis include 1) the malignant transformation of chronically inflamed cells, 2) epithelial hyperplasia, 3) the impaired clearance of carcinogens and, 4) different infections.

2.5. Infections

The infection by the Human Immunodeficiency Virus predisposes for the development of lung carcinomas. Once tobacco consume has been controlled, patients infected by the Human Immunodeficiency Virus present a hazard ratio of 3.6 for the development of bronchogenic carcinomas. Tobacco smoking remains the main risk factor for lung cancer in those patients. However immunosuppression and oncogenic virus co-infect contribute to increase this risk [38].

3. Pathology

Over 70% of lung cancers debut in and advanced, un-resectable stage, whose diagnosis is based on cytology and small tissue biopsies [39, 40]. Historically, lung cancers have been classified into small cell lung carcinoma (SCLC) and non-small cell lung carcinoma (NSCLC) according to differences in the tumor spread, response to treatment, and outcome.

An accurate histological definition of lung cancer is warranted in order to better define the therapeutic options [41]. In 2011, the International Association for the Study of Lung Cancer (IASLC)/ American Thoracic Society (ATS)/ European Respiratory Society (ERS) modified the lung adenocarcinoma classification, and altered the previous carcinoma classification by WHO in 2004. 2011 IASLC/ATS/ERS Classification of lung adenocarcinoma (Table 1) addressed the classification in resection specimens, and made suggestions according to tissue and cytology samples [42].

3.1. Preinvasive Lesions

The concept of preinvasive lesion has become a hot topic during the last decade due to the introduction of lung cancer early detection and lung cancer screening programs. The 2011 IASLC/ATS/ERS Classification of lung adenocarcinoma also included the concept of adenocarcinoma *in situ*.

a) Squamous dysplasia and carcinoma in situ:

During the carcinogenesis, normal bronchial mucosa suffers a multistep progress to be transformed into cancer, crossing through diverse preinvasive stages. They include hyperplasia, squamous metaplasia, dysplasia and carcinoma *in situ*, according to correlative molecular and morphologic changes. In the carcinoma *in situ* stage, the cytological atypia is noticeable alongside all the thickness of the epithelium, whereas the squamous dysplasia is classified in mild, moderate or severe depending on cytological atypia grade [43, 44].

b) Atypical adenomatous hyperplasia:

Atypical adenomatous hyperplasia is a focal proliferation of epithelial cells along the bronchioloalveolar tree, which size usually is shorter than 5 mm in diameter [45].

c) Adenocarcinoma in situ:

Adenocarcinoma *in situ* was recently added to the 2011 IASLC/ATS/ERS Classification, and histologically consist of less than 3 cm in diameter glandular proliferations with lepidic growth pattern [46, 47].

d) Diffuse idiopathic pulmonary neuroendocrine cell hyperplasia:

Diffuse idiopathic pulmonary neuroendocrine cell hyperplasia is an uncommon entity whose histology is characterized by neuroendocrine cell hyperplasia and tumorlets. It is often considered a preinvasive lesion for carcinoid tumors [48].

3.2. Squamous Cell Carcinoma

Squamous cell carcinoma represents 20% of lung cancers in the United States, and it is histologically characterized by the presence of intercellular bridges, squamous pearl formation, and cell keranitization.

The squamous cell carcinoma typically presented as a central tumor involving lobar and main bronchus. However, it could be peripheral in 50% of cases [49]. The squamous cell carcinoma can be sub-classified in papillary, clear cell, small cell, and basaloid subtypes [50, 51].

3.3. Adenocarcinoma

Adenocarcinoma accounts for 38% of lung cancers in the United States. The 2011 IASLC/ATS/ERS Classification of lung adenocarcinoma modified the previous one by WHO in 2004.

The 2011 IASLC/ATS/ERS Classification of lung adenocarcinoma introduced some new histology subtypes and developed formal criteria to diagnose lung cancer in small biopsies and cytology samples [42].

The Adenocarcinoma classification in resected specimens includes:

a) Minimally invasive adenocarcinoma:

Minimally invasive adenocarcinoma morphologic features include lepidic growth tumor 3 cm or less in diameter with 5 mm or less invasive component.

b) Invasive adenocarcinoma:

Lung adenocarcinoma could be differentiated into five groups depending on the predominant histological type: 1) lepidic predominant, 2) acinar, 3) papillary, 4) micropapillary (is recognized as a new subtype because of its poor prognosis), 5) solid with mucin predominant adenocarcinoma [52, 53].

3.4. Small Cell Carcinoma

In 2010, SCLC represented 14% of lung cancers in the United States [54]. SCLC uses to appear as a central peribronchial mass involving the surrounding tissues [55], and with an important lymph node involvement.

The histology of SCLC consists of round and fusiform shape cells with exiguous cytoplasm and unnoticed nucleoli. The 2004 WHO classification established two SCLC subtypes: SCLC (pure histology) and combined SCLC (mixture of any non-small cell type). SCLC is characterized by its aggressive course, an early metastatic spread, the presence of paraneoplastic syndromes, and a poor long-term response to chemotherapy.

3.5. Large Cell Carcinoma

Large cell carcinoma (LCC) accounts for approximately 3% of lung carcinomas in the United States [54]. LCCs are commonly found in the lung periphery as large necrotic tumors. LCC diagnosis use to be a diagnosis of exclusion, and small biopsies and cytology cannot exclude the presence of adenocarcinoma or squamous cell carcinoma components [41].

According to the 2004 WHO histological classification, LCC can be divided into: 1) large cell neuroendocrine carcinoma, 2) basaloid carcinoma, 3) lymphoepithelioma-like carcinoma, 4) clear cell carcinoma and, 5) large cell carcinoma with rhabdoid phenotype.

3.6. Typical and Atypical Carcinoid

Carcinoid tumors represent 1-2% of lung cancers [56]. Carcinoid tumors use to be centrally located with endobronchial involvement or to present periphery in a sub-pleural location. Histological features consist of moderate eosinophilic cytoplasm with finely granular chromatic pattern nuclei. Compared to typical carcinoids, atypical carcinoids have 2 and 10 mitoses per 2 mm^2 area of viable tumor or presence of necrosis.

Typical carcinoids have an excellent course once resected. Atypical carcinoids have higher rate of metastases, bigger size and lower disease free survival. The mortality rate for atypical carcinoid is approximately 30% [57].

4. Pathological Diagnosis in Lung Cancer

4.1. Cytopathology

The advent of the endoscopic ultrasonography and other imaging techniques associated with the fine needle aspirations has increased the diagnostic yield for lung cancer. Cytology has arisen as a safe, cost-effective and scarcely invasive technique, with a similar sensitivity and specificity than biopsy [58]. In the past, the diagnosis of malignancy was based on morphologic characteristics of the cells. Nowadays, immunohistochemistry and immunocytochemistry techniques based on the application of specific antibodies to detect specific antigens are routinely used to distinguish histologic subtypes of lung cancer. The development of techniques to detect molecular targets will contribute to improve the efficacy of cytology.

c) Sputum:

Induced sputum is the least invasive method to detect lung cancer, and it has been also applied to screen lung cancers in symptomatic smokers. Induced sputum has a high specificity, with a positive predictive value of 100%, and a negative predictive value of 15%. Sensitivity of an unique sputum is 45%. However, it is higher when the number of samples is increased, and in centrally located tumors. The accuracy of the cytology of sputum to diagnose and classify the lung cancer classification is low for adenocarcinoma (40%), but high for squamous cell carcinoma (77%) [59].

d) Bronchial brushing and wash:

Bronchial brushing is highly rentable in central located or endobronchial lung cancers. The sensitivity of the bronchial wash to detect lung cancer varies from 36 to 72%. However, when brushing and washing are combined with a biopsy, sensitivity rises from 68% to 88% [60, 61].

c) Bronchoalveolar lavage:

The sensitivity of bronchoalveolar lavage to detect lung cancer is 33% for tumors <2 cm, and 62% for tumors > 2 cm [62].

d) Pleural fluid:

Thoracentesis should be performed in those patients with a suspected lung cancer and pleural effusion. The cytological examination of pleural effusions is quick and minimally invasive. The sensitivity of cytology to confirm malignant pleural effusion is 50%, and ranges from 4 to 77% depending on the histological subtype and the baseline stage [63].

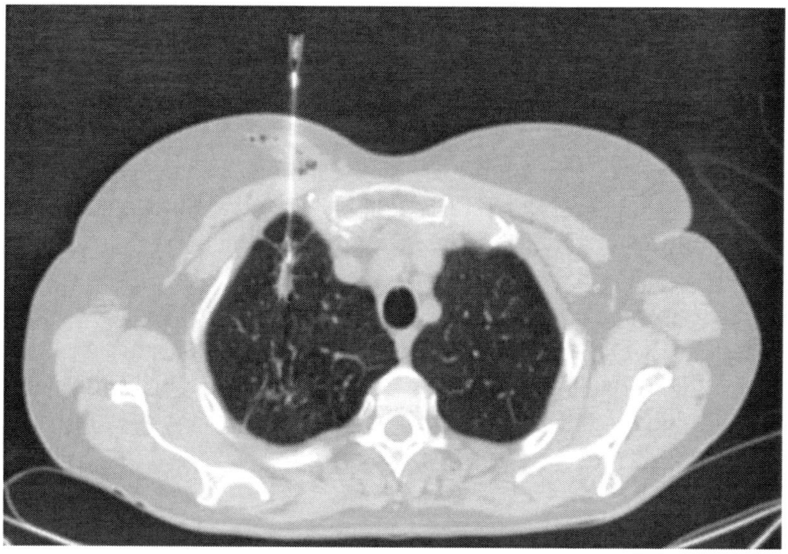

Figure 1. Coaxial technique for CT guided fine needle aspiration biopsy.

e) Fine needle aspiration cytology:

The development of imaging technologies during last decades has enabled great advances in cytopathology. The Multidetector computed tomography (CT-Scan) permitted the more precise assessment of lung lesions and provided a better biopsy planning. The CT-Scan is the standard imaging modality for guided transthoracic biopsies [64, 65]. CT-Scan is a cost-effective and available technique to biopsy deep located lesions with higher yield than transbronchial biopsy [66]. The coaxial technique is widely accomplished for CT-Scan guided biopsy, and consists of placing a CT-Scan guided needle pointed to the border of the target lesion (Figure 1). In order to verify the correct position of this introducer needle, a tissue sample is obtained with a fine biopsy needle. The opportunity to take several samples without needle repositioning decreases the percentage of complications. Sensitivity for fine needle aspiration ranges from 81 to 89%, and specificity from 75% to 100% [58].

Esophageal ultrasound (EUS) and endobronchial ultrasound (EBUS) are complementary and extremely precise techniques for lung cancer staging and diagnosis. EUS allows needle aspiration of lymph nodes stations 1L, 2L, 4L, 7, 8 and 9, with a sensitivity of 88% and specificity of 97% [67]. EBUS accesses to 1, 2R, 2L, 4R, 4L, 7, 10R, 10L and 11L stations, with a reported sensitivity of 93%, 9% false negative to detect lymph node involvement [68]. Mediastinoscopy was the gold standard for mediastinal staging until the advent of EUS and EBUS. Nowadays, mediastinoscopy is performed in fewer than 30% of surgical candidate lung cancer patients [69].

4.2. Establishing the Diagnosis of Lung Cancer

Only 1/3 of lung carcinomas are surgical candidates at the time of diagnosis. Tumor staging or comorbidity contra-indicate the surgery in the other 2/3, and they undergo chemotherapy, radiation or a combination of both in early stages, or receive palliative treatment only in the advanced stages.

The election of the most pertinent technique to perform biopsy has to be taken by a multidisciplinary tumor board with the collaboration of a pulmonologist, radiologist, thoracic surgeon, oncologist, and pathologist, and depend on the patient performance status, location and suspected stage of the tumor. The American College of Chest Physicians 3rd edition evidence based clinical practice guidelines [70, 71] (Table 2).

Table 2. Diagnosis of lung cancer. Modified from ACCP 3rd Edition evidence based clinical practice guidelines

CLINICALLY/RADIOLOGICALLY SUSPECTED LUNG CANCER	DIAGNOSTIC TECHNIQUE
Small cell lung cancer	Sputum cytology, thoracentesis, fine needle aspiration, bronchoscopy plus transbronchial needle aspiration
No extrathoracic metastatic disease and mediastinal involvement	Transbronchial fine needle aspiration, endoscopic ultrasound guided fine needle aspiration, endobronchial ultrasound guided fine needle aspiration, transthoracic fine needle aspiration or mediastinoscopy
Solitary extrathoracic site of metastasis	Fine needle aspiration of metastasis
Difficult to biopsy multiple distant metastasis	Diagnosis of primary lung lesion by least invasive method
Pleural effusion	Thoracentesis
Cytology negative pleural effusion	Pleural biopsy (surgical videothoracoscopy)
Peripheral lung nodule	Transthoracic needle aspiration, radial EBUS, electromagnetic navigation guided-bronchoscopy

References

[1] Jemal A, Bray F, Center MM, Ferlay J, Forman D. Global cancer statistics. *CA Cancer J. Clin.,* 2011; 61 (2): 69-90.

[2] Siegel R, Ward E, Brawley O, Jemal A. Cancer statistics, 2011: the impact of eliminating socioeconomic and racial disparities on premature cancer deaths. *CA Cancer J. Clin.,* 2011; 61 (4): 212-36.

[3] Parkin DM, Pisani P, Lopez AD, Masuyer E. At least one in seven cases of cancer is caused by smoking. Global estimates for 1985. *Int. J. Cancer,* 1994; 59 (4): 494-504.

[4] Wynder EL, Graham EA. Tobacco smoking as a possible etiologic factor in bronchiogenic carcinoma; a study of 684 proved cases. *J. Am. Med. Assoc.,* 1959; 143 (4): 329-36.

[5] Guindon GE, Boisclair D. Past, current and future trend in tobacco. Washington, DC: International Bank for Reconstruction and Development. *The World Bank,* 2009: 13-6.

[6] Verdecchia A, Franceschi S, Brenner H, Gatta G, Micheli A, Mangone L, Kunkler I. EUROCARE-4 Working Group. Recent cancer survival in Europe: a 2000-02 period analysis of EUROCARE 4 data. *Lancet Oncol.,* 2007; 8: 784-96.
[7] Kohler BA, Ward E, McCarthy BJ, et al. Annual report to the nation on the status of cancer, 1975-2007, featuring tumors of the brain and other nervous system. *J. Natl. Cancer Inst., 2011*; 103 (9): 714-36.
[8] Parkin DM, Bray F, Ferlay J, Pisani P. Global cancer statistics, 2002. *CA Cancer J. Clin.,* 2005; 55 (2): 74-108.
[9] Ou SH, Zell JA, Ziogas A, Anton-Culver H. Low socioeconomic status is a poor prognostic factor for survival in stage I nonsmall cell lung cancer and is independent of surgical treatment, race, and marital status. *Cancer,* 2008; 112 (9): 2011-20.
[10] Ou SH, Ziogas A, Zell JA. Prognostic factors for survival in extensive stage small cell lung cancer (ED-SCLC): the importance of smoking history, socioeconomic and marital statuses, and ethnicity. *J. Thorac. Oncol.,* 2009; 4 (1): 37-43.
[11] Pear R. Tobacco smoking and longevity. *Science.* 1938; 87 (2253): 216-7.
[12] Doll R, Hill AB. Smoking and carcinoma of the lung; preliminary report. *Br. Med. J.,* 1950; 2 (4682): 739-48.
[13] Wynder EL, Graham EA. Etiologic factors in bronchiogenic carcinoma with special reference to industrial exposures; report of eight hundred fifty-seven proved cases. *AMA Arch. Ind. Hyg. Occup. Med.,* 1951; 4 (3): 221-35.
[14] U.S. Department of Health and Human Services PHS, Centres of Disease and Prevention. The health consequences of smoking: a report of the Surgeon General, vol. 7829. Washington, DC: CDC Publication; 2004.
[15] Alberg AJ, Samet JM. Epidemiology of lung cancer. Chest. 2003; 123(suppl): 21S-49S.
[16] Jemal A, Ward E, Hao Y, Thun M. Trends in the leading causes of death in the United States, 1970-2002. *JAMA,* 2005; 294 (10): 1255-9.
[17] Harris JE, Thun MJ, Mondul AM, Calle EE. Cigarette tar yields in relation to mortality from lung cancer in the cancer prevention study II prospective cohort, 1982-8. *BMJ,* 2004; 328 (7431): 72.
[18] Loeb LA, Ernster VL, Warner KE, Abbotts J, Laszlo J. Smoking and lung cancer: an overview. *Cancer Res.,* 1984; 44 (12 Pt 1): 5940-58.
[19] Pisani P, Bray F, Parkin DM. Estimates of the world-wide prevalence of cancer for 25 sites in the adult population. *Int. J. Cancer,* 2002; 97 (1): 72-81.
[20] Smith CJ, Perfetti TA, Rumple MA, Rodgman A, Doolittle DJ. "IARC group 2A Carcinogens" reported in cigarette main-stream smoke. *Food Chem. Toxicol.,* 2000; 38 (4): 371-83.
[21] Smith CJ, Perfetti TA, Mullens MA, Rodgman A, Doolittle DJ. "IARC group 2B Carcinogens" reported in cigarette main-stream smoke. *Food Chem. Toxicol.,* 2000; 38 (9): 825-48.
[22] Akopyan G, Bonavida B. Understanding tobacco smoke carcinogen NNK and lung tumorigenesis. *Int. J. Oncol.,* 2006; 29 (4): 745-52.
[23] Hoffmann D, Djordjevic MV, Rivenson A, Zang A, Desai D, Amin S. A study of tobacco carcinogenesis. LI. Relative potencies of tobacco-specific N-nitrosamines as inducers of lung tumours in A/J mice. *Cancer Lett.,* 1993; 71 (1-3): 25-30.
[24] Belinsky SA, Devereux TR, Maronpot RR, Stoner GD, Anderson MW. Relationship between the formation of promutagenic adducts and the activation of the K-ras

protooncogene in lung tumors from A/J mice treated with nitrosamines. *Cancer Res.*, 1989; 49 (19): 5305-11.

[25] Rudin CM, Avila-Tang E, Samet JM. Lung cancer in never smokers: a call to action. *Clin. Cancer Res.*, 2009; 15 (18): 5622-5.

[26] Driscoll T, Nelson DI, Steenland K, Leigh J, Concha-Barrientos M, Fingerhut M, Prüss-Ustün A. The global burden of disease due to occupational carcinogens. *Am. J. Ind. Med.*, 2005; 48 (6): 419-31.

[27] Fingerhut M, Nelson DI, Driscoll T, et al. The contribution of occupational risks to the global burden of disease: summary and next steps. *Med. Lav.*, 2006; 97 (2): 313-21.

[28] Health Effects Institute. Asbestos in Public and Commercial Buildings: A Literature Review and a Synthesis of Current Knowledge. Cambridge, MA: Health Effects Institute, Asbestos Research Committee, Literature Review Panel; 1991.

[29] Doll R. Mortality from lung cancer in asbestos workers. *Br. J. Ind. Med.*, 1955; 12 (2): 81-6.

[30] Committee on the Biological Effects of Ionizing Radiation. Health Risks of Radon and Other Internally Deposited Alpha-Emitters: BEIR IV. Washington, DC: National Academy Press; 1988.

[31] Lubin JH, Boice JD Jr, Edling C, et al. Lung cancer in radon-exposed miners and estimation of risk from indoor exposure. *J. Natl. Cancer Inst.*, 1995; 87 (11): 817-27.

[32] Samet JM, Eradze GR. Radon and lung cancer risk: taking stock at the millennium. Environ Health Perspect. 2000; 108 (Suppl 4): 635-41.

[33] Samet JM. Residential radon and lung cancer: end of the story? *J. Toxicol. Environ. Health A*, 2006; 69 (7): 527-31.

[34] Lissowska J, Foretova L, Dabek J, et al. Family history and lung cancer risk: international multicentre case-control study in Eastern and Central Europe and meta-analyses. *Cancer Causes Control*, 2010; 21 (7): 1091-104.

[35] Turner MC, Chen Y, Krewski D, Calle E, Thun MJ. Chronic obstructive pulmonary disease is associated with lung cancer mortality in a prospective study of never smokers. *Am. J. Respir. Crit. Care Med.*, 2007; 176 (3): 285-90.

[36] Loganathan RS, Stover DE, Shi W, Venkatraman E. Prevalence of COPD in women compared to men around time of diagnosis of primary lung cancer. *Chest*, 2006; 129 (5): 1305-12.

[37] Hubbard R, Venn A, Lewis S, Britton J. Lung cancer and cryptogenic fibrosing alveolitis. A population-based cohort study. *Am. J. Respir. Crit. Care Med.*, 2000; 161 (1): 5-8.

[38] Kirk GD, Merlo C, O'Driscoll P, et al. HIV infection is associated with an increased risk for lung cancer, independent of smoking. *Clin. Infect. Dis.*, 2007; 45 (1): 103-10.

[39] Rekhtman N, Brandt SM, Sigel CS, et al. Suitability of thoracic cytology for new therapeutic paradigms in non-small cell lung carcinoma: high accuracy of tumor subtyping and feasibility of EGFR and KRAS molecular testing. *J. Thorac. Oncol.*, 2011; 6: 451-8.

[40] Travis WD, Rekhman N. Pathological diagnosis and classification of lung cancer in small biopsies and cytology: strategic management of tissue for molecular testing. *Semin Respir. Crit. Care Med.*, 2011; 32: 22-31.

[41] Travis WD, Brambilla E, Müller-Hermelink HK, Harris CC. Pathology and genetics: tumours of the lung, pleura, thymus and heart. Lyon (France): IARC; 2004.

[42] Travis WD, Brambilla E, Noguchi M. International Association for the Study of Lung Cancer/ American Thoracic Society/ European Respiratory Society International Multidisciplinary Classification of Lung Adenocarcinoma. *J. Thorac. Oncol.,* 2011; 6: 244-85.

[43] Travis WD, Brambilla E. Pathology of lung preneoplasia. In: Hirsch FR, Bunn PA, Kato H, et al. editors. Textbook of prevention and detection of early lung cancer; International Association for the Study of Lung Cancer. 1st edition. London and New York: Taylor & Francis; 2006: 75-89.

[44] Lantuéjoul S, Salameire D, Salon C, Brambilla E. Pulmonary preneoplasia-sequential molecular carcinogenetic events. *Histopathology,* 2009; 54: 43-54.

[45] Kitamura H, Kameda Y, Ito T, Hayashi H. Atypical adenomatous hyperplasia of the lung. Implications for the pathogenesis of peripheral lung adenocarcinoma. *Am. J. Clin. Pathol.,* 1990; 111: 610-22.

[46] Vazquez M, Carter D, Brambilla E, et al. International Early Lung Cancer Action Program Investigators. Solitary and multiple resected adenocarcinomas after CT screening for lung cancer: histopathologic features and their prognostic implications. *Lung Cancer,* 2009; 64: 148-54.

[47] Koike T, Togashi K, Shirato T, et al. Limited resection for non-invasive bronchioloalveolar carcinoma diagnosed by intraoperative pathologic examination. *Ann. Thorac. Surg.,* 2009; 88; 1106-11.

[48] Davies SJ, Gosney JR, Hansell DM, et al. Diffuse idiopathic pulmonary neuroendocrine cell hyperplasia: an under-recognised spectrum of disease. *Thorax,* 2007; 62: 248-52.

[49] Funai K, Yokose T, Ishii G, et al. Clinicopathologic characteristics of peripheral squamous cell carcinoma of the lung. *Am. J. Surg. Pathol.,* 2003; 27: 978-84.

[50] Maeshima AM, Maeshima A, Asamura H, Matsuno Y. Histologic prognostic factors for small-sized squamous cell carcinomas of the peripheral lung. *Lung Cancer,* 2006; 52: 53-8.

[51] Watanabe Y, Yokose T, Sakuma Y, et al. Alveolar space filling ratio as a favorable prognostic factor in small peripheral squamous cell carcinoma of the lung. *Lung Cancer,* 2011; 73 (2): 217-21.

[52] Tsutsumida H, Nomoto M, Goto M, et al. A micropapillary pattern is predictive of a poor prognosis in lung adenocarcinoma, and reduced surfactant apoprotein A expression in the micropapillary pattern is an excellent indicator of a poor prognosis. *Mod. Pathol.,* 2007; 20: 638-47.

[53] Maemondo M, Inoue A, Kobayashi K, et al. North-East Japan Study Group. Gefitinib or chemotherapy for non-small-cell lung cancer with mutated EGFR. *N. Engl. J. Med.,* 2010; 362: 2380-8.

[54] Altekruse SF, Kosary CL, Krapcho M, et al. SEER cancer statistics review. 1975-2007. National Cancer Institute; 2010.

[55] Kreisman H, Wolkove N, Quoix E. Small cell lung cancer presenting as a solitary pulmonary nodule. *Chest,* 1992; 101: 225-31.

[56] Travis WD, Travis LB, Devesa SS. Lung cancer. *Cancer,* 1995; 75: 191-202.

[57] Travis WD. Advances in neuroendocrine lung tumors. *Ann. Oncol.,* 2010; 21(Suppl 7): vii65-71.

[58] Yao X, Gomes MM, Tsao MS, Allen CJ, Geddie W, Sekhon H. Fine-needle aspiration biopsy versus core-needle biopsy in diagnosing lung cancer: a systematic review. *Curr. Oncol.,* 2012; 19: e16-27.

[59] Ammanagi AS, Dombale VD, Miskin AT, Dandagi GL, Sangolli SS. Sputum cytology in suspected cases of carcinoma of lung (sputum cytology a poor man's bronchoscopy!). Lung India. 2012; 29: 19-23.

[60] Karahalli E, Yimaz A, Turker H, Ozvaran K. Usefulness of various diagnostic techniques during fiberoptic bronchoscopy for endoscopically visible lung cancer: should cytologic examinations be performed routinely? *Respiration,* 2001; 68: 611-4.

[61] Van der Drift MA, Van der Wilt GJ, Thunnissen FB, Janssen JP. A prospective study of the timing and cost-effectiveness of bronchial washing during bronchoscopy for pulmonary malignant tumors. *Chest,* 2005; 128: 394-400.

[62] Schreiber G, McCrory DC. Performance characteristics of different modalities for diagnosis of suspected lung cancer: summary of published evidence. *Chest,* 2003; 123: 115S-28S.

[63] Bielsa S, Panades MJ, Egido R, et al. Accuracy of pleural fluid cytology in malignant effusions. *An. Med. Interna.,* 2008; 25: 173-7.

[64] Li H, Boiselle PM, Shepard JO, Trotman-Dickenson B, McLoud TC. Diagnostic accuracy and safety of CT-guided percutaneous needle aspiration biopsy of the lung: comparison of small and large pulmonary nodules. *AJR Am. J. Roentgenol.,* 1996; 167: 105-9.

[65] Oikonomou A, Matzinger FR, Seely JM, Dennie CJ, Macleod PJ. Ultrathin needle (25G) aspiration lung biopsy: diagnostic accuracy and complication rates. *Eur. Radiol.,* 2004; 14: 375-82.

[66] Ohno Y, Hatabu H, Takenaka D, Higashino T, Watanabe H, Ohbayashi C, Sugimura K. CT-guided transthoracic needle aspiration biopsy of small (< or = 20mm) solitary pulmonary nodules. *AJR Am. J. Roentgenol.,* 2003; 180: 1665-9.

[67] Micames CG, McCrory DC, Pavey DA, Jowell PS, Gress FG. Endoscopic ultrasound-guided fine-needle aspiration for non-small cell lung cancer staging: a systematic review and metaanalysis. *Chest,* 2007; 131 (2): 539-48.

[68] Gomez M, Silvestri GA. Endobronchial ultrasound for the diagnosis and staging of lung cancer. *Proc. Am. Thorac. Soc.,* 2009; 6 (2): 180-6.

[69] Little AG, Rusch VW, Bonner JA, Gaspar LE, Green MR, Webb WR, Stewart AK. Patterns of surgical care of lung cancer patients. *Ann. Thorac. Surg.,* 2005; 80 (6): 2051-6.

[70] Rivera PM, Mehta AC, Wahidi MM. Establishing the Diagnosis of Lung Cancer. *Chest,* 2013; 143(5): e142S-e165S.

[71] Goldstraw P, Crowley J, Chansky K, et al. International Association for the Study of Lung Cancer International Staging Committee; Participating Institutions. The IASLC lung cancer staging project: proposals for the revision of the TNM stage groupings in the forthcoming (seventh) edition of the TNM classification of malignant tumours. *J. Thorac. Oncol.,* 2007; 2: 706-14.

In: Fighting Lung Cancer through the HER Family …
Editor: Diego Márquez-Medina
ISBN: 978-1-63321-092-9

Chapter 2

Lung Cancer II. Conventional Treatment for Advanced Non-Small Cell Lung Cancer

Oscar Juan-Vidal, M.D., Ph.D. and Corina Escoin, M.D.
Medical Oncology Department, La Fe University Hospital of Valencia, Spain

Abstract

The presence or absence of a driver mutation (EGFR, ALK, etc.) for which a specific inhibitor is available has changed the initial treatment of advanced non-small cell lung cancer (NSCLC) patients. However, only a small group of patients (about 30%) will be candidates for this kind of personalized therapy. For other patients, the first-line treatment is a platinum-based doublet. In recent years, the efficacy or the toxicity of some drugs has been associated with histologic subtype, and this has led to a differential treatment for squamous and non-squamous lung cancer patients. Cisplatin/pemetrexed has shown a statistically superior overall survival (OS) than cisplatin/gemcitabine in patients with adenocarcinoma and large-cell carcinoma histology; whereas, bevacizumab has been associated with an increased risk of pulmonary hemorrhage in patients with squamous histology. For these reasons, pemetrexed and bevacizumab should not be used in patients with squamous histology and these patients should be treated with a combination of cisplatin or carboplatin with gemcitabine, vinorelbine, docetaxel or paclitaxel. On the other hand, the recommended first-line treatment for non-squamous NSCLC may be the cisplatin/pemetrexed or a platinum-based doubled plus bevacizumab, which has led to an increase in median OS exceeding 12 months.

Another important advance in the treatment of advanced NSCLC has also occurred in patients with non-squamous histology. The use of maintenance therapy in patients who obtain a response or stable disease after the completion of four to six cycles of chemotherapy has demonstrated an improvement in progression-free survival and OS. The use of good toxicity profile drugs such as pemetrexed and bevacizumab has made possible the maintenance therapy. In the PARAMOUNT trial, patients with response or stable disease after 4 cycles of cisplatin/pemetrexed were randomized to pemetrexed or placebo. Median OS was 13.9 months for patients treated with pemetrexed maintenance versus 11 months for placebo group. Furthermore, in the SAIL study, median OS was 18.8 months in the maintenance population.

In the choice of second-line therapy in patients with advanced NSCLC, multiple factors need to be considered including the presence of driver mutations, histology, clinical characteristics (performance status, age, comorbidity) and prior therapy. Pemetrexed use is also limited in this scenario for non-squamous histology patients. Docetaxel and erlotinib have shown efficacy in phase III trials. Combination chemotherapy regimens have not shown impact on OS.

1. Chemotherapy in the Era of Molecular Biology

Combination chemotherapy is the cornerstone of the initial treatment for most patients with advanced NSCLC. Whenever possible, it is recommended the determination of epidermal growth factor receptor (EGFR) activating mutations or anaplastic lymphoma kinase (ALK) rearrangements before the start of treatment in patients with advanced nonsquamous NSCLC, as well as never-smokers with squamous histology [1]. However, only a small percentage of these patients will benefit from targeted therapies. The presence of activating EGFR mutations is observed in approximately 17% of patients [2], who will benefit from initial treatment with erlotinib, gefitinib or afatinib. Furthermore, ALK rearrangement is less common (7%), but these patients should receive treatment with crizotinib. Although, according to the Lung Cancer Mutation Consortium [2], approximately 54% of NSCLC were shown to harbor driver mutations, for most of them a specific inhibitor is not yet available, and the best option for these patients should be the inclusion in a clinical trial or the standard treatment with chemotherapy. In this chapter we revised the conventional treatment with chemotherapy for patients without driver mutations.

Systemic chemotherapy using platinum-based doubled has demonstrated an improvement of overall survival (OS) compared with best supportive care in advanced NSCLC patients. A systematic review of the literature and meta-analysis incorporating individual data from 2714 patients enrolled on 16 randomized trials comparing chemotherapy with best supportive care [3], showed a statistically significant improvement in OS with chemotherapy (HR 0.77; 95% CI 0.71-0.83; p< 0.0001), equivalent to a relative increase in survival of 23% or an absolute improvement in survival of 9% at 12 months, increasing survival from 20% to 29%. Studies included in that meta-analysis were conducted before the identification of driver mutations and the use of specific inhibitors as first-line therapy. This survival benefit was independent of histology, performance status (PS) and age. American Society of Clinical Oncology (ASCO) [4], in patients with PS 0 or 1 recommended 4 to 6 cycles of platinum-based doublet as first-line therapy, while patients with PS 2 could be treated with single-agent chemotherapy, because data is insufficient to make a recommendation for or against a combination of two cytotoxic drugs. Non-platinum containing regimens may be used as alternative in patients with contraindications to receive platinum. Despite these recommendations from the ASCO, the benefit of platinum-based chemotherapy is small compared to a doublet without cisplatin. A meta-analysis from 4,792 patients included in 17 randomized trials comparing platinum-based doublets with nonplatinum-based doublets [5], found a slightly higher survival at one year favoring platinum-based doublets (RR 1.08, 95% CI 1.01–1.16; p= 0.03), better partial response (RR 1.11, 95% CI 1.02–1.21; p= 0.02), with a higher risk of anemia, nausea, and neurotoxicity. Cisplatin-based doublet regimens improved survival at 1 year (RR 1.16, 95% CI 1.06–1.27; p= 0.001), complete response (RR 2.29, 95% CI 1.08–4.88; p= 0.03), and partial response rate (RR 1.19, 95% CI 1.07–1.32; p= 0.002), with an increased risk of anemia, neutropenia, neurotoxicity and nausea. Conversely, carboplatin-based doublet regimens did not increase survival rate at 1 year (RR 0.95, 95% CI 0.85–1.07; p= 0.43). Therefore, in those patients where the initial treatment may not be selected depending on the molecular characteristics, the treatment option is chemotherapy, usually a platinum-based doublet (cisplatin or carboplatin) plus another active drug in NSCLC. For patients with nonsquamous histology, there is the possibility of adding bevacizumab.

2. Factors Influencing Choice of Treatment

Classically, the choice of first-line treatment in patients with advanced NSCLC was made based on clinical factors such as performance status (PS), age and comorbidities. Patients with PS 0-1 and no significant comorbidities were treated with a platinum-based doublet, either carboplatin or cisplatin. Several randomized trials comparing different combinations of cisplatin-based chemotherapy did not observe significant differences in survival between the regimens [6-10]. Schiller et al. [6] compared four regimens: cisplatin plus gemcitabine, paclitaxel, or docetaxel, and carboplatin plus paclitaxel, showing that the efficacy was similar in all of them in terms of response, median survival and survival at one and two years. These trials seemed to show that "plateau" with chemotherapy and classical treatment selection factors had been reached for patients with advanced NSCLC, with a median survival around 8-10 months and one-year survival of 30-40%.

2.1. Histology

In recent years, histology has become a new factor in the choice of the optimal agent to combine with a platinum compound. Several studies have established that nonsquamous histology is a predictor for better survival in patients treated with pemetrexed. In a phase III trial in which cisplatin/pemetrexed (CP) was compared with cisplatin/gemcitabine (CG) as first-line therapy, there was no significant differences in progression-free survival (PFS) and overall survival (OS) in the total population [11]. However, in a preplanned analysis, survival in patients with adenocarcinoma and large cell carcinoma was significantly prolonged with CP compared to CG (11.8 months versus 10.4 months; HR 0.81, 95% CI 0.70-0.84; p< 0.05). Conversely, patients with squamous histology had worse survival when they were treated with CP compared with CG (9.4 months versus 10.8 months; HR 1.23; 95% CI 1-1.51; p< 0.05). Similarly, the relationship between histology and efficacy has been shown both in a second-line trial and maintenance trial, demonstrating an increased activity for pemetrexed in patients with non-squamous histology [12, 13] (Table 1). Moreover, squamous histology NSCLC patients have shown increased toxicity with the use of bevacizumab, so bevacizumab use has been limited to nonsquamous histology patients. The initial phase II study compared the combination of carboplatin, paclitaxel and bevacizumab versus carboplatin and paclitaxel alone [14]; twenty patients with squamous histology were included, 6 of them had pulmonary hemorrhage, in 4 of them being fatal.

Table 1. Overall Survival of pemetrexed according to histology

	1st line	2nd line	Maintenance
	Cis-Gem vs Cis-Pem (HR)	Doc vs Pem (HR)	Plac vsPem (HR)
Non squamous	0.81*	0.78*	0.70*
Adenocarcinoma	0.84*	0.92	0.73*
Large cells	0.67	0.27*	0.98
NOS	1.08	0.57	0.61*
Squamous	1.23	1.56*	1.07

*HR: Hazard Ratio. *Statistically Significant (p<0.05)*

An association between the risk of pulmonary hemorrhage and squamous histology, central tumors next to large vessels, cavitation, or necrosis was observed. For this reason, squamous histology was excluded in phase III trials, and pulmonary hemorrhage grade ≥ 3 was reduced to less than 2% [15, 16]. Increased PFS (6.2 months versus 4.5 months; HR 0.66) and OS (12.3 months versus 10.3 months; HR 0.79) were shown in the Eastern Cooperative Oncology Group (ECOG) study [16]. The AVAiL study confirmed the benefit of cisplatin/gemcitabine plus bevacizumab versus cisplatin/gemcitabine in PFS (HR 0.75), however, the benefit in OS did not reach statistically significant difference [17]. Therefore, squamous histology is a selection factor for bevacizumab treatment to avoid toxicity.

2.2. Customized Chemotherapy

Another field of research to individualize treatment in patients with advanced NSCLC has been the pharmacogenomics, especially different genes involved in DNA repair that have been associated with sensitivity to certain drugs. ERCC 1 (excision repair cross-complementation group 1), RRM1 (ribonucleotide reductase messenger 1), BRCA 1 (breast cancer type 1) and RAP-90 (receptor-associated protein 80) are some of the proteins that have been associated with resistance or sensitivity to platinum, gemcitabine, vinka alkaloids and antimicrotubule agents. Lord et al. showed that low levels of ERCC mRNA were predictors of better response (58% versus 37%; p= 0.03) and longer survival (p= 0.009) to treatment with cisplatin [18]. These results have been corroborated by 2 meta-analyses, in which high levels of ERCC1 were associated with decreased survival and response to platinum-based chemotherapy in patients with advanced NSCLC [19, 20]. However, in a study conducted by the Spanish Lung Cancer Group (SLCG), 444 patients with advanced NSCLC were randomized to a control group treated with cisplatin and docetaxel or the experimental group (genotypic arm). In the genotypic arm, patients with low ERCC1 levels received docetaxel plus cisplatin, and those with high levels received docetaxel plus gemcitabine. Response rate was significantly higher in the genotypic arm (51.2% versus 39.3%), but no difference in OS was observed (9.8 versus 9.82 months). In the genotypic arm, patients with low ERCC1 levels showed higher response rates and survival than patients with high ERCC1 levels:

53.2% versus 43.8%, and 10.35 months versus 9.48 months, respectively, although these differences did not reach statistical significance [21].

High expression of RRM1 has been correlated with resistance to treatment with gemcitabine [22-25]. In a meta-analysis of 1243 patients from 18 studies, response rate to gemcitabine-containing regimen was significantly higher in patients with low/negative RRM1 (OR 0.31, 95% CI 0.21-0.45; p< 0.00001) [26]. However, in a prospective phase II study, patients with low RRM1 expression were treated with carboplatin/gemcitabine or docetaxel/gemcitabine, while patients with high levels of RRM1 were treated with carboplatin/docetaxel or docetaxel/vinorelbine. No correlation between the expression of RRM1 and response to treatment or survival was observed. Patients assigned to any of the 4 treatment regimens had the same results [27]. Prospective phase III trials to clarify whether RRM1 levels are predictors of response to treatment in patients with advanced NSCLC treated with gemcitabine-containing schemes are warranted. The low expression of BRCA1 mRNA was associated with a better outcome for patients treated with cisplatin and gemcitabine [28]. However, in a customized prospective phase III trial conducted by the SLCG, 279 patients were randomized to control arm (cisplatin/docetaxel) or experimental arm, in which patients received treatment according to their BRCA1 and RAP80 levels; BRCA1 and RAP80 were not predictive of PFS and OS [29].

3. First Line Chemotherapy for Advanced NSCLC

For patients with advanced NSCLC and good PS, initial systemic treatment generally consists of cisplatin or carboplatin based doublet, combined with an active cytotoxic agent (pemetrexed, docetaxel, paclitaxel, gemcitabine, vinorelbine), with or without bevacizumab.

Several randomized trials have compared chemotherapy versus best supportive care, but due to the small number of patients it is difficult to draw conclusions. Four meta-analyses of randomized trials have shown the benefits of platinum chemotherapy versus supportive treatment (Table 2).

Table 2. Meta-analysis of randomized trials of chemotherapy versus best supportive care in advanced NSCLC

Authors	Number of trials	Number of patients	Chemotherapy was associated to
Grilli [30]	6	635	1) 6 weeks benefit on survival 2) 24% reduction in the probability of death
Souquet [31]	7	706	1) Benefit on survival 3, 6 and 9 months. 2) Improvement in quality of life 3) Lower cost
Marino [32]	8	712	1) 20% benefit on i survival at 6 months. 2) 3 months benefit on median survival (from 3.9 to 6.7 months)
NSCLC Collaborative Group [3]	16	2,714	1) Relative 23% increase in survival 2) Absolute 9% improvement in 1-year survival (from 20% to 29%)

A survival [3, 30-32] and quality of life benefit were observed [30] in patients treated with platinum combinations. NSCLC Meta-Analyses Collaborative Group [3], as comment above, showed a significant benefit of chemotherapy (HR 0.77; 95% CI, 0.71-0.83; p= 0.0001), equivalent to a relative increase in survival of 23% or an absolute improvement in survival of 9% at 12 months, increasing survival from 20% to 29%. This benefit was independent of histology, PS and age. These results support the use of 4 to 6 cycles of platinum-based doublets as first line treatment for patients with advanced NSCLC.

The low survival benefit provided by chemotherapy has lead to a cost-benefit discussion about the necessity of treatment. A systematic review of randomized trials of treatment with new drugs concluded that although the benefit is small it seems that in patients with lung cancer it is cost-effective [33]. However, more recent studies have shown an additional survival benefit when platinum-based doublets were associated to biological agents such as bevacizumab or to cytotoxic maintenance treatment after the initial platinum-based chemotherapy.

3.1. Number of Cytotoxic Agents

Multiple randomized trials have compared cisplatin-containing combinations with single-agent therapy in patients with advanced NSCLC. In a meta-analysis published in 2004 that included 13,601 patients from 65 randomized trials, two-drug regimens compared to single agent chemotherapy significantly increased both response rate (26% versus 13%; OR 0.42; 95% CI 0.37-0.47; p< 0.001) and OS (1-year survival rate 35% versus 30%; OR 0.8; 95% CI 0,70-0.91; p< 0.001) [34]. The addition of a third cytotoxic drug to a two-drug combination improves response rates (OR 0.66; 95% CI 0.58-0.75; p< 0.001), but not 1-year survival (OR 1.01; 95% CI 0.85-1.21; p= 0.88). Toxicity was clearly increased with triplet regimen.

Currently, monochemotherapy as first-line treatment of advanced NSCLC is limited to patients who are not candidates to receive a platinum-based doublet due to poor PS, advanced age, comorbidities, etc.

3.2. Cisplatin versus Carboplatin

For patients with advanced NSCLC, cisplatin combinations have shown higher response rate compare to those using carboplatin. However, the impact on OS is small and, probably, not clinically meaningful in this group of palliative patients. Furthermore, carboplatin has a better toxicity profile and less negative impact on quality of life. As a result, carboplatin is considered the drug of choice in elderly patients, those with a poor PS or important comorbidities, in whom cisplatin is likely to be poorly tolerated.

A 2007 meta-analysis from 2,968 patients in 9 trials assessed the differences between carboplatin and cisplatin containing regimens for first line treatment of advanced NSCLC [35]. The objective response rate was higher for patients treated with cisplatin than for patients treated with carboplatin (30% versus 24%, respectively; OR 1.37; 95% CI 1.16-1.61; p< 0.001). In subset analyses, in patients with nonsquamous tumors and those treated with third-generation chemotherapy (paclitaxel, docetaxel o gemcitabine), carboplatin-based chemotherapy was associated with a statistically significant increase in mortality (HR 1.12;

95% CI 1.01-1.23 and HR 1.11; 95% CI 1.01-1.21, respectively). Cisplatin-based chemotherapy was associated with more severe nausea and vomiting and nephrotoxicity, while carboplatin combinations caused more severe thrombocytopenia.

Moreover, a phase III clinical trial that enrolled 1,363 advanced NSCLC patients showed that the use of full-dose carboplatin (AUC 6) might reduce the difference in overall survival compared to cisplatin-based chemotherapy schemes [36]. In this trial patients were randomly assigned to gemcitabine combined with cisplatin 50 mg/m^2, cisplatin 80 mg/m^2 and carboplatin AUC 6; median survival for the three arms were 8.3, 9.5 and 10 months, respectively.

Therefore, although the number of responses increased with combination with cisplatin, the impact on survival and better toxicity profile of carboplatin makes this valid option for patients with advanced NSCLC.

3.3. Weekly versus Three-Week Interval Schemes

Weekly administration at lower doses may reduce toxicity maintaining the efficacy. This aspect was examined in a phase III trial that compared the efficacy and tolerability of first-line treatment with weekly paclitaxel/carboplatin or every there weeks administration in 883 advanced NSCLC patients [37]. Patients were randomly assigned to: arm A, weekly paclitaxel 100 mg/m^2 and carboplatin AUC 2, for 6-8 weeks; and arm B, paclitaxel 200 mg/m^2 and carboplatin AUC 6 every 21 days. No statistically significant differences in response rate (38% versus 33%), time to progression (median 6.1 versus 7.2 months), or OS (8.9 versus 9.5 months) were observed. The chemotherapy was well tolerated in both schedules. However, grade 3/4 sensory neuropathy occurred more frequently in the tri-weekly schedule (9.1% versus 4.4%), whereas grade 3/4 diarrhea occurred more frequently in the weekly schedule (4.2% versus 1.1%).

3.4. Nonplatinum Regimens

Although platinum-based doublets are the first-line chemotherapy accepted by most of the oncology scientific societies [4, 38, 39], the benefit obtained with them is small compared with nonplatinum schemes.

A meta-analysis that included 4,792 patients from 17 randomized trial compared the efficacy and toxicity non-platinum-based with platinum-based doublet regimens given as first-line treatment for NSCLC [5]. The use of platinum-based doublet regimens was associated with a slightly higher survival at 1 year (RR 1.08, 95% CI 1.01-1.16; p= 0.03), better partial response (RR 1.11, 95% CI 1.02-1.21; p= 0.02), with a higher risk of anemia, nausea, and neurotoxicity. When the trials were analyzed according to the platinum compound used, cisplatin-based doublet regimens improved survival at 1 year (RR 1.16, 95% CI 1.06-1.27; p= 0.001), complete response (RR 2.29, 95% CI 1.08-4.88; p= 0.03), partial response (RR1.19, 95% CI 1.07-1.32; p= 0.002) with an increased risk of anemia, neutropenia, neurotoxicity and nausea. Conversely, carboplatin-based doublet regimens did not increase survival rate at 1 year (RR 0.95, 95% CI 0.85-1.07; p= 0.43). There was a statistically significant difference between the efficacy of cisplatin and carboplatin (p=0.05).

For patients who are not candidates for a platinum-containing regimens, nonplatinum schemes such as gemcitabine/docetaxel, gemcitabine/paclitaxel, gemcitabine/vinorelbine, paclitaxel/vinorelbine and pemetrexed-gemcitabine may offer similar benefit.

4. First Line Chemotherapy in Advanced NSCLC according to Histology

As discussed above, histology is one of the factors influencing the choice of treatment; patients with non-squamous histology tumors have a different treatment to those who have squamous histology. For this reason, definition of histological type is crucial to select the adequate treatment, immunohistochemistry is a useful tool to differentiate between squamous and non-squamous, and minimize the number of patients classified as *non-other specified* (NOS).

4.1. Treatment of Patients with Nonsquamous Histology Tumors

a) Cisplatin-pemetrexed

In a noninferiority phase III study, 1,725 chemotherapy naive patients with stage III or IV and an Eastern Cooperative Oncology Group PS 0 to 1, were randomized to receive cisplatin 75 mg/m^2 on day 1 and gemcitabine 1250 mg/m^2 on days 1 and 8 or cisplatin 75 mg/m^2 and pemetrexed 500 mg/m^2 on day 1 every 3 weeks for up to 6 cycles [11]. OS was the same in both therapeutic arms (median survival 10.3 months versus 10.3 months). However, OS was statistically longer for cisplatin/pemetrexed versus cisplatin/gemcitabine in 847 patients with adenocarcinoma (12.6 months versus 10.9 months, respectively). Cisplatin/pemetrexed showed significantly lower grade 3 or 4 neutropenia, anemia, thrombocytopenia ($p< 0.001$), febrile neutropenia ($p< 0.002$) and alopecia ($p< 0.001$). Conversely, grade 3 or 4 nausea ($p< 0.004$) was more common.

b) Carboplatin-paclitaxel-bevacizumab

Angiogenesis is a complex process that leads to the activation, proliferation and migration of endothelial cells and their assembly for the formation of new capillaries from existing vessels. The clinical significance of angiogenesis in human tumors is shown in several studies, which have shown a relationship between tumor microvessel density and prognosis. High microvessel density was correlated with a worse disease-free survival and overall survival in different types of cancer. The prototype of pro-angiogenic factor involved in most physiological and pathological processes is the vascular endothelial growth factor A, commonly referred to as VEGF, which is secreted by the majority of tumors. Initially, it was thought that the VEGF receptor (VEGFR) was only found in endothelial cells and that its stimulation played a crucial role in proliferation, the formation of new vessels and capillary permeability; however, recent investigations have demonstrated that VEGFR is also expressed in cancer cells of most human tumors, including lung cancer, and may mediate proliferation and tumor invasion. Several studies have shown the expression of VEGF in patients with NSCLC to be an independent predictor besides conventional prognostic factors for PFS and OS [40-43]. For these reasons the inhibition of angiogenesis by blocking factors such as VEGF constitutes an attractive approach for cancer treatment. Bevacizumab is a humanized monoclonal antibody with high affinity to VEGF, blocking the binding of all isoforms of VEGF to its receptors.

There have been two large randomized phase III trials of chemotherapy with or without bevacizumab in patients with advanced NSCLC (Table 3). The ECOG conducted a phase III trial (E4599) comparing carboplatin and paclitaxel (N= 444) with or without bevacizumab 15 mg/kg (N= 434) in patients with advanced or recurrent NSCLC of non-squamous histology [16]. Patients received up to 6 cycles of chemotherapy with carboplatin and paclitaxel with or without bevacizumab in the absence of disease progression. In the bevacizumab arm, bevacizumab was continued as maintenance therapy until progression or intolerable toxicity. Both OS and PFS were significantly better for patients treated with bevacizumab plus chemotherapy compared with chemotherapy alone: 12.3 months versus 10.3 months (HR 0.79; 95% CI 0.67-0.92; p= 0.003) for OS and 6.2 months versus 4.5 months (HR 0.66; 95% CI 0.57- 0.77; p< 0.001) for PFS, respectively. The correlation of biomarkers with survival was studied; there was no correlation with the levels of VEGF or basic fibroblast growth factor with survival, only patients who had low baseline levels of intercellular adhesion molecule showed significantly better survival [44].

In the other randomized phase III trial conducted in Europe and Canada (AVAstin in lung cancer: AVAiL), 1043 patients with non-squamous advanced NSCLC were randomly assigned to cisplatin and gemcitabine alone (N= 347), cisplatin and gemcitabine plus bevacizumab 7.5 mg/kg (N= 345) or cisplatin and gemcitabine plus bevacizumab 15 mg/kg (N= 351) [15]. Chemotherapy was administered for up to 6 cycles in the absence of progression followed by bevacizumab until disease progression in both bevacizumab arms.

Table 3. Phase III trials comparing chemotherapy versus chemotherapy plus bevacizumab

	ECOG [16] **N= 878**	**AVAiL [15, 17]** **N= 1043**
Chemotherapy ± bevacizumab	Carboplatin-paclitaxel (444) ± BVZ 15 mg/Kg (434)	Cisplatin-gemcitabine (347) ± BVZ 7.5 mg/Kg (345) ± BVZ 15 mg/Kg (351)
OS (months)	10.3 12.3 HR 0.79; p= 0.003	13.1 13.4 13.6 A vs. B HR 0.93, p= 0.420 A vs. C 1.03, p= 0.761
PFS (months)	4.5 6.2 HR 0.66, p< 0.001)	6.1 6.7 6.5 A vs. B HR 0.75; p= 0.003) A vs. C HR 0.82, p= 0.03

A significant improvement in PFS, the primary endpoint, was seen in the bevacizumab arms: 6.7 months for low-dose bevacizumab (HR 0.75; p= 0.003) and 6.5 months for high-dose bevacizumab (HR 0.82; p= 0.03), compared with 6.1 months for the chemotherapy alone arm. However, OS did not significantly increase with bevacizumab (HR 0.93; 95% CI 0.78-1.11; p= 0.42 and HR 1.03; 95% CI 0.86-1.23; p= 0.761) for the 7.5 and 15 mg/kg groups, respectively, versus placebo [17].

Soria et al. have recently published a meta-analysis of randomized trials comparing first-line bevacizumab plus platinum-based chemotherapy with chemotherapy alone for inoperable locally advanced, recurrent or metastatic NSCLC. Four trials were included: the 2 phase III trial commented before and 2 phase II trials (AVF-0757g and JO199907) [45]. In total 2194 patients were analyzed, 1313 patients treated with bevacizumab and 881 patients with chemotherapy alone. The addition of bevacizumab to chemotherapy significantly increased both OS (HR 0.9; 95% CI 0.81-0.99; p= 0.03) and PFS (HR 0.72; 95% CI 0.66-0.79; p< 0.001) compared with the use of chemotherapy alone. Bevacizumab showed a significantly greater effect on OS in patients with adenocarcinoma versus other histology (p= 0.02). By contrast, the addition of bevacizumab increased risk of proteinuria ≥3, hypertension, hemorrhagic events, neutropenia and febrile neutropenia.

In spite of this slight increase in toxicity, bevacizumab is well tolerated. The SAiL study is a phase IV trial designed to assess the safety and efficacy of first line bevacizumab combined with standard chemotherapy regimens in clinical practice [46]. The incidence of clinically significant (grade ≥3) toxicity was generally low; thromboembolism occurred in 172 (8%) patients, hypertension in 125 (6%), bleeding in 80 (4%), proteinuria in 67 (3%) and pulmonary hemorrhage in 15 (1%). Mortality due to adverse events was of 3%, with thromboembolism (1%) and bleeding (1%) as the most common causes. Although evidence of CNS metastases was an exclusion criterion in SAiL, some patients with asymptomatic CNS metastases could have been enrolled, since brain imaging was not mandated before enrolment. Of the 281 patients who were assessed as having CNS metastases during the course of the study, only five (2%) had CNS bleeding.

In summary, for advanced NSCLC patients with good PS and nonsquamos histology, platinum-based doublet plus bevacizumab get better response rate, PFS and OS compared with chemotherapy alone.

c) Chemotherapy Plus Cetuximab

Cetuximab has been studied in two large phase III trials combined with platinum-based doublet as initial therapy for advanced NSCLC patients.

In the FLEX trial [47], 1,125 chemotherapy-naive patients with wet stage III or IV NSCLC and EGFR-expression were randomly assigned to cisplatin 80 mg/m^2 on day 1 and vinorelbine 25 mg/m^2 on days 1 and 8 plus cetuximab at a starting dose of 400 mg/m^2 intravenous infusion on day 1, and from day 8 onwards at 250 mg/m^2 per week, or just chemotherapy. Cetuximab was continued after the end of chemotherapy until disease progression or unacceptable toxicity. Patients who received chemotherapy plus cetuximab survived longer than those in the chemotherapy-alone group (median 11.3 months versus 10.1 months; HR 0.871; 95% CI 0.762-0.996; p= 0.044). Response rate was statistically higher for patients treated with cetuximab (36% versus 29%). However, there was no statistically significant difference in PFS (median 4.8 months in both groups). Patients receiving cetuximab had increased toxicity (acne-like rash, febrile neutropenia, diarrhea and infusion-related reactions).

In the BMS-099 phase III trial [48], 676 chemotherapy-naive patients with stage IIIB (pleural effusion) or IV NSCLC, without restrictions by histology or epidermal growth factor receptor expression, were randomly assigned to carboplatin AUC 6 combined with docetaxel 75 mg/m^2 or paclitaxel 225 mg/m^2, with or without cetuximab (load dose of 400 mg/m^2 on day 1 followed by 250 mg/m^2 weekly). Cetuximab was continued after the end of chemotherapy until disease progression or unacceptable toxicity. The addition of cetuximab to chemotherapy did not meet the primary endpoint (PFS) compared to chemotherapy alone (median 4.4 months versus 4.2 months with chemotherapy alone; HR 0.9, 95% CI 0.76-1.07). The increase in OS with the cetuximab-based regimen was not statistically significant (9.7 months versus 8.4 months; HR 0.89, 95% CI 0.75-1.05).

A third trial is ongoing, the SWOG-0819; patients are randomly assigned to carboplatin/paclitaxel/bevacizumab with or without cetuximab.

d) Patients with PS 2

ASCO guidelines recommend the use of single-agent chemotherapy in patients with a PS 2 [4]. However, more recent data suggest that combination regimens may be advantageous in patients with PS 2 who could tolerate such therapy.

A multicenter, randomized phase III study for first-line treatment of PS 2 patients was conducted in Italy (CAPPA-2 study) [49]. Patients with advanced NSCLC and PS 2 were randomized to receive gemcitabine or cisplatin plus gemcitabine every 3 weeks. Unfortunately, the study was stopped early after the enrolment of 57 patients due to the slow accrual. Median OS was 3 months with single-agent gemcitabine and 5.9 months with cisplatin plus gemcitabine (HR 0.52, 95% CI 0.28-0.98; p= 0.039). Combination chemotherapy produced longer PFS (median 1.7 months versus 3.3 months; HR 0.49, 95% CI 0.27-0.89; p= 0.017) and higher response rate (4% versus 18%; p= 0.19), without substantial increase in toxicity.

In other multicenter phase III trial, 205 patients with advanced NSCLC and PS 2 and non-squamous histology (after amendment) were randomized to pemetrexed alone or carboplatin/pemetrexed every 3 weeks. In the intent-to-treat population, the median PFS was 2.8 months for pemetrexed and 5.8 months for carboplatin/pemetrexed (HR 0.46, 95% CI 0.35-0.63; p< 0.001), and the median OS was 5.3 months for pemetrexed and 9.3 months for carboplatin/pemetrexed (HR 0.62; 95% CI 0.46-0.83; p= 0.001). One-year survival rates were 21.9% and 40.1%, respectively. A subsequent analysis, excluding patients with squamous cell carcinoma (N= 14) and unknown histology (N= 10), showed similar results [50]. Although, hematologic toxicity was more common in combination arm it was mild. However, there were four documented treatment-related deaths in the combination arm (3.9%).

In conclusion, combination chemotherapy with carboplatin plus pemetrexed improves OS compared to single agent pemetrexed in advanced NSCLC patients with PS 2 with tolerable toxicity.

Table 4. Phase III trials comparing combinations of new drugs in advanced NSCLC

References	Chemotherapy	RR (%)	mOS (m)	1-year OS (%)
Kelly [51]	CDPP-VNR	26	8	36
	CBDCA-PTX	28	8	35
Schiller [6]	CDDP-PTX	21	7,8	36
	CBDCA-PTX	15	8,2	35
	CDDP-DTX	17	7,4	31
	CDDP-GEM	21	8,1	38
Scagliotti [9]	CDPP-VNR	30	9,5	37
	CDDP-GEM	30	9,8	37
	CBDCA-PTX	32	9,9	43
Fosella [52]	CDPP-VNR	24,5	10,1	41
	CDDP-DTX	31,6	11,3	46
	CBDCA-DTX	23,9	9,4	38

CBDCA carboplatin; CDDP cisplatin; DTX docetaxel; GEM gemcitabine; mOS median overall survival; PTX paclitaxel; RR overall response rate; VNR vinorelbine; 1-year OS= survival at 1 year

4.2. Treatment of Patients with Squamous Tumors

Platinum-based doublets are the standard treatment for patients with squamous histology tumors. Different studies have compared whether any of these combinations are more effective than others (Table 4). Patients of all histology were included in these studies.

In the SWOG group trial [51], cisplatin/vinorelbine combination is equivalent in both response rate and OS to carboplatin/paclitaxel. Although the authors concluded that carboplatin/paclitaxel is associated to better tolerance and acceptance for the patients, no differences was observed in quality of life between the two arms.

One of the most relevant studies was conducted by the ECOG [6], in which 4 chemotherapy combinations (cisplatin/paclitaxel, carboplatin/paclitaxel, cisplatin/docetaxel and cisplatin/gemcitabine) were compared. The response rate and survival did not differ significantly between patients assigned to receive cisplatin and paclitaxel and those assigned to receive any of the three experimental regimens. Treatment with cisplatin and gemcitabine was associated with a significantly longer time to the progression of disease than was treatment with cisplatin and paclitaxel.

In the Italian Lung Cancer Project study, 612 patients were randomized in equal proportion to one of the three treatment arms: cisplatin/gemcitabine, carboplatin/paclitaxel or cisplatin/vinorelbine [9]. There were no differences in overall survival, time to disease progression, or time to treatment failure.

The TAX-326 trial is the biggest study published until now, 1,218 patients with stage IIIB to IV NSCLC were randomly assigned to receive docetaxel/cisplatin (DC), docetaxel/carboplatin (DCb) or vinorelbine/cisplatin (VC). The study was designed to compare each of the docetaxel combinations with the standard arm VC. Patients treated with DC had a higher median survival (11.3 months versus 10.1 months for VC), response rate and quality of life than patients treated with VC. Median survival (9.4 months versus 9.9 months for VC) and response (23.9%) with DCb were similar to those results for VC [52].

The analysis of the previous studies shows that no differences in efficacy exist among any of the platinum combinations used. Toxicity profile is more favorable for carboplatin combinations and these have greater acceptance. Any cisplatin or carboplatin doublet combined with active cytotoxic agents is accepted for the treatment of patients with advanced/metastatic NSCLC with good PS.

Recently, pemetrexed has joined to the active agents to combine with platinum. In the study mentioned above, Scagliotti et al. compared cisplatin/gemcitabine with cisplatin/pemetrexed [11]. OS was the same in both treatment arms (10.3 months). In a preplanned subanalysis, the treatment efficacy was assessed according to the histologic subtype. In patients with squamous cell histology treatment with cisplatin/gemcitabine was associated with a longer median survival than was treatment with cisplatin/pemetrexed (10.8 months versus 9.4 months, respectively). The use of pemetrexed is limited to patients with nonsquamous histology tumors.

5. Maintenance Therapy

Maintenance therapy is defined as the prolongation of treatment after a specified number of cycles in patients in whom the tumor has been controlled. In patients with NSCLC this represents the continuation of treatment after the recommended 4-6 cycles of a platinum-based combination [4], until unacceptable toxicity or disease progression. The aim of maintenance treatment is to prolong survival and improve quality of life. When the agents used in maintenance are the same drugs included in the first-line combination or the drugs have a similar mechanism of action it is called maintenance therapy or consolidation therapy, whereas when the drug used in the maintenance phase has a different mechanism of action it is usually referred to as "early second-line treatment" [53].

For years, studies on NSCLC have not shown benefits in terms of OS with the prolongation of chemotherapy [54] (Table 5). Some of these studies had methodological limitations or did not have enough power to detect differences; in addition, the chemotherapy regimens used were too toxic for maintenance treatment and less effective when compared with current treatment options. In most of these trials a significant number of patients progressed during induction therapy and only a small number is included in the maintenance phase. On the trials by Westeel et al. [55], Belani et al. [56] and Brodowicz et al. [57], all patients received a platinum-based doublet during the induction phase and only 32%, 32% and 59%, of the patients, respectively, underwent randomization to maintenance therapy or observation.

While the 3-month improvement in overall survival with early docetaxel did not reach significance [58], the use of pemetrexed as “early second-line therapy" showed a statistically significant benefit in survival [13]. In this phase III trial conducted by Ciuleanu et al., 663 patients with NSCLC stage IIIB or IV who had not progressed on four cycles of platinum-based chemotherapy were randomly assigned (2:1 ratio) to receive pemetrexed plus best supportive care or placebo plus best supportive care until disease progression. Pemetrexed significantly PFS (4.3 months versus 2.6 months; HR 0.50, 95% CI 0.42–0.61; p< 0.0001) and OS (13.4 months versus 10.6 months; HR 0.79, 95% CI 0.65–0.95; p= 0.012) compared with placebo. Subanalysis of efficacy of maintenance pemetrexed by histology was performed, and only patients with non-squamous histology have shown statistically significant benefit in both PFS (HR 0.44, 95% CI 0.36–0.55) and OS (HR 0.77, 95% CI 0.56–0.88) compared with squamous histology (HR 0.69, 95% CI 0.49–0.98; and HR 1.07, 95% CI 0.77–1.5, respectively).

The meta-analysis of Soon et al., that included these studies showed a significant improvement in DFS (HR 0.75, 95% CI 0.69-0.81; p< 0.00001) and a modest improvement in survival (HR 0.92; 95% CI 0.86-0.99; p= 0.03) with the prolongation of chemotherapy [59]. However, this meta-analysis has its limitations because it only included studies with cytotoxic agents, it is based on published results and not individual data, and the heterogeneity of trials designs.

Two recent randomized trials with the new agent docetaxel and pemetrexed have reopened the debate on maintenance therapy [13, 58]. Fidias et al. [58] treated 566 patients with advanced NSCLC with 21-days cycles of gemcitabine plus carboplatin. After four cycles, 309 patients (54%) without evidence of disease progression were randomly assigned to immediate treatment with single agent docetaxel for up to six cycles or to observation with docetaxel treatment when disease progression occurred. Median PFS for immediate docetaxel (5.7 months) was significantly greater (p< 0.0001) than for delayed docetaxel (2.7 months). However, median OS for immediate docetaxel (12.3 months) was greater than for delayed docetaxel (9.7 months), the difference was not statistically significant (p< 0.0853).

Table 5. Classical randomized trials of maintenance therapy

Study	Phase	N Induction/ Randomized	Induction	Maintenance	OS (m)	1-year OS (%)	TTP (m)
Westeel [55]	III	573/181 OR	MIC (4)	VNR versus Observation	12.3 12.3	42 51	5 3
Belani [56]	II	401/130 CR, PR, SD	CBDCA + PTX (3)	Weekly PTX versus Observation	18.8 15	72 60	9.5 7.3
Brodowicz [57]	III	354/215 CR, PR, SD	CDDP + GMZ	BMZ versus Observation	13 11	NR	6.6 5

CBDCA Carboplatin; **CDDP** Cisplatin; **CR** complete response; **GMZ** Gemcitabine; **MIC** Mitomicin C, Ifosfamide, CDDP; **NR** no reported; **OR** objective response; **PR** partial response; **PTX** Paclitaxel; **SD** stable disease; **VNR** Vinorelbine.

The phase III PARAMOUNT trial was published after the meta-analysis of Soon et al., and it the largest trial of continuation maintenance therapy. This trial evaluated pemetrexed maintenance in patients with non-squamous NSCLC who had disease control after four cycles of cisplatin/pemetrexed. In total, 939 patients with stage IIIB or IV non-squamous NSCLC entered in the induction phase and 539 (57%) patients who had complete or partial response, or stable disease were randomly assigned (2:1 ratio) to receive maintenance therapy with either pemetrexed 500 mg/m^2 every 21 days plus best supportive care or placebo plus best supportive care until disease progression. Pemetrexed significantly increased PFS from 2.8 months for the placebo group to 4.4 months ($p < 0.0001$). There was a significant reduction in the risk of disease progression in the pemetrexed group over the placebo group (HR 0.62, 95% CI 0.49–0.79; $p < 0.0001$) [60]. With a follow-up of 24 months, a statistically significant 22% reduction in the risk of death (HR 0.78; 95% CI 0.64-0.96; $p = 0.0195$) was observed with the pemetrexed therapy. Median OS was 13.9 months for patients treated with pemetrexed maintenance versus 11 months for placebo group [61].

Recently, studies with agents against molecular targets, such as erlotinib, an epidermal growth factor (EGFR) tyrosine kinase inhibitor, or bevacizumab, have shown an increase in PFS when they are used as maintenance therapy after four cycles of frontline chemotherapy [62, 63]. The role of erlotinib maintenance is revised in other chapters; here, we review the role of bevacizumab as maintenance therapy in patients with NSCLC.

In the two large randomized phase III trials comparing chemotherapy with or without bevacizumab in patients with advanced NSCLC (E4599 and AVAiL) [15, 16], PFS were significantly better for patients treated with bevacizumab plus chemotherapy compared with chemotherapy alone. In both trials, bevacizumab was administered at the beginning of treatment concurrently with chemotherapy, but bevacizumab was continued as maintenance therapy after completing the predefined number of cycles of chemotherapy. Therefore, it is difficult to assess how much of the benefit observed is due to the phase of concurrent administration of chemotherapy and how much to the maintenance treatment. Mezger et al. conducted an analysis of the AVAiL study to assess the results of the bevacizumab maintenance therapy after completion of chemotherapy. PFS was measured from the last day of the last cycle to disease progression or death. The use of bevacizumab as a single agent in maintenance therapy is associated with a benefit in PFS, the median PFS was 3.2 months (95% CI 3-5) for the chemotherapy alone arm, 4.6 months (95% CI 4-6) for the chemotherapy plus bevacizumab 7.5 mg/kg arm and 4.6 months (95% CI 4-5) for the chemotherapy plus bevacizumab 15 mg/kg arm supporting the use of bevacizumab until disease progression [64].

Two studies have assessed the effectiveness of maintenance bevacizumab in NSCLC patients in clinical practice. The SAIL study was a phase IV study undertaken to assess the safety and efficacy of combined first-line standard chemotherapy with bevacizumab in patients with non-squamous NSCLC in clinical practice [46]. A total of 2,212 patients with advanced, metastatic or recurrent non-squamous NSCLC were recruited during two years in this open-label, single group, phase IV study from centers in 40 countries. Patients received bevacizumab (7.5 or 15 mg/kg every 3 weeks) plus standard chemotherapy for up to six cycles, followed by single-agent bevacizumab until disease progression. Bevacizumab as maintenance therapy was administered in 1,332 patients (60.2%) of the overall SAIL population. Dansin et al. reported a subanalysis of the SAiL study according to whether patients received maintenance bevacizumab [65]. The primary endpoint was the safety profile of bevacizumab. Adverse events of special interest were more frequent in the maintenance population than in the non-maintenance population (73% versus 62.8%, respectively). However, a low incidence of clinically significant adverse events (grade ≥ 3) was observed in the maintenance population compared with the non-maintenance population (16.9% and 23.5%, respectively). The most common adverse events of special interest were grade 1–2 epistaxis, hypertension, and proteinuria in both populations; more severe adverse events of special interest (e.g., thromboembolism, gastrointestinal perforation and congestive heart failure) were more frequently reported in the non-maintenance population. Grade 3 bleeding had a low incidence; less than 5% in both groups and it was mainly limited to epistaxis. As per protocol guidance, permanent discontinuation of bevacizumab was more common in the non-maintenance population than in the maintenance population (21% versus 4.5%, respectively). This SAiL subanalysis demonstrated that bevacizumab maintenance therapy was well tolerated. Median time to progression was 8.9 months and median OS was 18.8 months in the maintenance population, and 4.5 months and 8.3 months in the non-maintenance population.

Ravelo et al. reported a retrospective study using electronic medical records of advanced non-squamous NSCLC patients receiving first-line chemotherapy plus bevacizumab in an outpatient community setting in 20 US states to evaluate the potential association between bevacizumab treatment to progression and OS and PFS [66]. Of the 498 patients identified, 403 patients were eligible for analysis: 154 patients (38%) received bevacizumab until disease progression and 249 patients (63%) did not. PFS and OS were significantly longer for patients receiving bevacizumab therapy to progression compared with those who did not receive bevacizumab (10.3 months versus 6.5 months for PFS, and 20.9 months versus 10.2 months for OS, respectively). In this study, advanced non-squamous NSCLC patients receiving continued VEGF suppression with bevacizumab had more favorable clinical outcomes relative to patients who discontinued bevacizumab when chemotherapy was completed.

The non-randomized nature of both studies precludes establishing the causal relationship between maintenance bevacizumab and improved clinical outcomes, and could be explained by patient selection bias. However, in both studies, patients treated with bevacizumab had an OS of about 20 months, which is more favorable than in the majority of studies in this population. This data opens the door to the search for criteria for identifying patients who may benefit from maintenance therapy with bevacizumab.

5.1. Combinations of Bevacizumab with other Drugs As Maintenance Therapy

a) Bevacizumab and Erlotinib

Angiogenesis is a complex process involving the possible interaction of different pathways in tumor development. It is interesting, at least from a theoretical point of view, to act on different pathways involved in tumor growth to increase antitumor activity. The aim of the ATLAS study was to assess whether the simultaneous blocking of the VEGF and EGFR pathways increased antitumor activity. After four cycles of chemotherapy with a platinum doublet plus bevacizumab, patients were randomized to maintenance treatment with a combination of bevacizumab and erlotinib or bevacizumab alone [62]. Frontline chemotherapy was initiated in 1,160 patients, 786 patients (66%) completed all four cycles without progression and were randomized. PFS was the primary endpoint and statistical improvement was observed in patients treated with bevacizumab and erlotinib as maintenance therapy compared to patients treated with bevacizumab alone: 4.8 months versus 3.8 months, respectively (HR 0.72; 95% CI 0.59-0.88; p= 0.0012). The number of patients who received treatment to progression was similar in both groups (50% versus 55%), indicating that the addition of erlotinib in maintenance therapy is not an obstacle to receiving further treatment to progression. The PFS improvement was seen across multiple subgroups, including those defined by gender, histology, age, and smoking status. No new safety data was observed, with the exception of rash and diarrhea that were superior in the group of patients treated with erlotinib and bevacizumab.

b) Bevacizumab and Pemetrexed

Cisplatin-pemetrexed as first-line treatment in advanced NSCLC in a randomized phase III trial showed improvement in OS when compared with cisplatin-gemcitabine in the subgroup of patients with non-squamous histology (11.8 months versus 10.4 months; HR 0.81, 95% IC 0.70-0.94) [11]. As mentioned above, in another phase III trial, compared with standard of care, maintenance pemetrexed after a non-pemetrexed-based first-line regimen improved PFS (4.3 months versus 2.6 months; HR 0.5; p< 0.001) and OS (13.4 months versus 10.6 months; HR 0.79; p= 0.012) [60, 61]. Considering the benefit obtained with the combination of bevacizumab plus chemotherapy in first line treatment and maintenance bevacizumab in phase III trials, testing the combination of cisplatin-pemetrexed with bevacizumab seems an interesting approach. Data from phase II trial showed that maintenance with bevacizumab and pemetrexed was associated with acceptable toxicity and relatively long survival (14.1 months) [67]. On this basis, the AVAPERL1 study is designed to investigate whether continuing pemetrexed with bevacizumab maintenance further improves clinical outcomes over bevacizumab alone following induction treatment with bevacizumab-cisplatin-pemetrexed [68]. In total, 376 patients with advanced non-squamous NSCLC received first-line therapy with bevacizumab 7.5 mg/kg, cisplatin 75 mg/m^2, and pemetrexed 500 mg/m^2 once every 3 weeks for four cycles. Two hundred and fifty three patients (67.3%) were randomly assigned to receive single-agent bevacizumab or bevacizumab plus pemetrexed. At a median follow-up of 8.1 months, PFS from random assignment was significantly improved in the bevacizumab plus pemetrexed arm (median 3.7 months versus 7.4 months; HR 0.48, 95% CI, 0.35-0.66; p< 0.001). In the OS analysis from time to random assignment, there was a benefit to the two-drugs regimen, but it was not statistically significant: 12.8 months (range 0-16 months) in the bevacizumab arm and was not yet reached (range 0.1-16.2 months) in the bevacizumab plus pemetrexed arm. (HR 0.75, 95% CI 0.47-1.19; p= 0 .219).

Finally, in the phase III POINTBREAK study [69], 939 patients with non-squamous advanced NSCLC were randomly assigned to: experimental arm, pemetrexed carboplatin plus bevacizumab for up to four 21-day cycles, followed by pemetrexed plus bevacizumab for maintenance; or the control arm, paclitaxel combined with carboplatin and bevacizumab for up to four 21-day cycles, followed by bevacizumab for maintenance. No differences in OS were observed (median OS 12.6 months versus 13.4 months; HR 1; p= 0.949). In an exploratory analysis of the maintenance population, median OS was 17.7 months for experimental group and 15.7 months for control group.

With the results of these two studies the impact in OS of the association of pemetrexed and bevacizumab as maintenance treatment has not been defined.

6. Second Line Treatment in Advanced NSCLC

In the choice of second-line treatment in patients with advanced NSCLC should take into account the presence of activating mutations, drugs received in the first line and time from the end of the previous chemotherapy, histology (squamous versus non-squamous) and clinical factors (age, performance status, comorbidities, etc.).

Nowadays, 3 drugs have shown their utility as second line therapy in advanced NSCLC in phase III trials: docetaxel, pemetrexed and erlotinib. The role of second line erlotinib in patients with or without EGFR mutation is addressed in other chapters, so here we will discuss the utility of docetaxel and pemetrexed.

6.1. Docetaxel

Docetaxel is a classical cytotoxic drug widely used in the treatment regimens for advanced NSCLC and its use is not limited by histological subtype. Overall, docetaxel is indicated in patients with NSCLC with squamous histology and those with non-squamous histology whose initial chemotherapy schedule included pemetrexed.

In a phase III trial, 104 patients with PS 0-2 and stage IIIB-IV NSCLC previously treated with one or more platinum-based chemotherapy regimens were randomized to receive treatment with docetaxel (100 mg/m^2 or 75 mg/m^2 every 21 days) or best supportive care [70]. Of 84 patients with measurable lesions, six (7.1%) achieved partial responses. Time to progression was longer for docetaxel patients than for best supportive care patients (10.6 weeks versus 6.7 weeks, respectively; $p< 0.001$), as was median survival (7 months versus 4.6 months; $p= 0.047$). However, the difference in median survival was more significant for patients treated with docetaxel 75 mg/m^2 compared with patients who received best supportive care alone (7.5 months versus 4.6 months, respectively; $p= 0.01$); as was also 1-year survival (37% versus 11%, respectively; $p= 0.003$). No statistically significant difference in survival was seen between the docetaxel 100 mg/m^2 and BSC arms ($p= 0.78$). Grade 3 or 4 hematologic toxicities were common in chemotherapy arms; especially in treated with docetaxel 100 mg/m^2, three patients died in the context of febrile neutropenia.

This study prospectively investigated quality of life and showed statistically significant differences in patient-rated pain scores in favor of docetaxel overall ($p= 0.005$) or docetaxel 100 mg/m^2 ($p= 0.003$) compared to BSC. There was also significantly less deterioration in the global quality of life score in patients treated with docetaxel ($p< 0.01$) [71].

A meta-analysis published in 2007 by Di Maio et al. compared the administration of docetaxel every 3 weeks with a weekly schedule second-line treatment of advanced NSCLC [72]. Five trials were eligible for meta-analysis for a total of 865 patients: 433 patients had received docetaxel every 3 weeks and 432 patients weekly docetaxel. PS was 0 in 81%, and 1 in 91% of the patients had received previous platinum containing regimens. Median survival was similar in both treatment groups (27.4 weeks and 26.1 weeks for patients treated every 3 weeks or weekly, respectively). The most striking finding was related to toxicity; weekly docetaxel was associated with a lower frequency of grade 3-4 neutropenia and febrile neutropenia, whereas no significant differences were observed for other hematological toxicities and for nonhematological toxicities.

6.2. Pemetrexed

Hanna et al. conducted a phase III trial in which 571 patients with advanced NSCLC previously treated with one chemotherapy line were randomized to receive pemetrexed (500 mg/m^2) or docetaxel (75 mg/m^2), both every 3 weeks [12]. There were no differences in overall response rate (9.1% and 8.8% for pemetrexed and docetaxel, respectively). Median PFS was 2.9 months for each arm, and median survival time was 8.3 months versus 7.9 months (p= not significant) for pemetrexed and docetaxel, respectively. The 1-year survival rate for each arm was 29.7%. Patients receiving docetaxel were more likely to have grade 3 or 4 neutropenia (40.2% versus 5.3%; p< 0.001), febrile neutropenia (12.7% versus 1.9%; p< 0.001), and hospitalizations for neutropenic fever (13.4% versus 1.5%; p< 0.001) or hospitalizations due to other drug related adverse events (10.5% versus 6.4%; p= 0.092).

An analysis of differential efficacy of pemetrexed according to histology was done in this second-line study and the phase III study of pemetrexed and cisplatin versus cisplatin plus gemcitabine in chemotherapy-naive patients [11]. Nonsquamous patients treated with pemetrexed-based therapy experienced longer survival than the comparators (median 9.3 months versus 8 months; HR 0.78 and 0.84, respectively) whereas squamous patients had shorter survival (6.2 months versus 7.4 months; HR 1.56 and 1.23, respectively). Therefore, the indication of pemetrexed, both for first and for second line therapy, is limited to NSCLC patients with non-squamous histology [73].

6.3. Combination Chemotherapy

Combination chemotherapy as second line treatment does not appear to improve OS compared to single agent chemotherapy. In a meta-analysis of 847 patients from 6 trials, OS was not significantly different between arms (p= 0.32) [74]. Median OS was 37.3 weeks for patients treated with a doublet and 34.7 weeks for patients treated with single agent (HR 0.92, 95% CI 0.79-1.08). Response rate was 15.1% with doublet and 7.3% with single-agent (p= 0.0004). Median PFS was 14 weeks for doublet and 11.7 weeks for single agent (HR 0.79, 95% CI 0.68-0.91; p= 0.0009). Patients treated with doublet chemotherapy had significantly more grade 3 to 4 hematologic (41% versus 25%, p= 0.0001) and grade 3 to 4 nonhematologic toxicity (28% versus 22%, p= 0.034).

In a recent phase II trial comparing the efficacy of pemetrexed versus carboplatin/pemetrexed in patients previously treated with platinum-based chemotherapy, no difference was observed in PFS (median 3.6 months versus 3.5 months; HR 1.05, 95% CI, 0.81-1.36; p= 0.706), OS (median 9.2 months versus 8.8 months; HR 0.97, 95% CI 0.73-1.30; p= 0.834); or response rate (12.6% versus 12.5%; OR 1.01, 95% CI 0.47-2.17; p= 0.980) [75].

The use of combinations chemotherapy regimens in the second line is only indicated for patients with advanced NSCLC whose tumors contain a targeted mutation and have progressed to the initial treatment with targeted agents.

Conclusion

Therapy directed against molecular targets is the first-line choice for patients who have activating mutations of EGFR or ALK translocations. However, less than 30% of patients may benefit from these treatments. In the rest, outside of clinical trials, chemotherapy with platinum-based doublets is the standard treatment. In recent years, the biggest change that has occurred in the management of advanced NSCLC is the differential treatment according to the histological subtype (squamous versus non-squamous). Pemetrexed has shown to be effective only in the non-squamous carcinoma, whereas bevacizumab is associated with an increased risk of bleeding in squamous cell carcinoma. The use of these drugs in first-line and maintenance has allowed an increase in the survival of NSCLC patients with non-squamous histology until 14-18 months.

References

[1] NCCN Clinical Practice Guidelines in Oncology. National Comprensive Cancer Network. http://www.nccn.org/professionals. Version 2.2104.

[2] Lung Cancer Mutation Consortium. http://www.golcmc.com/about-mutation. Updated October 18, 2013

[3] NSCLC Meta-Analyses Collaborative Group. Chemotherapy in addition to supportive care improves survival

[4] Azzoli CG, Baker S Jr, Temin S, et al: American Society of Clinical Oncology clinical practice guideline update on chemotherapy for stage IV non–small-cell lung cancer. *J. Clin. Oncol.* 2009; 27: 6251-66.

[5] Rajeswaran A, Trojan A, Burnand B, Giannelli M. Efficacy and side effects

[6] Schiller JH, Harrington D, Belani C, et al. Comparison of four chemotherapy regimens for advanced non-small-cell lung cancer. *N. Engl. J. Med.* 2002; 346: 92-8.

[7] Alberola V, Camps C, Provencio M, et al. Cisplatin plus gemcitabine versus a cisplatin-based triplet versus nonplatinum sequential doublets in advanced non-small-cell lung cancer: a Spanish lung cancer group phase III randomized trial. *J. Clin. Oncol.* 2003; 21: 3207-13.

[8] Smit EF, Van Meerbeeck JPAM, Lianes P, et al. Three-arm randomized study of two cisplatin–based regimens and paclitaxel plus gemcitabine in advanced non-small-cell lung cancer: A phase III trial of the European Organization for Research and Treatment of Cancer Lung Cancer Group- EORTC 08975. *J. Clin. Oncol.* 2003; 21: 3909-17.

[9] Scagliotti GV, De Marinis F, Rinaldi M, et al. Phase III randomized trial comparing three platinum-based doublets in advanced non-small-cell lung cancer. *J. Clin. Oncol.* 2002; 20: 4285-91.

[10] Georgoulias V, Papadakis E, Alexopoulos A, et al. Platinum-based and non-platinum-based chemotherapy in advanced non-small-cell lung cancer: a randomised multicentre trial. *Lancet.* 2001; 357: 1478-84.

[11] Scagliotti GV, Pariskh P, von Pawel J, et al. Phase III study comparing cisplatin plus gemcitabine with cisplatin plus pemetrexed in chemotherapy non-small-cell lung cancer. *J. Clin. Oncol.* 2008; 25: 3543-51.

[12] Hanna N, Shepherd FA, Fosella FV, et al. Randomized phase III trial of pemetrexed versus docetaxel in patients with non-small-cell lung cancer previously treated with chemotherapy. *J. Clin. Oncol.* 2004; 22: 1589-97.

[13] Ciuleanu T, Brodowitcz T, Zielinski C, et al. Maintenance pemetrexed plus best supportive care v placebo plus best supportive care for non-small-cell lung cancer: a randomised, double-blind, phase 3 study. *Lancet.* 2009; 374: 432-40.

[14] Johnson DH, Fehrenbaccher L, Novotny WF, et al. Randomized phase II trial comparing bevacizumab plus carboplatin and paclitaxel with carboplatin and paclitaxel alone in previously untreated locally advanced or metastatic non-small-cell lung cancer. *J. Clin. Oncol.* 2004; 22: 2184-91.

[15] Reck M, von Pawel J, Zatloukal P, et al. Phase III trial of cisplatin plus gemcitabine with either placebo or bevacizumab as first-line therapy for non-squamous non-small-cell lung cancer: AVAiL. *J. Clin. Oncol.* 2009; 27: 1227-34.

[16] Sandler A, Gray R, Perry MC, et al. Paclitaxel-carboplatin alone or with bevacizumab for non-small-cell lung cancer. *N. Engl. J. Med.* 2006; 355: 1542-2550.

[17] Reck M, von Pawel J, Zatloukal P, et al. Overall survival with cisplatin-gemcitabine and bevacizumab or placebo as first-line therapy for non-squamous non-small-cell lung cancer: result from a randomized phase III trial (AVAiL). *Ann. Oncol.* 2010; 21: 1804-9.

[18] Lord RV, Brabender J, Gandara D, et al. Low ERCC1 expression correlates with prolonged survival after cisplatin plus gemcitabine chemotherapy in non-small cell lung cancer. *Clin. Cancer Res.* 2002; 8 (7): 2286-91.

[19] Hubner R, Riley RD, Billinghan LJ, Sanjay P. Excision Repair Cross-Complementation Group 1 (ERCC1) Status and Lung Cancer Outcomes: A Meta-Analysis of Published Studies and Recommendations. *Plos One.* 2011; 6 (10): e25164.

[20] Jiang J, Liang X, Zhou X, Huang R, Chu Z, Zhan Q. ERCC1 expression as a prognostic and predictive factor in patients with non-small cell lung cancer: a meta-analysis. *Mol. Biol. Rep.* 2012; 39: 6933-42.

[21] Cobo M, Isla D, Massuti B, et al. Customizing Cisplatin Based on Quantitative Excision Repair Cross-Complementing 1 mRNA Expression: A Phase III Trial in Non–Small-Cell Lung Cancer. *J. Clin. Oncol.* 25: 2747-54.

[22] Rosell R, Danenberg KD, Alberola V, et al. Ribonucleotide Reductase Messenger RNA Expression and Survival in Gemcitabine/Cisplatin-Treated Advanced Non-Small Cell Lung Cancer Patients. *Clin. Cancer Res.* 2004; 10: 1318-25.

[23] Bepler G, Kusmartseva I, Sharma S, Gautam A, Cantor A, Sharma A, Simon G. RRM1 modulated in vitro and in vivo efficacy of gemcitabine and platinum in non-small-cell lung cancer. *J. Clin. Oncol.* 2006; 24 (29): 4731-7.

[24] Souglakos J, Boukovinas I, Taron M, et al. Ribonucleotide reductase subunits M1 and M2 mRNA expression levels and clinical outcome of lung adenocarcinoma patients treated with docetaxel/gemcitabine. *Br. J. Cancer.* 2008; 98 (10): 1710-5.

[25] Ceppi P, Volante M, Novello S, et al. ERCC1 and RRM1 gene expressions but not EGFR are predictive of shorter survival in advanced non-small-cell lung cancer treated with cisplatin and gemcitabine. *Ann. Oncol.* 2006; 17: 1818-25.

[26] Gong W, Zhang X, Wu J, et al. RRM1 expression and clinical outcome of gemcitabine-containing chemotherapy for advanced non-small-cell lung cancer: A meta-analysis. *Lung Cancer.* 2012; 75: 374-80.

[27] Simon G, Sharma A, Li X, et al. Feasibility and efficacy of molecular analysis-directed individualized therapy in advanced non-small-cell lung cancer. *J. Clin. Oncol.* 2007; 25: 2741-6.

[28] Taron M, Rosell R, Felip E, et al. BRCA1 mRNA expression levels as an indicator of chemoresistance in lung cáncer. *Hum. Mol. Genet.* 2004; 13: 2443–9.

[29] Rosell R, Moran T, Cobo M, et al. The Spanish Lung Cancer Group (SLCG) BRCA1-RAP80 Expression Customization (BREC) randomized phase III trial of customized chemotherapy in advanced non- small-cell lung cancer (NSCLC) patients with wild-type epidermal growth factor receptor (EGFR) (NCT00617656/GECP-BREC). International Association for the Study of Lung Cancer. 15th World Conference on Lung Cancer, 2013. Abstract 1157.

[30] Grilli R, Oxman AD, Julian JA. Chemotherapy for advanced non-small-cell lung cancer: How much benefit is enough? *J. Clin. Oncol.* 1993; 11: 1866-72.

[31] Souquet PJ, Chauvin F, Boissel JP, Cellerino R, Cormier Y, Ganz PA, et al. Polychemotherapy in advanced non small cell lung cancer: a meta-analysis. *Lancet.* 1993; 342: 19-21.

[32] Marino P, Pampallona S, Preatroni A, Cantoni A, Invernizzi F. Chemotherapy vs supportive care in advanced non-small-cell lung cancer. Results of a meta-analysis of the literature. *Chest.* 1994; 106: 861-5.

[33] Clegg A, Scott DA, Hewitson P, Sidhu M, Waugh N. Clinical and cost effectiveness of paclitaxel, docetaxel, gemcitabine and vinorelbine in non-small celll luna cancer: a systematic review. *Thorax.* 2002; 57: 20-8.

[34] Delbaldo C, Michiels S, Syz N, et al. Benefits of adding a drug to a single-agent or a 2-agent chemotherapy regimen in advanced non-small-cell lung cancer: a meta-analysisis. *JAMA.* 2004; 2929: 470-84.

[35] Ardizzoni A, Boni L, Tiseo M, et al. Cisplatin- versus carboplatin-based chemotherapy in first-line treatment of advanced non-small-cell lung cancer: an individual patient data meta-analysis. *J. Natl. Cancer Inst.* 2007; 99: 847-57.

[36] Ferry D, Billingham L, Harrett H, et al. British Thoracic Oncology Group trial, BTOG2: randomized phase III clinical trial of gemcitabine combined with cisplatin 50 mg/m2 versus cisplatin 80 mg/m2 versus carboplatin AUC6 in advanced NSCLC (abstract 2219). *J. Thorac. Oncol.* 2011; 6: S274.

[37] Schuette W, Blankenburg T, Guschall W, et al. Multicenter randomized trial for stage IIIB/IV non-small-cell lung cancer using evety-3-week *versus* weekly paclitaxel/carboplatin. *Clin. Lung Cancer.* 2006; 7: 338-43.

[38] Peters S, Adjei AA, Gridelli C., et al. Metastatic non-small-cell lung cancer (NSCLC): ESMO Clínical Practice Guidelines for diagnosis, treatment and follow-up. *Ann. Oncol.* 2012: 23 (S7): vii56-vii64.

[39] Camps C, Felip E, García-Campelo R, et al. SEOM clinical guidelines for the treatment of non-small cell lung cancer (NSCLC) 2013. *Clin. Transl. Oncol.* 2013; 15 (12): 977-84.

[40] Volm M, Koomagi R, Mattern J. Prognosis value of vascular endothelial growth factor and its receptor Flt-1 in squamous cell lung cancer. *Int. J. Cancer.* 1997; 74: 64-8.

[41] Imoto H, Okasi T, Taga S, et al. Vascular endotelial growth factor expression in non-small-cell lung cáncer: prognosis significance in squamous cell carcinoma. *J. Thorac. Cardiovasc. Surg.* 1998; 115: 1007-14.

[42] Fontanini G, Vignati S, Boldrini L, et al. Vascular endothelial growth factor is associated with neovascularization and influences progression of non-small cell lung carcinoma. *Clin. Cancer Res.* 1997; 3: 861-5.
[43] Zhan P, Wang J, Xiao-jing LV, et al. Prognostic value of vascular endothelial growth factor expression in patients with lung cancer. A systematic review with meta-analysis. *J. Thorac. Oncol.* 2009; 4: 1094-103.
[44] Dowlati A, Gray R, Johnson DH, et al. Prospective correlative assessment of biomarkers in E4599 randomized phase II/III trial of carboplatin and paclitaxel (+/-) bevacizumab in advanced non-small cell lung cancer (NSCLC). *J. Clin. Oncol.* 2006; 24: 7027.
[45] Soria JC, Mauguen A, Reck M, et al. Systematic review and meta-analysis of randomised, phase II/III trials adding bevacizumab to platinum-based chemotherapy as first-line treatment in patients with advanced non-small-cell lung cancer. *Ann. Oncol.* 2013; 24: 20-30.
[46] Crinò L, Dansin E, Garrido P, et al. Safety and efficacy of first-line bevacizumab-based therapy in advanced non-squamous non-small-cell lung cancer (SAiL, MO19390): a phase 4 study. *Lancet Oncol.* 2010; 11: 733-40.
[47] Pirker R, Pereira JR, Szczesna A, et al. Cetuximab plus chemotherapy in patients with advanced non-small cell lung cancer (FLEX): an open-label randomized phase III trial. *Lancet.* 2009; 373: 1525-31.
[48] Lynch TJ, Patel T, Dreisbach L, et al. Cetuximab and first-line taxane/carboplatin chemotherapy in advanced non-small-cell lung cancer: results of the randomized multicenter phase III trial BMS 099. *J. Clin. Oncol.* 2010; 38: 911-7.
[49] Morabito A, Gebbia V, Di Maio M, et al. Randomized phase III trial of gemcitabine and cisplatin versus gemcitabine alone in patients with advanced non-small cell lung cancer and a performance status of 2: the CAPPA-2 study. *Lung Cancer.* 2013; 81 (1): 77-83.
[50] Zukin M, Barrios CH, Pereira JR, et al. Randomized phase III trial of single-agent pemetrexed versus carboplatin and pemetrexed in patients with advanced non-small-cell lung cancer and Eastern Cooperative Oncology Group performance status of 2. *J. Clin. Oncol.* 2013; 31 (23): 2849-53.
[51] Kelly K, Crowley J, Bunn PA Jr, Presant CA, Grevstad PK, Moinpour CM, et al. Randomized phase III trial of paclitaxel plus carboplatin versus vinorelbine plus cisplatin in the treatment of patients with advanced non-small cell lung cancer: a Southwest Oncology Group trial. *J. Clin. Oncol.* 2001; 19: 3210-8.
[52] Fossella F, Pereira JR, von Pawel J, et al. Randomized, multinational, phase III study of docetaxel plus platinumcombinations versus vinorelbine plus cisplatin for advanced non-small-cell lung cancer: the TAX 326 study group. *J. Clin. Oncol.* 2003; 21 (16): 3016-24.
[53] Gridelli C, Maione P, Rossi A, et al. Potential treatment options after first-line chemotherapy for advanced NSCLC: maintenance treatment or early second-line? *Oncologist.* 2009; 14: 137-47.
[54] Owonikoko TK, Ramalingam SS, Belani C. Maintenance therapy for advanced non-small cell lung cancer: Current status, controversies, and emerging consensus. *Clin. Cancer Res.* 2010; 16: 2496-504.

[55] Westeel V, Quoix E, Moro-Sibilot D, et al. Randomized Study of Maintenance Vinorelbine in Responders With Advanced Non – Small-Cell Lung Cancer. *J. Natl. Cancer Inst.* 2005; 97: 499-506.

[56] Belani CP, Barstis J, Perry MC, et al. Multicenter, Randomized Trial for Stage IIIB or IV Non–Small-Cell Lung Cancer Using Weekly Paclitaxel and Carboplatin Followed by Maintenance Weekly Paclitaxel or Observation. *J. Clin. Oncol.* 2003; 21: 2933-9.

[57] Brodowicz T, Krzakowski M, Zwitter M,et al. Cisplatin and gemcitabine first-line chemotherapy followed by maintenance gemcitabine or best supportive care in advanced non-small cell lung cancer: a phase III trial. *Lung Cancer.* 2006; 52: 155-63.

[58] Fidias PM, Dakhil SR, Lyss AP, et al. Phase III study of immediate compared with delayed docetaxel after fron-line therapy with gemcitabine plus carboplatin in advanced non-small-cell lung cancer. *J. Clin. Oncol.* 2009; 27: 591-8.

[59] Soon YY, Stockler MR, Askie LM, Boyer MJ. Duration of chemotherapy for advanced non-small-cell lung cancer: A systematic review and meta-analysis of randomized trials. *J. Clin. Oncol.* 2009; 27: 3277-83.

[60] Paz-Ares L, de Marinis F, Dediu M, et al. Maintenance therapy with pemetrexed plus best supportive care versus placebo plus best supportive care after induction therapy with pemetrexed plus cisplatin for advanced non-squamous non-small-cell lung cancer (PARAMOUNT): a double-blind, phase 3, randomised controlled trial. *Lancet Oncol.* 2012; 13 (3): 247-55.

[61] Paz-Ares LG, de Marinis F, Dediu M, et al. PARAMOUNT: Final overall survival results of the phase III study of maintenance pemetrexed versus placebo immediately after induction treatment with pemetrexed plus cisplatin for advanced nonsquamous non-small-cell lung cancer. *J. Clin. Oncol.* 2013; 31 (23): 2895-902.

[62] Cappuzzo F, Ciuleanu L, Stelmakh S, et al., on belhalf of the SATURN Investigators. Erlotinib as maintenance treatment in advanced non-small-cell lung cancer: a multicentre, randomised, placebo-controlled phase 3 study. *Lancet Oncol.* 2010; 11: 521-9.

[63] Johnson BE, Kabbinavar F, Fehrenbacher L, et al. ATLAS: randomized, double-blind, placebo-controlled, phase IIIB trial comparing bevacizumab therapy with or without erlotinib, after completion of chemotherapy, with bevacizumab for first-line treatment of advanced non-small-cell lung cancer. *J. Clin. Oncol.* 2013; 31: 3926-34.

[64] Mezger J, von Pawel J, Reck M, et al. Bevacizumab (Bv) single-agent maintenance following Bv-based chemotherapy in patients with advanced non-small cell lung cancer (NSCLC): Results from an exploratory analysis of the AVAiL study. *J. Clin. Oncol.* 2009; 27: e19001.

[65] Laskin j, Hirsh V, Cheng AC, et al. Final safety data from patients (pts) who received maintenance (mnt) bevacizumab (bv) in the mo19390 (SAiL) trial: first-line bv plus chemotherapy (ct) in advanced or recurrent non-small cell lung cancer (NSCLC). *Ann. Oncol.* 2010; 21 (suppl 8): 428.

[66] Ravelo A, Nadler E, Yu E, et al. Bevacizumab (BV) treatment (TX) to progression (BTP): outcomes from a US community practice Network. *Ann. Oncol.* 2010; 21 (suppl 8): 431.

[67] Patel JD, Hensing TA, Rademaker A, et al. Phase II study of pemetrexed and carboplatin plus bevacizumab with maintenance pemetrexed and bevacizumab as first-

line therapy for nonsquamous non-small-cell lung cancer. *J. Clin. Oncol.* 2009; 27: 3284-9.

[68] Barlesi F, Schepereel A, Rittmeyer A, et al. Randomized Phase III Trial of Maintenance Bevacizumab With or Without Pemetrexed After First-Line Induction With Bevacizumab, Cisplatin, and Pemetrexed in Advanced Nonsquamous Non–Small-Cell Lung Cancer: AVAPERL (MO22089). *J. Clin. Oncol.* 2013; 31: 3004-11.

[69] Patel JD, Socinski MA, Garon EB, et al. PointBreak: A Randomized Phase III Study of Pemetrexed Plus Carboplatin and Bevacizumab Followed by Maintenance Pemetrexed and Bevacizumab Versus Paclitaxel Plus Carboplatin and Bevacizumab Followed by Maintenance Bevacizumab in Patients With Stage IIIB or IV Nonsquamous Non–Small-Cell Lung Cancer. *J. Clin. Oncol.* 2013; 31:4349-57.

[70] Shepherd FA, Dancey J, Ramlau R, et al. Prospective randomized trial of docetaxel versus best supportive care in patients with non-small-cell lung cancer previously treated with platinum-based chemotherapy. *J. Clin. Oncol.* 2000; 18: 2095-103.

[71] Dancey J, Shepherd FA, Gralla RJ, Kim YS. Quality of life assessment of second-line docetaxel versus best supportive care in patients with non-small-cell lung cancer previously treated with platinum-based chemotherapy: results of a prospective, randomized phase III trial. *Lung Cancer.* 2004; 43: 183-94.

[72] Di Maio M, Perrone F, Chiodini P, et al. Individual patient data meta-analysis of docetaxel administered once every 3 weeks compared with once every week second-line treatment of advanced non-small-cell lung cancer. *J. Clin. Oncol.* 2007; 25: 1377-82.

[73] Scagliotti G, Hanna N, Fossella F, et al. The differential efficacy of pemetrexed according to NSCLS histology: a review of two phase III studies. *Oncologist.* 2009; 14: 253-63.

[74] Di Maio M, Chiodini P, Georgoulias V, et al. Meta-analysis of single-agent chemotherapy compared with combination chemotherapy as second-line treatment of advanced non-small-cell lung cancer. *J. Clin. Oncol.* 2009; 27: 1836-43.

[75] Ardizzoni A, Tiseo M, Boni L, et al. Pemetrexed versus pemetrexed and carboplatin as second-line chemotherapy in advanced non-small-cell lung cancer: results of the GOIRC 02-2006 randomized phase II study and pooled analysis with the NVALT7 trial. *J. Clin. Oncol.* 2012; 30: 4501-7.

In: Fighting Lung Cancer through the HER Family ...
Editor: Diego Márquez-Medina

ISBN: 978-1-63321-092-9

Chapter 3

Biology I. Human Epidermal Growth Factor Receptors in Health and Tumor Cells

M. Ángeles Montero-Fernández, M.D., Ph.D.
Histopathology Department, Royal Brompton and
Harefield NHS Trust, Imperial College of London, UK

Abstract

Surgical resection remains the treatment of choice of selected patients with lung cancer to achieve good results. In the last decade, advances in the understanding of molecular alterations in lung cancer have improved survival and quality of life of selected patients. Among the most important findings, the determination of activating mutations in the receptor tyrosine kinase, and the possibility of treating a poor prognosis cancer, have created new expectations. All of these changes have made the role of the pathologist more relevant. From the preoperative diagnosis, staging, intraoperative evaluation and extension of the disease as well as the study of the margins of resection. Changes in the latest classifications, advances in immunohistochemistry, discovery of molecular alterations and, identification of prognostic and response to therapy markers, have forced the pathologist to change their way of work. Actually, pathologists are part of multi-disciplinary work teams that integrate clinical, radiological and pathological data to improve patient management. Furthermore, continuous advances in genomics and proteomics are creating new and exciting expectations in the knowledge of early diagnosis and new gene therapies, which are expected to be applied in a near future to increase survival, reduce recurrences and improve quality of life in lung cancer patients.

1. Introduction

In the last decade, advances in the understanding of molecular alterations in lung cancer have improved survival and quality of life of selected patients. Among the most important findings, the determination of activating mutations in the receptor tyrosine kinase, and the possibility of treating a cancer that until now had been considered virtually untreatable, have created new expectations. Despite progress, it is still unknown mutational status in 50% of cases, and therapeutic targets can be used in only 20% of lung cancers.

2. Basic Knowledge in Small Doses

2.1. Cell Communication

Communication between cells is vital for the maintenance of its own homeostasis. Cells link up with nearby cells, what so called local communication, by means of cell junctions, superficial receptors, chemical messengers or changes in the physical environment and with cells in other organs or long distance communication, mainly produced by hormones.

Local communication is characterized by a direct intercellular contact through cell junctions, which directly connect the cytoplasm of adjacent cells or via direct contact between membranes bound cell surface molecules, a process called cell to cell recognition. This type of local signaling is important in embryonic development and immune response. In many other cases, local signaling is induced by messenger molecules, which are secreted by the signaling cells. These are called local regulators. One class of local regulators is growth factors (GF), which comprise compounds that stimulate growth and division of local target cells. Numerous cells can simultaneously receive and respond to GF produced by a single cell. This type of local signaling is called paracrine signaling.

Long distance signaling is yield by hormones. In hormonal signaling, also known as endocrine signaling, specialized cells release hormone molecules, which travel the circulatory system to other parts of the body, where they reach their target cells that can recognize and respond to their stimuli.

Cell signaling is a well-recognized three-step process. The first one is called reception, in which the cell detects the signaling molecule or ligand coming from outside the cell. This signal is detected when the ligand binds the receptor protein located at the cell´s surface or inside the cell. The second step is the transduction, which is the process that converts the signal into an intracellular event that induce a specific response and the third step is the response, which activates any cellular activity.

2.2. Tyrosine Kinase Receptors

Most ligands bind to specific sites on receptor transmembrane proteins, which transmit the information from the extracellular environment to the inside of the cell by changing the shape or aggregating when a specific ligand binds to it. One of the three major types is the receptor tyrosine kinase.

Tyrosine Kinase receptors (TKRs) belong to a major class of plasma membrane receptors characterized by having an enzymatic activity. The cytoplasmic domain of the receptor functions as a tyrosine kinase, an enzyme that catalyzed the transfer of a phosphate group from an ATP to the amino acid tyrosine on a substrate protein. Before the ligand binds, the receptor exists as an individual unit, a monomer. The binding of the ligand induces association between two monomers, forming a complex known as a dimer.

Dimerization activates the tyrosine kinase region of each monomer. Each tyrosine kinase adds a phosphate from an ATP molecule to a tyrosine on the tail of each monomer, and activates the receptor. This activation induces the transduction pathway, leading to a cellular response (Figure 1) [1].

3. The Epidermal Growth Factors Receptors in Normal Cells

The epidermal growth factor receptor (EGFR) belongs to the ErbB family of receptor tyrosine kinases which includes four members: EGFR or Her1/ErbB1, Her2/Erb-2, Her3/Erb-3 and Her4/Erb-4 [2].

All these transmembrane proteins have an extracellular ligand-binding domain, a single hydrophobic transmembrane domain and a cytoplasmic tyrosine kinase-containing domain, which is activated after binding with peptide growth factors of the EGF-family of proteins [3].

Erb-B2 has no known ligands, but can stabilize EGFR in a conformation that potentiates dimerization and phosphorylation in the absence of ligand. Erb-B3 was considered to be kinase dead, but retains the ability to transphosphorylate its own intracellular domain [4] and form a very active signaling complex with other EGFR TKR, especially ErbB2.

In addition to cross-talks between members of the EGRF/Erb family, there is evidence of significant interactions with other TKR such as c-MET and IGFR-1R, and it is possible that such alternative signaling pathways are linked to resistance to targeted therapies [5].

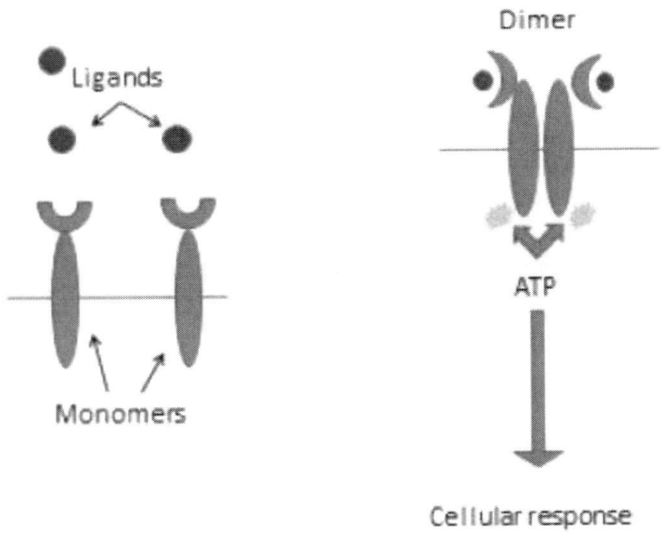

Figure 1. The binding of the ligand induces dimerization, phosphorylation and activation of the receptor. This activation induces the transduction pathway and the cellular response.

4. Ligands

There are up to 13 recognized ligands of the EGFR family: EGF itself, Transforming factor-α (TGF-α), amphiregulin, heparin-binding EGF, β-cellulin, epigen, neuregulin 1-6, and epiregulin. EGF and TGF-α are the key EGFR binding ligands.

It is well known that the EGFR signaling pathways mediate a wide range of cellular responses such as evasion of apoptosis, self-sufficient growth, and insensitivity to anti-growth signals, sustained angiogenesis, tissue invasion and metastasis upon ligand binding activation. The EGFR pathways are also regulated by feed-back loops, thereby, activation induces an increase of cellular production of ligands and increase of receptor internalization [6]. EGF-like growth factors can be produced either by the same cells that express EGFRs in an autocrine secretion fashion or by the surrounding cells in a paracrine secretion fashion [7].

5. Downstream Signaling

Ligand binding induces conformational rearrangements of the receptors to expose the interaction loop, promoting association of both homodimers and heterodimers, followed by internalization and/or phosphorylation events. EGFR activates two major intracellular signaling pathways: the PI3 Kinase-AKT/protein kinase B-mammalian target of rapamycin (mTOR) cascades, which regulates anti-apoptotic and pro-survival cascades and the Ras-Raf-MEK (MAPK), which on the other hand, controls gene transcription, G1/S cell-cycle progression and cellular proliferation.

These pathways are also modulated by other proteins such as c-mesenchymal-epithelial transition factor (c-MET), insulin-like growth factor 1 receptor (IGF-1R), LKB1 and the echinoderm microtubule-associated protein-like 4/anaplastic lymphoma kinase (EML4-ALK) fusion proteins. EGFR also activates other cascades as the phospholipase C-protein kinase (PKC) and Janus Kinase/signal transducers and activators of transcription of nuclear factors (STAT) pathways [6].

The ligands induce not only cell proliferation but also alter adhesion and motility, protect against apoptosis at the cellular level, and promote invasion and angiogenesis at the physiological level [8].

6. Growth Factors in Tumor Microenvironment

Communication is not only limited to the interaction between cells but also with extracellular matrix (ECM) and stromal cells. These two components of the microenvironment can module cell growth and differentiation. These interactions are quite specific and it has been known that changes in the microenvironment accompany the transformation process. This is often indicated by increased of fibroblast proliferation and extensive ECM remodeling in neoplastic areas [9]. EGFR is expressed in almost all types of stromal cells [2], therefore, sustained activation of the EFGR signaling in non-malignant cells in tumor microenvironment might influence the behavior of transformed cells and can play an important role in tumor progression.

It is well recognized that overexpression of the EGFR and amplification of its signal is an oncogenic common feature in a variety of human cancers including renal, breast, glioma, ovarian, non-small cell lung, prostate, pancreatic and head and neck cancers [3], but these alterations are not common in other tumor types, which may indicate that activation of EGFR is regulated by other physiological events instead of amplification and mutations. Among these physiological processes, hypoxia is the most relevant [9]. Hypoxia is the result from the imbalance between the cancer cell proliferation and the ability of the vasculature to supply enough oxygen to the tumor [10]. Actually, it had been demonstrated an up-regulation of EGFR protein in human cell lines induced by hypoxic microenvironment [11]. Furthermore, investigations had demonstrated an important relation between microenvironment hypoxia and up-regulation of EGFR in tumor cells without alterations of the receptor.

Immunohistochemical analysis of resected tumor had shown an increase of EGFR expression in areas close to necrotic areas, a histological marker of tumor hypoxia [12]. Moreover, hypoxia increases the motility of cancer cells facilitating tumor metastasis, through inhibition of cell-cell adhesion and increase of the migratory ability [13].

There have been numerous studies focusing on the study of EGFR signaling in the pathogenesis of metastasis. In this respect, interesting results have been obtained in the metastasis of colon cancers [14], breast [15] and esophagus [16] via direct implication of EGFR signaling, as well as in induction of osteolytic lesions in the osseous metastasis [17].

7. EGFR in Lung Cancer

Aberrant activation of the EGFR pathway is thought to be produced at least by three different mechanisms in lung cancer: a) increased production of ligands by cancer cells, b) increased expression of membrane EGF receptors, and c) activating mutations of the *EGFR* gene [6, 18]. EGFR is frequently overexpressed in NSCLC and it has been associated with poor prognosis [19, 20]. Total EGFR protein is detectable in 10 to 85% of patients with NSCLC depending on the methods of assessment, including immunohistochemistry, fluorescence in-situ hybridization and chromogenic in-situ hybridization (FISH/CISH) and mutational analysis.

Somatic mutations in exons 18 to 21 of the tyrosine kinase domain of the EGFR had been shown to correlate with response to tyrosine kinase inhibitors (TKI). They occur in approximately 10% of Western and up to 50% in Asian patients. In fact, several clinical traits such as female gender, never smoker, Asian ethnicity and adenocarcinoma histology were found to be associated with increased response to EGFR-TKI and the presence of *EGFR* mutations. The most common are in-frame deletions in exon 19 (45%), followed by missense mutations in exon 21 (41%). Genetic mutations in the gene encoding proteins involved in the EGFR signaling cascade (Kras, HER2, BRAF, PI3K, LKB1, SHP2) seem to be mutually exclusive somatic mutations and are negative predictors of tumor response to EGFR-TKI. Acquired resistance to EGFR-TKI has been associated most frequently with mutation T790M (Figure 2). *EGFR* gene amplification is detected in some *EGFR* mutated tumors and is reported to be associated with disease progression [21]. EGFR protein levels can be detected using several methods, which comprise radioactive-labeled ligand binding, competitive immunoassay, western blotting and immunohistochemistry (IHC).

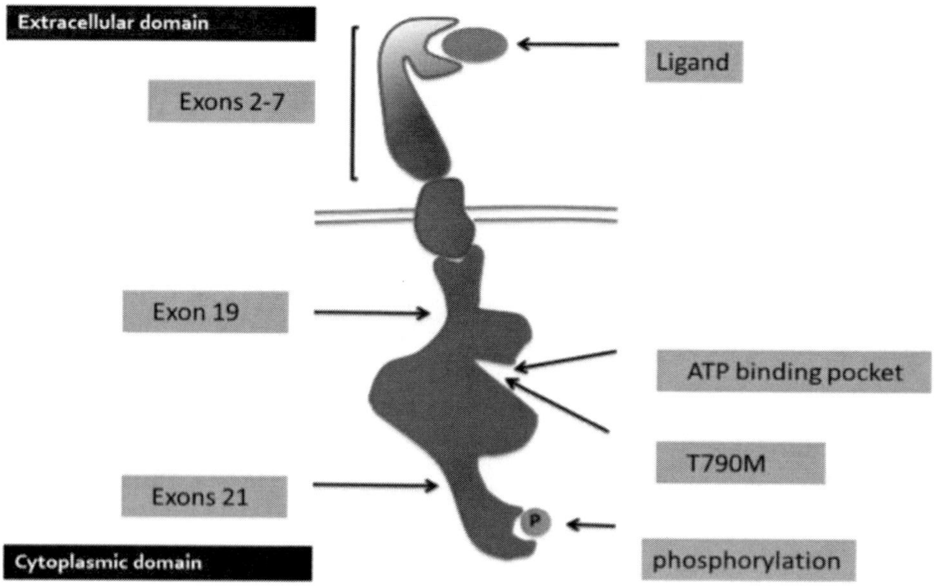

Figure 2. Epidermal growth factor receptor. Most frequent exons with driver mutations.

All these technologies, excluding IHC require expensive and complex laboratory equipment and their sensitivity may vary with the quality of the extracted DNA, tumor cellularity, and contamination with non-mutated allele [6, 22]. IHC detection of EGFR protein levels has been inconsistent in predicting response to EGFR-TKIs. Moreover, greater response has been observed in tumors harboring activating *EGFR* TK domain mutations, mainly exon 19 in-frame deletion and exon 21 missense mutations. To overcome some of these limitations, mutation-specific antibodies have been developed to detect mutant EGFR by IHC and are under validation. IHC is a cost-effective and simple method universally used in pathology laboratories, which can reduce drastically turn-around times to perform the tests [22].

8. Pulmonary Pre-Invasive Lesions

Three pulmonary pre-invasive lesions have been recognized in the recent WHO classification: squamous bronchial dysplasia and carcinoma in-situ as precursors of squamous cell and basalioid carcinoma, atypical adenomatous hyperplasia of peripheral adenocarcinoma and diffuse idiopathic pulmonary neuroendocrine cell hyperplasia of typical carcinoids. So far, it has not been identified the precursor for small cell carcinoma.

The mere recognition of the existence of a precursor lesion indicates a multistage progression model mainly for squamous carcinomas and peripheral adenocarcinomas.

In 1995, Noguchi and colleagues developed an interesting independent classification for small and peripheral adenocarcinomas, less than 2 cm in size, consisting in six tumors subtypes, A to G [23]. Types A and B comprised small size tumors with pure lepidic pattern and without or with alveolar collapse and fibrosis respectively.

The rest of sub-types showed different degree of invasion. Among A and B sub-types, nodal metastasis were never present and these tumors had a 100% 5-year free survival if they were completely resected.

Nowadays, both tumors are considered adenocarcinoma in-situ in the recent WHO 2011 classification, and interestingly *EGFR* mutations had been found in both of them, as well as in the non-malignant peripheral airways in the vicinity of invasive peripheral adenocarcinomas. This indicates that mutation is an early event in tumor development [24, 25].

Atypical adenomatous hyperplasia (AAH) is a discrete lesion, single or multiple, less than 5 mm in diameter, and situated at the periphery of the respiratory bronchioles (Figure 3A). It comprises a proliferation of mild to moderate atypical type II pneumocytes, lining the distal small airways from the alveoli to the respiratory bronchioles. Typically lacks interstitial inflammation and fibrosis. Intranuclear inclusions, increase of nuclear size and nuclear tufts are also seen, but they differ from true papillae with stromal cores typical of papillary adenocarcinoma or atypical intraalveolar tufts seen in micropapillary adenocarcinomas.

Differentiate AAH from adenocarcinoma in-situ (AIS) is sometimes difficult, mainly in small biopsies. AIS is mainly considered when the lesion measures more than 10 mm and less than 30 mm, and displays higher nuclear atypia or pleomorphism than AAH (Figure 3B and C).

AAH is frequently observed (up to 40%) in the peripheral lung parenchyma of patients with lung adenocarcinoma unlike the lower incidence (less than 4%) in patients without cancer [26]. These lesions are found as pure ground glass opacity in the lung periphery on computed tomography, but even when multiple, do not influence the prognosis of patients with adenocarcinoma [27].

9. Phenotype and EGFR Mutation Status Correlation

Mucinous adenocarcinoma has been consistently described as TTF1 Negative, EGFR negative and *Kras* mutation positive [28], but genetic abnormalities can be seen in different histologies, and in the same tumor.

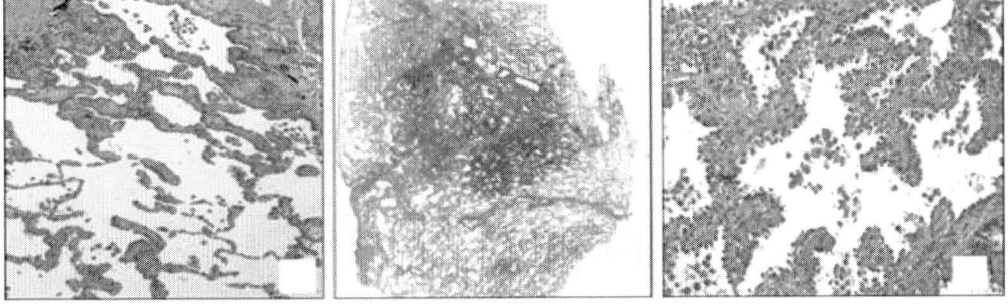

a b c

Figure 3. (A) atypical adenomatous hyperplasia, less than 5 mm lesion, with mild type II pneumocyte atypia. (B) Adenocarcinoma in-situ, less than 20 mm lesion with moderate to severe type II pneumocyte atypia (C).

Favorable responses (20% of the patients) had been obtained in adenocarcinomas with predominant lepidic and papillary patterns [29, 30] treated with genitinib [31] but *EGFR* mutational status and adenocarcinoma subtype has been an issue of intense debate [21]. Most frequently, adenocarcinomas with *EGFR* mutations show acinar, papillary and micropapillary patterns (Figure 4A and B). The presence of *EGFR* mutations in squamous cell carcinoma is a subject to debate. Interesting works have been made that stress the low frequency of mutations in pure squamous carcinomas [32] and in the absence of role of *EGFR* mutations in EGFR-TKIs prediction of efficacy [33]. On the other hand, adenosquamous carcinoma is a rare type of lung carcinoma, comprising 0.4 to 4% of non-small cell type. It is characterized by a mixture of both adeno and squamous carcinoma and *EGFR* mutations usually present with the same frequency as adenocarcinomas. Of noted, *EGFR* mutations can be found in both components, adeno and squamous (Figure 4C and D).

Another explanation for the detection of *EGFR* mutations in squamous cell carcinomas is the solid growth pattern adenocarcinoma. This variant, usually corresponds to poorly differentiated adenocarcinoma, whose histologic diagnosis requires the use of IHC or molecular techniques given the close morphological similarity [34].

Large cell carcinoma is defined as a non-small cell carcinoma lacking morphological differentiation as either adenocarcinoma or squamous carcinoma. It is suspected to represent an end-stage of poor differentiation of these tumor types. Some authors have observed that a high percentage of these tumors can be classified by IHC as variants of adenocarcinomas more frequently, squamous cell carcinomas, undifferentiated carcinomas and those with neuroendocrine differentiation.

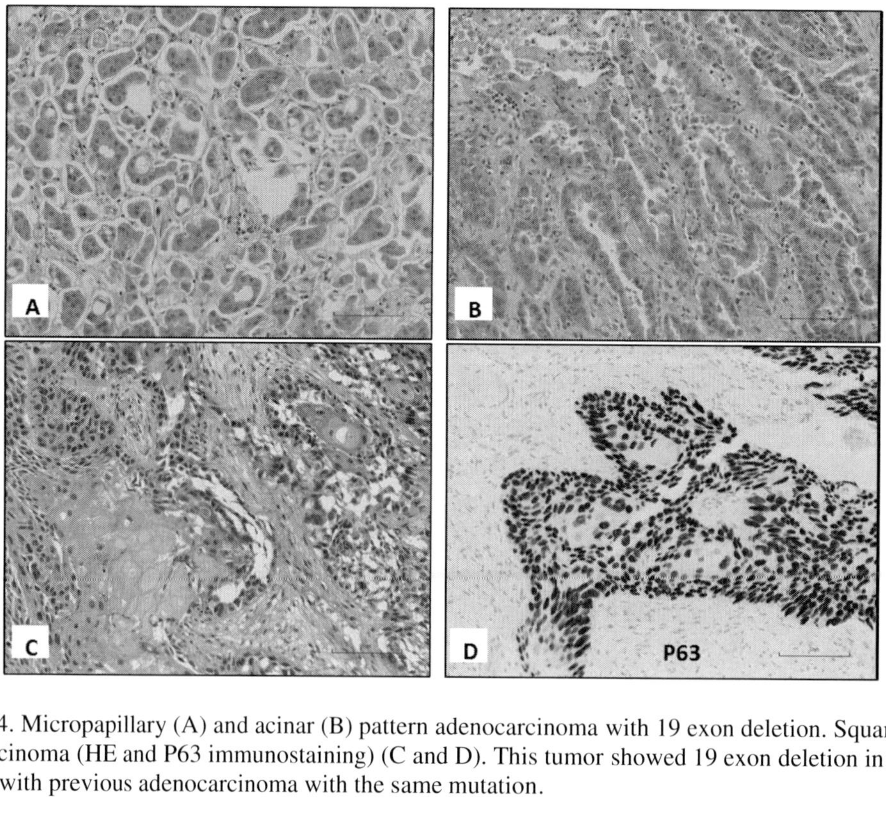

Figure 4. Micropapillary (A) and acinar (B) pattern adenocarcinoma with 19 exon deletion. Squamous cell carcinoma (HE and P63 immunostaining) (C and D). This tumor showed 19 exon deletion in a patient with previous adenocarcinoma with the same mutation.

Stratifiying these tumors according to their immunoprofile and driver mutations may impact drastically in the choice of the adequate gene therapy [35, 36].

Conclusion

Surgical resection remains the treatment of choice of selected patients with lung cancer to achieve good results. However, the role of the pathologist has changed with the latest advances in therapy. Nowadays, pathologists play an important role in lung cancer patient management: From the preoperative diagnosis, staging, intraoperative evaluation and extension of the disease as well as the study of the margins of resection. Changes in the latest classifications, advances in immunohistochemistry, discovery of molecular alterations and, identification of prognostic and response to therapy markers, have forced the pathologist to change their way of work. Actually, pathologists are part of multidisciplinary work teams that integrate clinical, radiological and pathological data to improve patient management.

Continuous advances in genomics and proteomics are creating new and exciting expectations in the knowledge of early diagnosis and new gene therapies, which are expected to be applied in a new future to increase survival, reduce recurrences and improve quality of life in lung cancer patients.

References

[1] Reece, J. B., Urry, L. A., Cain, M. L., Wasserman, S. A., Minorsky, P. V., Jackson, R. B. *Campbell Biology*. 9th edition. US: Pearson Education Inc; 2011.

[2] Normanno, N., Gullick, W. J. Epidermal growth factor receptor tyrosine kinase inhibitors and bone metastases: different mechanism of action for a novel therapeutic application? *Endocr. Relat. Cancer*. 2006; 13: 3-6.

[3] Olayioye, M. A., Neve, R. M., Lane, H. A., Hynes, N. E. The Erb signaling network: receptor heterodimerization in development and cancer. *Embo J.* 2000; 19: 3159-67.

[4] Shi, F., Telesco, S. E., Liu, Y., Radhakrishnan, R., Lemmon, M. A. ErbB3/HER 3 intracellular domain is competent to bind ATP and catalyze autophosphorylation. *Proc. Natl. Acad. Sci. US*. 2010; 107: 7692-7.

[5] Jin, Q., Esteva, F. J. Cross-talk between ErbB/Her family and the type I insulin-like growth factor receptor signaling pathway in breast cancer. *J. Mammary gland boil. neoplasia*. 2008; 13: 485-98.

[6] Gazdar, A. F. Epidermal growth factor receptor inhibition in lung cancer: the evolving role of individualized therapy. *Cancer Metastasis Rev*. 2012; 29 (1): 37-48.

[7] Yarden, Y. The EGFR family and its ligands in human cancer. Signaling mechanisms and therapeutic opportunities. *Eur. J. Cancer*. 2001; 37 (Suppl. 4): S3-S8.

[8] Eccles, S. A. The epidermal growth factor receptor/Erb-B/HER family in normal and malignant breast biology. *Int. J. Dev. Biol*. 2011; 55: 685-96.

[9] Zhang, X., Nie, D., Chakrabarty, S. Growth factors in tumour microenvironment. *Front Biosci*. 2012; 15: 151-65.

[10] Vaupel, P. The role of hypoxia-induced factors in tumour progression. *Oncologist.* 2004; 9 (Suppl. 5): 10-7.
[11] Franovic, A., Gunaratnam, L., Smith, K., Robert, I., Patten, D., Lee, S. Translational up-regulation of the EGFR by tumor hipoxia provides a nonmutational explanation for its overexpression in human cancer. *Proc. Natl. Acad. Sci. US.* 2007; 104: 13092-7.
[12] Harris, A. L. Hipoxia-a key regulatory factor in tumour growth. *Nat. Rev. Cancer.* 2002; 2: 38-47.
[13] Wang, T., Nikki, T., Goto, A., et al. Hipoxia increases motility of lung adenocarcinoma cell line A549 via activation of the epidermal growth factor receptor pathway. *Cancer Sci.* 2007; 98: 506-11.
[14] Sasaki, T., Nakamura, T., Rebhun, R. B., et al. Modification of the primary tumour microenvironment by transforming growth factor alpha-epidermal growth factor receptor signaling promotes metastasis in an orthotopic colon cancer model. *Am. J. pathol.* 2008; 173: 205-16.
[15] Pu, J., McCaig, C. D., Cao, L., Zhao, Z., Segall, J. E., Zhao, M. EGF receptor signaling is essential for electric field-directed migration of breast cancer cells. *J. Cell Sci.* 2007; 120: 3395-403.
[16] Wei, Q., Chen, L., Sheng, L., Nordgren, H., Wester, K., Carlsson, J. EGFR, HER 2 and HER 3 expression in esophageal Primary tumours and corresponding metastases. *Int. J. Oncol.* 2007; 31: 493-9.
[17] De Luca, A., Carotenuto, A., Rachiglio, A., et al. The role of EGFR in tumour micro-environment. *J. Cell Physiol.* 2008; 214: 559-67.
[18] Ciardiello, F., Tortora, G. EGFr antagonists in cancer treatment. *N. Engl. J. Med.* 2008; 358 (11): 1160-74.
[19] Hirsch, F. R., Varela-Garcia, M., Bunn, P. A., Jr, et al. Epidermal growth factor receptor in non-small-cell lung carcinomas: correlation between gene copy number and protein expression and impact on prognosis. *J. Clin. Oncol.* 2003; 21 (20): 3798-807.
[20] Ohsaki, Y., Tanno, S., Fujita, Y., et al. Epidermal growth factor receptor expression correlates with poor prognosis in non-small cell lung cancer patients with p53 over-expression. *Oncol. Rep.* 2000; 7 (3): 603-7.
[21] Chirieac, L. R., Dacic, S. Targeted therapies in lung cancer. *Surg. Pathol.* 2010; 3: 72-82.
[22] Allo, G., Bandarchi, B., Yanagawa, N., et al. EGFR mutation-specific immunohisto-chemical antibodies in lung adenocarcinoma. *Histopathology.* 2013. doi: 10.1111/his. 12331. [Epub. ahead of print].
[23] Noguchi, M., Morakawa, A., Kawasaki, M., et al. Small adenocarcinoma of the lung. *Cancer* 1995; 75 (12): 2844-52.
[24] Junichi, S., Shinichi, T., Shuji, I., et al. Sequential molecular changes during multistage pathogenesis of small peripheral adenocarcinomas of the lung. *J. Thorac. Oncol.* 2008; 3 (4): 340-7.
[25] Lantuéjoul, S., Salameire, D., Salon, C., Brambilla, E. Pulmonary pre-neoplasia-sequential molecular carcinogenetic events. *Histopathology.* 2009; 54: 43-54.
[26] Chapman, K. D., Kerr, K. M. The association between atypical adenomatous hyper-plasia and primary lung cancer. *Br. J. Cancer.* 2000; 83: 632-6.
[27] Sukuzi, K., Nagai, K., Yoshida, J., et al. The prognosis of resected lung carcinoma associated with atypical adenomatous hyperplasia: a comparison of the prognosis of

well-differentiated adenocarcinoma associated with atypical adenomatous hyperplasia and intrapulmonary metastasis. *Cancer*. 1997; 79: 1521-6.

[28] Finberg, K. E., Sequist, L., Joshi, V., et al. Mucinous differentiation correlates with absence of EGFR mutation and presence of KRAS mutation in lung adenocarcinomas with bronchioloalveolar features. *J. Mod. Diagn*. 2007; 9 (3): 320-6.

[29] Miller, V. A., Kris, M. G., Shan, N. Bronchioloalveolar pathology subtype and smoking history predict sensitivity to genitinib in advanced non-small-cell lung cancer. *J. Clin. Oncol.* 2004; 22 (6): 1103-9.

[30] Miller, V. A., 2008, Piely, G. J., Zakowski, M. F. Molecular characteristics of bronchioloalveolar carcinoma and adenocarcinoma. Bronchioloalveolar subtype, predict response to erlotinib. *J. Clin. Oncol*. 2008; 26 (9): 1472-8.

[31] West, H. L., Franklin, W. A., McCoy, J. Genitinib therapy in advanced bronchioloalveolar adenocarcinoma. Southwest Oncology group Study S0126. *J. Clin. Oncol.* 2006; 24 (12): 1807-13.

[32] Fang, W., Zhang, J., Liang, W., et al. Efficacy of epidermal growth factor receptor-tyrosine kinase inhibitors for Chinese patients with squamous cell carcinoma of lung harbouring EGFR mutation. *J. Thorac. Dis*. 2013; 5 (5): 585-92.

[33] Fiala, O., Pesek, M., Finek, J., et al. Gene mutations in squamous cell NSCLC: insignificance of EGFR, KRAS and PIK3CA mutations in prediction of EGFR-TKI treatment efficacy. *Anticancer Res*. 2013; 33 (4): 1705-11.

[34] Paik, P. K., Varghese, A. M., Sima, C. S., et al. Response to erlotinib in patients with EGFR mutant advanced non-small cell lung cancers with a squamous or squamous-like component. *Mol. Cancer Ther*. 2012; 11 (11): 2535-40.

[35] Reckhtman, N., Tafe, L. J., Chaft, J. E., et al. Distinct profile of driver mutations and clinical features in immunomarker-defined subsets of pulmonary large cell carcinoma. *Mod. Pathol.* 2013; 26 (4): 511-22.

[36] Rossi, G., Mengoli, M. C., Cavazza, A., et al. Large cell carcinoma of the lung: clinically oriented classification integrating immunohistochemistry and molecular biology. *Virchows Arch.* 2014; 464 (1): 61-8.

In: Fighting Lung Cancer through the HER Family ...
Editor: Diego Márquez-Medina
ISBN: 978-1-63321-092-9

Chapter 4

Biology II. Etiology and Histology of Lung Cancer According to the Presence of Alterations in the Human Epidermal Growth Factor Family of Receptors

Diego Márquez-Medina, M.D., Ph.D.
Medical Oncology Department, Arnau of Vilanova University Hospital of Lleida, Spain

Abstract

Over 35 histologically different malignancies are gathered under the name lung cancer. These different histological patterns originate tumors with a different molecular expression and a diverse clinical behavior. We review those clinical and pathological phenomena eventually associated to alterations in the human epidermal growth factor family of surface receptors. Clinical (race, female gender, histology, age, and smoke habit) and molecular of response to tyrosine kinase inhibitors of the epidermal growth factor receptor are exhaustively discussed. Those etiological factors that could be related to the development of lung cancers harboring alterations in the human epidermal growth factor family of receptors are considered too.

1. Background

Lung cancer is a very common and lethal malignancy. In 2011, over 226,000 and 24,400 new cases were diagnosed in the United States of America, and the European Economic Community, respectively, provoking over 160,000 and 20,000 deaths, respectively [1, 2].

Lung cancer should not be considered a unique disease. The 2012 World Health Organization classification [3] distinguishes 37 subtypes of histologically different malignancies gathered under the name lung cancer, whose main subtypes include: 1) lung adenocarcinomas ranging from pre-invasive, to in situ, minimally invasive, and invasive adenocarcinomas, which could present a lepidic, acinar, papillary, micropapillary, and solid predominant pattern; 2) squamous cell carcinoma with papillary, small-cell, clear-cell, and basaloid varieties; 3) large-cell carcinomas; 4) small-cell; and neuroendocrine lung cancers; 5) mixed and pleomorphic carcinoma with sarcomatous characteristics; and 6) carcinomas of salivary gland origin.

Those different histological patterns originate tumors with a very distinct clinical behavior. For instance, lung squamous carcinomas tend to be centrally located and present a lower metastatic capacity than lung adenocarcinomas, which are predisposed to be peripheral and easily metastasized to lung, pleura, bone, suprarenal glands, and central nervous system. Moreover, molecular characteristics of the tumor cell such as sensitizing mutations of the epidermal growth factor receptor (EGFR) or anaplastic lymphoma kinase translocations also depend on the histology and define the different behavior, response, outcome, and etiology of the disease. The present chapter is intended to review clinical and pathological phenomena eventually associated to alterations in the human epidermal growth factor family of surface receptors.

2. Clinical and Molecular Predictors of Response to Tyrosine Kinase Inhibitors of the EGFR

Over 80% of non-small cell lung cancers (NSCLC) overexpress EGFR. However, most patient with NSCLC do not respond to gefitinib or erlotinib, reversible inhibitors of the inner tyrosine kinase portion of the EGFR (EGFR-TKI). In the ISEL trial [4-7], gefitinib obtained only 8% of response rate and failed to demonstrate a survival benefit over placebo in previously treated un-selected advanced NSCLC (5.6 months versus 5.1 months; p= 0.087). However, a significant survival benefit was observed when gefitinib was administered to Asian (9.5 months versus 5.5 months; p= 0.01), and never-smoker patients (8.9 months versus 6.1 months; p= 0.012), and a tendency to a better survival was noticed when it was applied to lung adenocarcinoma (6.3 months versus 5.4 months; p= 0.089). Furthermore, in the BR.21 trial [8-12], erlotinib obtained a significant survival benefit over placebo in pre-treated un-selected advanced NSCLC (6.7 months versus 4.7 months; p< 0.001) yet the response rate hardly reached 8.9%. Instead, response rate was higher in women (14.4% versus 6%; p= 0.006), never-smokers (24.7% versus 3.9%; p< 0.001), Asian patients (18.9% versus 7.5%; p= 0.02), and lung adenocarcinomas (13.9% versus 4.1%; p< 0.001). As a result, the importance of all those clinical characteristics to predict response to EGFR-TKI were confirmed.

Molecular alterations lie beneath those items and are the basis of the better response to EGFR-TKI in specific subsets of patients. The *EGFR* gene amplification, EGFR over-expression, and the presence of sensitizing conformational *EGFR* mutations have been exhaustively explored as predictive factors for a higher effect of EGFR-TKI. Thus, c*onformational sensitizing EGFR-mutations were confirmed to be the better predictive marker of benefit from EGFR-TKI in the IPASS,* INTEREST, and BR.21 trials, as well as in different prospective and retrospective series around the world.

3. Clinical and Pathological Features Associated to the Presence of Molecular Predictors of Response to EGFR-TKI

3.1. Race

The proportion of sensitizing EGFR-mutations is higher among Asian patients [13-16]. Taiwanese, Korean, Chinese, and Japanese series [17-21] report an incidence of 46% to 64.2% in lung adenocarcinomas and never-smoker patients.

The frequency of sensitizing EGFR-mutant patients decreases from East to West. A Malaysian series (N= 812) [22] including multiethnic lung adenocarcinomas reported the presence of sensitizing *EGFR*-mutations in 39.5% of cases, with a tendency for a higher incidence in Chinese than Malaysian or Indian patients (40.8% versus 37.2% versus 33.3%, respectively; p= 0.591). In India, the proportion of sensitizing *EGFR*-mutations (N= 907) was 23% [23].

As for Arabian and Mediterranean patients the incidence of *EGFR*-mutations was determined to be lower. The overall frequency of sensitizing *EGFR*-mutations among Moroccan lung adenocarcinomas was 21% (N= 137) [24], and 16.6% among Spanish patients (N= 2,105) [25].

In America, the rate of sensitizing *EGFR*-mutations was higher in Asian descents with lung cancer than in Caucasian patients (30% vs. 15%, respectively). A series including NSCLCs from different Latin American countries (N= 1,150) indicated a higher incidence of sensitizing *EGFR*-mutation in Peruvian patients (67% versus 33.2%), which could be connected to migratory fluxes or genomic influences [26].

The proportion of sensitizing *EGFR*-mutations in North American Hispanic and Caucasian patients (16.9%) was similar [26, 27], and most series also provided a similar incidence of sensitizing *EGFR*-mutations in African American and Caucasian patients with lung cancer. Cote et al. [29] reported an overall *EGFR*-mutation rate of 13.9%, without significant differences between African American and Caucasian patients (N= 144) (11.9% versus 15.6%, p = 0.53). Similarly, The Memorial Sloan-Kettering Cancer Center accounted for a similar incidence of *EGFR*-mutations between Afro American and Caucasian NSCLC patients (N= 476) (19% versus 13%, p = 0.11) [30]. The Abramson Cancer Center of Philadelphia (N= 497) [31] reported an overall sensitizing *EGFR*-mutation rate of 13.9% in North American NSCLC, with a leaning to a lower incidence in African American than in Caucasians ones (4.8% vs. 13.7%; p= 0.06). In addition, Leidner et al. (N= 151) [32] found a lower incidence of sensitizing *EGFR*-mutations in African American than in Caucasian NSCLC patients (2% versus 17%; p= 0.022).

Nevertheless, the nature of those sensitizing *EGFR*-mutations seems to be the same in all those ethnic groups, and the percentage of exon 19, 21, and 20 mutations in Asian (54%, 44%, and 4%, respectively), Caucasian (51%, 31%, and 0%, respectively), North African (69%, 21%, and 7%, respectively), and Hispanic patients (42.8%, 14.3%, and 28.6%) does not differ excessively. The proportion of uncommon *EGFR*-mutations [33] has been suggested to be more frequent in African American patients (51% versus 32%; p= 0.018).

3. 2. Gender

Female gender has been extensively associated with a higher incidence of sensitizing EGFR-mutations. The Memorial Sloan-Kettering Cancer Center (N= 2,142) [34], and the Spanish Lung Cancer Group (N= 2,105) [25] reported a significant higher incidence among women with lung adenocarcinoma (19% versus 26%, and 8.2% versus 30%, respectively). This higher proportion of sensitizing *EGFR*-mutations in NSCLC samples of female patients has been related to the presence of estrogen receptors [35, 36], although the significance of this phenomenon has not been defined [17, 21].

3.3. Age

Age is a consistent but not commonly considered predictive factor for sensitizing *EGFR*-mutations. A significantly higher incidence of sensitizing *EGFR*-mutations was reported in elderly Japanese (N= 1,262) [37], regardless of gender. Among Korean women with 98 gefitinib-treated NSCLC (N= 98) [18], sensitizing *EGFR*-mutations were also higher in older patients (70% versus 39%; OR 4.03; p= 0.003). In Spanish patients (N= 2105) [25], age increased the presence of sensitizing *EGFR*-mutations from 13.9% in younger than 56.7 years, to 15.5% in those between 56.7 and 69.1 years, and to 22.2% in older than 69 years patients.

3.4. Histology

a) Lung adenocarcinoma

Multiple works revealed that a*denocarcinomas present a higher incidence of sensitizing EGFR-mutations in any ethic group***.** Moreover, the proportion of sensitizing *EGFR*-mutations varies according to the histologic subset of lung adenocarcinoma. *Sensitizing EGFR-mutations are higher in hobnail, broncholoalveolar, and micropapilar subtypes.* The Spanish Lung Cancer Group (N= 2,105) [25] reported that sensitizing *EGFR*-mutations increased from 17.1% in lung adenocarcinoma to 23.1% in formerly known bronchioloalveolar carcinomas. An Australian series (N= 69) [38] indicated a higher proportion of sensitizing *EGFR*-mutation in tumors with an acinar and micropapillary predominant pattern than in the whole population (44% versus 38% versus 29%, respectively). In North American Hispanic patients [26-28], over 85% of *EGFR*-mutations were also found in acinar NSCLC with lepidic or papillary component.

Concerning Asian patients, a series of Korean resected or biopsied NSCLC (N= 382) [39] reported a higher incidence of sensitizing *EGFR*-mutations in tumors with bronchioloalveolar or papillary component, that increased from 51.3% in the whole series to 67.6% in tumors with mixed acinar and bronchioloalveolar pattern, and to 65.2% in those with mixed papillary and acinar pattern. On the other hand, *EGFR*-mutations rate decreased to 38.2% in tumors with mixed solid and acinar pattern, to 30.4% in tumors with micropapillary and acinar pattern, and to 13.3% in tumors with acinar and mucinous bronchioloalveolar pattern.

Sensitizing *EGFR*-mutations has been also reported to increase in NSCLC expressing the thyroid transcription factor 1 (17.7% versus 1.4%; p< 0.001), a well-known marker for lung adenocarcinoma, in both Asian and European patients [30-40].

b) Squamous carcinomas

The incidence of sensitizing *EGFR*-mutations in squamous carcinomas depends on the presence and proportion of mixed adenocarcinoma component. It has been suggested to be the same as in adenosquamous carcinomas and conventional adenocarcinoma (13%), and lower in pure squamous carcinomas [41]. A Czech (N= 223) [42] and a Taiwanese series [43] indicated a similar 7.2% and 7.4% incidence of sensitizing *EGFR*-mutations is squamous carcinomas, whereas a Japanese series (N= 249) [44] reported a higher 13% incidence. However, some tumors in this series were positive for thyroid transcription factor-1 suggesting the presence of adenocarcinoma component. Another Japanese series (N= 89) [45] with presumed pure squamous carcinomas reported 5.6% *EGFR*-mutation rate. Two samples really corresponded to non-pure squamous carcinomas, and the final rate of *EGFR*-mutations lowered to 3.4%. *Nevertheless, the presence of sensitizing EGFR-mutations also predicts a higher benefit from EGFR-TKI lung squamous carcinomas.*

c) Other NSCLC and small cell lung cancer

Sensitizing EGFR-mutations were reported in 11.5% of large cell carcinomas from Spanish patients [25].

The incidence of sensitizing EGFR-mutations in small cell lung cancers is really scarce, and tends to occur in tumors with a combined histology. It has been reported to be only 2.6% in Taiwanese patients (N= 75) [46]. *In Korean [47] and Japanese patients (N= 122) [48], the frequency of sensitizing EGFR-mutations has been reported to be 4%.* Nevertheless, in *this Japanese study,* all the patients presented histologically mixed tumors and *EGFR*-mutations were existent in both adenocarcinoma and small cell components.

4. Etiology of EGFR-Mutant Lung Cancers

4.1. Smoke

Tobacco smoke is related to over 90% of NSCLC. However, only a limited percentage of smoker patients develop lung cancer, likewise lung cancer is also possible in non-smoker patients confirming the existence of any other etiologic agents such as genetic alterations, exposure to chemical substances, exposure to ionic radiations, the presence of previous lung scars, and virus infections such as cytomegalovirus, John Cunningham virus, or the simian vacuolating virus.

Never and long-term formerly smokers have been associated with a higher incidence of *EGFR*-mutant NSCLC in *Latin American, African*, Malaysian (54.8% versus 20.7%; p< 0.001), Indian (29.4% versus 15.3%), Caucasian, and East Asian patients *(46.3% vs. 23.3%; p= 0.047).*

The Memorial Sloan-Kettering Cancer Center (N= 2,142) [34, 49] reported that the incidence of sensitizing *EGFR*-mutations is higher in never-smoker than smoker patients (43% versus 11%), although it rose from 6% in current smokers, to 15% in former smokers, and to 52% in never smokers with lung adenocarcinoma, and increasing the smoking-free years raise the possibility of *EGFR*-mutations in former-smokers. The Spanish Lung Cancer Group [25] also found a progressive reduction in the incidence of *EGFR*-mutations from 37.7% in never-smoker, to 9.5% in former smokers, and to 5.8% in current smokers with NSCLC.

a) Smoke and KRAS-mutations

On the other hand, smoke-related Kirsten ras oncogene homolog gene (KRAS) mutations seem to be exclusive with sensitizing *EGFR*-mutations. *KRAS*-mutations were encountered in 20-30% lung adenocarcinomas, and were more common among smokers patients (p< 0.01) in the TRIBUTE trial [50, 51]. The Memorial Sloan Kettering Cancer Center (N= 3,026) [49, 52] reported that the incidence of *KRAS-mutations is higher in lung adenocarcinomas samples from smoker patients when compared to never smoker ones (34% versus 6%), and it rises from 15% in never smokers, to 22% in former smokers, and to 25% in current smokers with lung adenocarcinomas.* The Korean Yonsei Cancer Center (N= 229) [19] reported a 3.5% of *KRAS*-mutations in NSCLC from never-smoker patients that were mutually exclusive with sensitizing *EGFR*-mutations.

b) Smoke and radiologic alterations

Similarly, EGFR-mutant NSCLCs do not tend to be presented in pulmonary areas with those radiologic alterations that have been classically associated with cigarette smoking. Sekine el al. [53] observed that *EGFR*-mutant NSCLCs associated with less emphysematous and interstitial changes than tumors wild type (p= 0.005), even in smoker patients. Furthermore, other Japanese series (N= 555) [54] provided that interstitial lung disease was less common in patients with *EGFR*-mutant adenocarcinoma (0.004% versus 0.097%; p< 0.001). Therefore, sensitizing *EGFR*-mutations seems to be less common in tumors with ground-glass pattern in both Western *and Asian patients [55, 56].*

4.2. Hereditary Cancer

To date, genes conferring susceptibility to lung cancer have not been demonstrated although a genetic origin for some lung cancers is highly suspected. Lung cancer risk is higher in non-smoker members of families with lung cancers diagnosed in young or many afflicted members [57], and in patients with the Li-Fraumeni syndrome. The Harvard Medical School (N= 230) [58] accounted for a family history of lung cancer in 18% of never smoker NSCLC, and a high 42% incidence of sensitizing *EGFR*-mutations among them. In this series, family aggregation was significantly more common among *EGFR*-mutant patients (41.5%). Similarly, a Shanghai series (N= 538) [59] noted that sensitizing *EGFR*-mutations were more common in NSCLC patients with a family history of cancer (p= 0.031) or lung cancer (p= 0.008).

4. 3. Infections

a) Mycobacterium tuberculosis

The pulmonary infection by Mycobacterium tuberculosis has also been classically related to the development of lung adenocarcinomas, and NSCLC patients with antecedents of tuberculous scars present a higher incidence of sensitizing *EGFR*-mutations [60]. This finding accords with a Chinese series of *EGFR*-mutant lung adenocarcinomas (N= 191) [61] that revealed the clinical history of pulmonary tuberculosis in 8.9%, old radiologic lesions of pulmonary tuberculosis in 37.7%, and scar carcinomas in 7.3% of them. The incidence of sensitizing *EGFR*-mutations, especially exon 19 deletions, was higher in patients with old radiologic lesions of pulmonary tuberculosis (p= 0.018).

b) Human immunodeficiency virus

Infection by human immunodeficiency virus increases the risk of lung carcinoma (HR 3.6) once smoking is controlled. Immunosuppression and oncogenic virus co-infection contribute to the increment of the incidence of lung cancer [62].

c) Human papillomavirus

Human papillomavirus (HPV) infection has been related to the development of lung malignancies. However, although HPV traces have been successively reported in lung cancer samples, no definitive association between both events has been confirmed in Caucasian patients.

HPV belong to the wide Papillomaviridae family, host- and tissue-tropic non-enveloped DNA viruses that infect different animals [63, 64]. Over 120 HPV subtypes affect humans, infecting selectively specific tissues such us skin, mouth, airways, genital mucosa, and anus. Most of HPV subtypes are cleared up by the immune system. Persistent HPV infection could induce the proliferation of epithelium cells and produce warts, benign tumors or cancers. Over 5% of human malignancies are attributable to HPV, the most important infectious cause of cancer, and HPV-16, 18, 31, 33, 35, 39, 45, 51, 52, 56, 58, 59, 68, 73, and 82 subtypes are considered clearly carcinogenic [65]. Urogenital malignancies had been classically related to high-risk sexually transmitted HPV subtypes, and current literature also suggests an eventual relationship between HPV infection and the development of malignancies distant from the genital area such as oropharyngeal, esophagus, and lung cancers [66, 67].

The HPV infection rate in lung cancer samples widely ranges depending on geography [68, 69]. On the one hand, European series [70-76] including over 3100 NSCLCs indicate a very low HPV infection rate that goes from 0 to 5%, and rise to 14-20% in some Italian series [72, 73]. On the other hand, the HPV infection rate clearly increases in Asian patients [77-80], as it is evidenced in three meta-analyses [75]. The first one (N= 4,508) [68] reported 16% HPV infection rate in Western patients and 35.7% in Asian patients. The second one (N= 2,435) [69] reached 7.1% HPV infection rate in Western patients and 20.4% in Asian patients.

The impact of histology in the HPV infection rate is controversial. Some European series [81] did not detect differences in the HPV infection rate according to histology, although a French series [82] reported a higher HPV infection rate in lung adenocarcinomas than in any other histology (11% versus 25%). As for Asian patients, a West Chinese series [83] reported a higher HPV infection rate in lung squamous carcinomas (16.2% versus 51.4%), whereas a Japanese series [84] did not find significant differences in respect of histology (10% versus 9%). A higher HPV infection rate in lung adenocarcinomas (30% versus 7%) was found throughout another Japanese series [85].

Many authors [75, 86-90] have shown a higher HPV infection rate in Asian, elderly, female, non-smoker patients with lung adenocarcinomas, the same population with an increased incidence of sensitizing *EGFR*-mutations. Likewise, a better outcome has been reported in both HPV-infected or *EGFR*-mutant NSCLC patients [56, 57].

Recent investigations suggest that the HPV infection rate could depend on the *EGFR* status. Baba et al. [87] reported a higher HPV infection rate in gefitinib-responder NSCLC (75% versus 0%), a Spanish series [73] suggested a direct relationship between HPV infection and the presence of sensitizing *EGFR*-mutations. Finally, Kato et al. [91] confirmed the higher HPV infection rate of Japanese NSCLC harboring sensitizing *EGFR*-mutations (38% versus 7%; p= 0.021), as well as Tung et al. [92] who also detected a higher incidence of sensitizing *EGFR*-mutations in Taiwanese patients with HPV E6-positive NSCLC (41% versus 20%; p= 0.006).

5. Other Alterations in the Family of Human Epidermal Growth Factor Receptors

5.1. EGFR-Amplification and EGFR-Overexpression

The EGFR gene amplification and the receptor over-expression have been analyzed as predictive factors for a higher benefit from EGFR-TKI. In the ISEL trial (N= 222) [4-7], 43.2% of patients with EGFR-amplification presented a higher response rate to gefitinib (3.5% versus 16.4%; p< 0.05) and a survival benefit (HR 0.61). In the phase-II ONCOBELL trial (N= 42) [93], second or first line gefitinib obtained a better response rate (68% versus 9.1%; p< 0.001) and a longer time to progression (7.6 vs. 2.7 months; p= 0.02) in patients with EGFR-amplification. In the phase-III BR.21 trial (N= 91) [8-12], erlotinib increased the response rate (4.8% versus 21.4%; p= 0.02), and reached a survival benefit (HR 0.44) in patients with EGFR-amplification.

The EGFR over-expression was explored as a predictor of response to EGFR-TKI in retrospective series, the ISEL, BR.21, and TRIBUTE trials. Two retrospective series (N= 158) [20] reported that the gefitinib response rate increased from 5% to 21%, and from 3.7% to 17.3%, respectively, in 59% and 46% patients with EGFR over-expression. In the ISEL trial (N= 379), gefitinib increased the response rate (1.5% versus 8.2%; HR 0.77) of 70% of patients with EGFR over-expression. In the BR.21 trial (N= 638) [8-12], the response rate to erlotinib used to be higher in patients with EGFR over-expression (3.8% versus 11.3%; p= 0.1). A sub-analysis of the BR.21 trial (N= 325) confirmed a benefit on response rate (4% versus 11%), quality of life, and survival (p= 0.02) when erlotinib was administered to 57% of patients with EGFR over-expression.

In the same way that EGFR-mutations, both EGFR amplified and overexpressed tumors are more common lung adenocarcinomas, although they do not vary so widely according to race, smoking habit, and gender. *A higher proportion of EGFR-amplification have been reported in African American patients (51% versus 32%; p= 0.018) [29-33], and* they have also been found in EGFR-mutant small cell lung cancers with adenocarcinoma component, but detected in the adenocarcinoma component only [48].

Nevertheless, the presence of sensitizing EGFR-mutations is the most reliable predictive factor of benefit from EGFR-TKI. In the IPASS trial (N= 1,217) [94], first line gefitinib obtained a higher response rate and progression free survival in Asian patients with EGFR-amplified (HR 0.66 versus 1.24) or EGFR-mutant NSCLC (HR 0.77 versus 1.38). However, progression free survival decreased when EGFR-amplification was not accompanied by EGFR-mutation (HR 3.85). In the INTEREST trial (N= 1,316) [95], gefitinib obtained the better *progression free survival* in patients harboring sensitizing EGFR-mutations only, and not in those with EGFR-amplification or over-expression. In the BR.21 trial, the response rate to erlotinib increased from 2.4% to 20% in patients with EGFR-amplification, from 3.8% to 11.3% in patients with EGFR over-expression, and from 9% to 33% in patients with sensitizing EGFR-mutations when compared to the whole population. Similarly, the HR for overall survival increased from 0.85 to 0.44 (p= 0.008) in patients with EGFR-amplification, from 0.93 to 0.68 (p= 0.02) in EGFR over-expression, and from 0.73 to 0.77 in EGFR-mutant patients. Finally, in a Korean series (N= 92) of erlotinib treated NSCLC [20], EGFR-amplification was found in 40.9% of patients, EGFR over-expression in 72%, and sensitizing EGFR-mutations 26.1% of cases. There was a significant association between EGFR-mutations and -amplification, and both markers predicted a benefit from erlotinib in response rate (58.3% versus 16.2%; p< 0.001; and 41.7% versus 17.3%; p= 0.012, respectively), time to progression (8.6 months versus 2.5 months; p= 0.003; and 5.8 versus 1.8 months, p< 0.001, respectively), and overall survival (not reached versus 10.8 months; p= 0.023; and not reached versus 10.1 months; p= 0.033, respectively). However, the presence of sensitizing EGFR-mutations was the only significant molecular predictor for survival in the multivariate analysis.

5.2. *HER2*-Mutations

The Memorial Sloan-Kettering Cancer Center [96] noted *HER2*-mutations in 6% of *EGFR*, *KRAS*, and *ALK* negative lung adenocarcinomas, and those *HER2*-mutations seem to be more common in never-smoker patients (p< 0.0001), with no relation to gender, race, or stage. HER2 over-expression has been reported in 10% of NSCLC, regardless of gender [97]. This percentage rises to 20% in a retrospective Italian series (N= 40) [98] including resected brochioloalveolar carcinomas, especially in those with a mucinous pattern (46% versus 7%; p= 0.014).

Acknowledgments

The author would like to thank Svetozara Georgieva Hristova for her collaboration and convenient suggestions in language style and review.

References

[1] Jemal A, Bray F, Center MM, Ferlay J, Ward E, Forman D.2. Siegel R. Global cancer statistics. *CA Cancer J. Clin.,* 2011; 61 (2): 69-90.

[2] Siegel R, Naishadham D, Jemal A. Cancer statistics, 2012. *CA Cancer J. Clin.,* 2012; 62 (1): 10-29.

[3] Travis WD, Bambrilla E, Noguchi M, et al. International Association for the Study of Lung Cancer. American Thoracic Society. European Respiratory Society International Multidisciplinary Classification of Lung Adenocarcinoma. *J. Thorac. Oncol.,* 2011; 6 (2): 244-85.

[4] Chang A, Parikh P, Thongprasert S, et al.Gefitinib (IRESSA) in patients of Asian origin with refractory advanced non-small cell lung cancer: subset analysis from the ISEL study. *J. Thorac. Oncol.,* 2006; 1 (8): 847-55.

[5] Hirsch FR, Varella-Garcia M, Bunn PA Jr, et al. Molecular predictors of outcome with gefitinib in a phase III placebo-controlled study in advanced non-small-cell lung cancer. *J. Clin. Oncol.,* 2006; 24 (31):5034-42.

[6] Hirsch FR, Dziadziuszko R, Thatcher N, et al. Epidermal growth factor receptor immunohistochemistry: comparison of antibodies and cutoff points to predict benefit from gefitinib in a phase 3 placebo-controlled study in advanced nonsmall-cell lung cancer. *Cancer,* 2008; 112 (5): 1114-21.

[7] Thatcher N, Chang A, Parikh P, et al. Gefitinib plus best supportive care in previously treated patients with refractory advanced non-small-cell lung cancer: results from a randomised, placebo-controlled, multicentre study (Iressa Survival Evaluation in Lung Cancer). *Lancet,* 2005; 366 (9496): 1527-37.

[8] Zhu CQ, da Cunha Santos G, Ding K, et al. Role of KRAS and EGFR as biomarkers of response to erlotinib in National Cancer Institute of Canada Clinical Trials Group Study BR.21. *J. Clin. Oncol.,* 2008; 26: 4268-75.

[9] Cioffi P, Marotta V, Fanizza C, Giglioni A, Natoli C, Petrelli F, Grappasonni I. Effectiveness and response predictive factors of erlotinib in a non-small cell lung cancer unselected European population previously treated: a retrospective, observational, multicentric study. *J. Oncol. Pharm Pract.,* 2013; 19 (3): 246-53.

[10] Health Quality Ontario. Epidermal Growth Factor Receptor Mutation (EGFR) Testing for Prediction of Response to EGFR-Targeting Tyrosine Kinase Inhibitor (TKI) Drugs in Patients with Advanced Non-Small-Cell Lung Cancer: An Evidence-Based Analysis. *Ont. Health Technol Assess Ser.,* 2010; 10 (24): 1-48.

[11] Clark GM, Zborowski DM, Santabarbara P, et al. Smoking history and epidermal growth factor receptor expression as predictors of survival benefit from erlotinib for patients with non-small-cell lung cancer in the National Cancer Institute of Canada Clinical Trials Group study BR.21. *Clin. Lung Cancer,* 2006; 7 (6): 389-94.

[12] Shepherd FA, Rodrigues Pereira J, Ciuleanu T, et al. Erlotinib in previously treated non-small-cell lung cancer. *N. Engl. J. Med.,* 2005 Jul 14;353(2):123-32.

[13] Tsao MS, Saturada A, Cutz JC, et al. Erlotinib in lung cancer-molecular and clinical predictors of outcome. *N. Engl. J. Med.,* 2005; 353:133-44.

[14] Agarwala A, Fisher W, Bruetman D, et al. Gefitinib plus celecoxib in chemotherapy-naïve patients with stage IIIB/IV non-small cell lung cancer: a phase II study from the Hoosier Oncology Group. *J. Thorac. Oncol.,* 2008; 3 (4): 374-9.

[15] Wu JY, Yu CJ, Yang CH, et al. First or Second-Line Therapy With Gefitinib Produces Equal Survival in Non Small Cell Lung Cancer. *Am. J. Respir. Crit. Care Med.,* 2008; 178 (8): 847-53.

[16] Tiseo M, Gridelli C, Cascinu S, et al. An expanded access program of erlotinib (Tarceva) in patients with advanced non-small cell lung cancer (NSCLC): Data report from Italy. *Lung Cancer,* 2009; 64 (2): 199-206.

[17] Bell DW, Brannigan BW, Matsuo K, et al. Increased Prevalence of EGFR-Mutant Lung Cancer in Women and in East Asian Populations: Analysis of Estrogen-Related Polymorphisms. *Clin. Cancer Res.,* 2008; 14: 4079-84.

[18] Choi YH, Lee JK, Kang HJ, et al. Association between age at diagnosis and the presence of EGFR mutations in female patients with resected non-small cell lung cancer. *J. Thorac. Oncol.,* 2010; 5: 1949-52.

[19] Kim HR, Shim HS, Chung JH, et al. Distinct clinical features and outcomes in never-smokers with nonsmall cell lung cancer who harbor EGFR or KRAS mutations or ALK rearrangement. *Cancer,* 2012; 118 (3): 729-39.

[20] Ahn MJ, Park BB, Ahn JS, et al. Are there any ethnic differences in molecular predictors of erlotinib efficacy in advanced non-small cell lung cancer? *Clin. Cancer Res.,* 2008; 14: 3860-6.

[21] Chen KY, Hsiao CF, Chang GC, et al. EGFR polymorphisms, hormone replacement therapy and lung adenocarcinoma risk: analysis from a genome-wide association study in never-smoking women. *Carcinogenesis,* 2013; 34: 612-9.

[22] Liam CK, Wahid MI, Rajadurai P, Cheah YK, Ng TS. Epidermal growth factor receptor mutations in lung adenocarcinoma in Malaysian patients. *J. Thorac. Oncol.,* 2013; 8 (6): 766-72.

[23] Chougule A, Prabhash K, Noronha V, et al. Frequency of EGFR Mutations in 907 Lung Adenocarcioma Patients of Indian Ethnicity. *PLoS One,* 2013; 8 (10): e76164.

[24] Errihani H, Inrhaoun H, Boukir A, et al. Frequency and type of epidermal growth factor receptor mutations in moroccan patients with lung adenocarcinoma. *J. Thorac. Oncol.,* 2013; 8 (9): 1212-4.

[25] Rosell R, Moran T, Queralt C, et al. Screening for Epidermal Growth Factor Receptor Mutations in Lung Cancer. *N. Engl. J. Med.,* 2009;361 (10): 958-67.

[26] Arrieta O, Cardona AF, Federico Bramuglia G, et al. Genotyping non-small cell lung cancer (NSCLC) in Latin America. *J. Thorac. Oncol.,* 2011; 6 (11): 1955-9.

[27] Zhang W, McQuitty EB, Olsen R, et al. EGFR Mutations in US Hispanic Versus Non-Hispanic White Patients With Lung Adenocarcinoma. *Arch. Pathol. Lab. Med.,* 2013. [Epub ahead of print].

[28] McQuitty E, Zhang W, Hendrickson H, Tio FO, Jagirdar J, Olsen R, Cagle P. Lung Adenocarcinoma Biomarker Incidence in Hispanic Versus Non-Hispanic White Patients. *Arch. Pathol. Lab. Med.,* 2013 Jun 26. [Epub ahead of print].

[29] Cote ML, Haddad R, Edwards DJ, et al. Frequency and Type of Epidermal Growth Factor Receptor Mutations in Americans with Non-small Cell Lung Cancer. *J. Thorac. Oncol.,* 2011; 6: 627-30.

[30] Reinersman JM, Johnson ML, Riely GJ, et al. Frequency of EGFR and KRAS mutations in lung adenocarcinomas in African Americans. *J. Thorac. Oncol.,* 2011; 6: 28-31.

[31] Bauml J, Mick R, Zhang Y, et al. Frequency of EGFR and KRAS mutations in patients with non small cell lung cancer by racial background: do disparities exist? *Lung Cancer,* 2013; 81 (3): 347-53.

[32] Leidner RS, Fu P, Clifford B, et al. Genetic abnormalities of the EGFR pathway in African American Patients with non-small-cell lung cancer. *J. Clin. Oncol.,* 2009; 27 (33): 5620-6.

[33] Harada T, Lopez-Chavez A, Xi L, Raffeld M, Wang Y, Giaccone G. Characterization of epidermal growth factor receptor mutations in non-small-cell lung cancer patients of African-American ancestry. *Oncogene,* 2011; 30 (15): 1744-52.

[34] D'Angelo SP, Pietanza MC, Johnson ML, et al. Incidence of EGFR exon 19 deletions and L858R in tumor specimens from men and cigarette smokers with lung adenocarcinomas. *J. Clin. Oncol.,* 2011; 29: 2066-70.

[35] Mazières J, Rouquette I, Lepage B, et al. Specificities of lung adenocarcinoma in women who have never smoked. *J. Thorac. Oncol.,* 2013; 8 (7): 923-9.

[36] Rouquette I, Lauwers-Cances V, Allera C, et al. Characteristics of lung cancer in women: importance of hormonal and growth factors. *Lung Cancer,* 2012; 76 (3): 280-5.

[37] Ueno T, Toyooka S, Suda K, et al. Impact of age on epidermal growth factor receptor mutation in lung cancer. *Lung Cancer,* 2012; 78 (3): 207-11.

[38] Russell PA, Barnett SA, Walkiewicz M, Wainer Z, et al. Correlation of mutation status and survival with predominant histologic subtype according to the new IASLC/ATS/ERS lung adenocarcinoma classification in stage III (N2) patients. *J. Thorac. Oncol.,* 2013; 8: 461-8.

[39] Sun PL, Seol H, Lee HJ, et al. High incidence of EGFR mutations in Korean men smokers with no intratumoral heterogeneity of lung adenocarcinomas: correlation with histologic subtypes, EGFR/TTF-1 expressions, and clinical features. *J. Thorac. Oncol.,* 2012; 7: 323-30.

[40] Vallee A, Sagan C, Le Loupp AG, Bach K, et al. Detection of EGFR gene mutations in non-small cell lung cancer: Lessons from a single-institution routine analysis of 1,403 tumor samples. *Int. J. Oncol.,* 2013; 43: 1045-51.

[41] Tochigi N, Dacic S, Nikiforova M, et al. Adenosquamous carcinoma of the lung: a microdissection study of KRAS and EGFR mutational and amplification status in a western patient population. *Am. J. Clin. Pathol.,* 2011; 135: 783-9.

[42] Fiala O, Pesek M, Finek J, et al. Gene mutations in squamous cell NSCLC: insignificance of EGFR, KRAS and PIK3CA mutations in prediction of EGFR-TKI treatment efficacy. *Anticancer. Res.,* 2013; 33: 1705-11.

[43] Lee Y, Shim HS, Park MS, Kim JH, Ha SJ, Kim SH, Cho BC. High EGFR gene copy number and skin rash as predictive markers for EGFR tyrosine kinase inhibitors in patients with advanced squamous cell lung carcinoma. *Clin. Cancer Res.,* 2012; 18 (6): 1760-8.

[44] Hata A, Katakami N, Yoshioka H, et al. How sensitive are epidermal growth factor receptor-tyrosine kinase inhibitors for squamous cell carcinoma of the lung harboring EGFR gene-sensitive mutations? *J. Thorac. Oncol.,* 2013; 8: 89-95.

[45] Miyamae Y, Shimizu K, Hirato J, et al. Significance of epidermal growth factor receptor gene mutations in squamous cell lung carcinoma. *Oncol. Rep.*, 2011; 25 (4): 921-8.

[46] Shiao TH, Chang YL, Yu CJ, et al. Epidermal growth factor receptor mutations in small cell lung cancer: a brief report. *J. Thorac. Oncol.*, 2011; 6: 195-8.

[47] Kim YT, Kim TY, Lee DS, et al. Molecular changes of epidermal growth factor receptor (EGFR) and KRAS and their impact on the clinical outcomes in surgically resected adenocarcinoma of the lung. *Lung Cancer,* 2008; 59 (1): 111-8.

[48] Tatematsu A, Shimizu J, Murakami Y, et al. Epidermal growth factor receptor mutations in small cell lung cancer. *Clin. Cancer Res.*, 2008; 14: 6092-6.

[49] Dogan S, Shen R, Ang DC, et al. Molecular epidemiology of EGFR and KRAS mutations in 3,026 lung adenocarcinomas: higher susceptibility of women to smoking-related KRAS-mutant cancers. *Clin. Cancer Res.*, 2012; 18: 6169-77.

[50] Wu CC, Hsu HY, Liu HP, et al. Reversed mutation rates of KRAS and EGFR genes in adenocarcinoma of the lung in Taiwan and their implications. *Cancer,* 2008; 113 (11): 3199-208.

[51] Hirsch FR, Varella-Garcia M, Dziadziuszko R, et al. Fluorescence in situ hybridization subgroup analysis of TRIBUTE, a phase III trial of erlotinib plus carboplatin and paclitaxel in non-small cell lung cancer. *Clin. Cancer Res.*, 2008; 14 (19): 6317-23.

[52] Herbst RS, Prager D, Hermann R, et al. TRIBUTE: a phase III trial of erlotinib hydrochloride (OSI-774) combined with carboplatin and paclitaxel chemotherapy in advanced non-small-cell lung cancer. *J. Clin. Oncol.*, 2005; 23 (25): 5892-9.

[53] Riely GJ, Kris MG, Rosenbaum D, et al. Frequency and distinctive spectrum of KRAS mutations in never smokers with lung adenocarcinoma. *Clin. Cancer Res.*, 2008; 14: 5731-4.

[54] Sekine A, Tamura K, Satoh H, et al. Prevalence of underlying lung disease in smokers with epidermal growth factor receptor-mutant lung cancer. *Oncol. Rep.*, 2013; 29 (5): 2005-10.

[55] Fujimoto D, Tomii K, Otoshi T, Kawamura T, et al. Preexisting interstitial lung disease is inversely correlated to tumor epidermal growth factor receptor mutation in patients with lung adenocarcinoma. *Lung Cancer,* 2013; 80: 159-64.

[56] Glynn C, Zakowski MF, Ginsberg MS. Are there imaging characteristics associated with epidermal growth factor receptor and KRAS mutations in patients with adenocarcinoma of the lung with bronchioloalveolar features? *J. Thorac. Oncol.*, 2010; 5: 344-8.

[57] Hsu KH, Chen KC, Yang TY, et al. Epidermal growth factor receptor mutation status in stage I lung adenocarcinoma with different image patterns. *J. Thorac. Oncol.*, 2011; 6: 1066-72.

[58] Matakidou A, Eisen T, Houlston RS. Systematic review of the relationship between family history and lung cancer risk. *Br. J. Cancer,* 2005; 93 (7): 825-33.

[59] Gaughan EM, Cryer SK, Yeap BY, Jackman DM, Costa DB. Family history of lung cancer in never smokers with non-small-cell lung cancer and its association with tumors harboring EGFR mutations. *Lung Cancer,* 2013; 79 (3): 193-7.

[60] He Y, Li S, Ren S, et al. Impact of family history of cancer on the incidence of mutation in epidermal growth factor receptor gene in non-small cell lung cancer patients. *Lung Cancer,* 2013; 81 (2): 162-6.

[61] Park JA, Park HJ, Lee JS, Ha JO, Lee GK, Park BK, Ghim TT. Adenocarcinoma of lung in never smoked children. *Lung Cancer,* 2008; 61 (2): 266-9.
[62] Luo YH, Wu CH, Wu WS, et al. Association between tumor epidermal growth factor receptor mutation and pulmonary tuberculosis in patients with adenocarcinoma of the lungs. *J. Thorac. Oncol.,* 2012; 7: 299-305.
[63] Kirk GD, Merlo C, O'Driscoll P, et al. HIV infection is associated with an increased risk for lung cancer, independent of smoking. Clin Infect Dis. 2007; 45 (1): 103-10.
[64] Lange CE, Favrot C, Ackermann M, Gull J, Vetsch E, Tobler K. Novel snake papillomavirus does not cluster with other non-mammalian papillomaviruses. *Virol. J.,* 2011; 8: 436.
[65] Bernard HU, Burk RD, Chen Z, van Doorslaer K, Hausen Hz, de Villiers EM. Classification of papillomaviruses (PVs) based on 189 PV types and proposal of taxonomic amendments. *Virology,* 2012; 401 (1): 70-9.
[66] Parkin DM. The global health burden of infection-associated cancers in the year 2002. Int. J. *Cancer,* 2006; 118 (12): 3030–44.
[67] D'Souza G, Kreimer AR, Viscidi R. Case-control study of human papillomavirus and oropharyngeal cancer. *N. Engl. J. Med.,* 2007; 356 (19): 1944–56.
[68] Ridge JA, Glisson BS, Lango MN, et al. Head and Neck Tumors in Pazdur R, Wagman LD, Camphausen KA, Hoskins WJ (Eds) Cancer Management: A Multidisciplinary Approach. 11 ed. 2008.
[69] Klein F, Amin Kotb WF, Petersen I. Incidence of human papilloma virus in lung cancer. *Lung cancer,* 2009; 65 (1): 13–8.
[70] Srinivasan M, Taioli E, Ragin CC. Human papillomavirus type 16 and 18 in primary lung cancers--a meta-analysis. *Carcinogenesis,* 2009; 30 (10): 1722-8.
[71] al-Ghamdi AA, Sanders CM, Keefe M, Coggon D, Maitland NJ. Human papillomavirus DNA and TP53 mutations in lung cancers from butchers. *Br. J. Cancer,* 1995; 72 (2): 293-7.
[72] Coggon D, Pannett B, Pippard EC, Winter PD. Lung cancer in the meat industry. *Br. J. Ind. Med.,* 1989; 46 (3): 188-91.
[73] Koshiol J, Rotunno M, Gillison ML, et al. Assessment of human papillomavirus in lung tumor tissue. *J. Natl. Cancer Inst.,* 2011; 103 (6): 501-7.
[74] Márquez-Medina D, Gasol-Cudós A, Taberner-Bonastre MT, Samamé Pérez-Vargas JC, Salud-Salvia A, Llombart-Cussac A. Human papillomavirus in Non-Small-Cell Lung Cancer: The impact of EGFR mutations and the response to erlotinib. Arch. *Bronconeumol.,* 2013; 49 (2): 79–8.
[75] Syrjänen KJ. HPV infections and lung cancer. J Clin Pathol. 2002; 55 (12): 885-91.
[76] Syrjänen K, Silvoniemi M, Salminen E, et al. Detection of human papillomavirus genotypes in bronchial cancer using sensitive multimetrix assay. *Anticancer. Res.,* 2012; 32: 625-31.
[77] Galvan A, Noci S, Taverna F, Lombardo C, Franceschi S, Pastorino U, Dragani TA. Testing of human papillomavirus in lung cancer and non-tumor lung tissue. *BMC Cancer,* 2012; 12: 512.
[78] Iwakawa R, Kohno T, Enari M, Kiyono T, Yokota J. Prevalence of human papillomavirus 16/18/33 infection and p53 mutation in lung adenocarcinoma. *Cancer Sci.,* 2010; 101 (8): 1891-6.

[79] Jain N, Singh V, Hedau S, et al. Infection of human papillomavirus type 18 and p53 codon 72 polymorphism in lung cancer patients from India. *Chest,* 2005; 128 (6): 3999-4007.

[80] Lim WT, Chuah KL, Leong SS, Tan EH, Toh CK. Assessment of human papillomavirus and Epstein-Barr virus in lung adenocarcinoma. *Oncol. Rep.,* 2009; 21 (4): 971-5.

[81] Zafer E, Ergun MA, Alver G, Sahin FI, Yavuzer S, Ekmekci A. Detection and typing of human papillomavirus in non-small cell lung cancer. *Respiration,* 2004; 71 (1): 88-90.

[82] Miasko A, Niklińska W, Nikliński J, Chyczewska E, Naumnik W, Chyczewski L. Detection of human papillomavirus in non-small cell lung carcinoma by polymerase chain reaction. *Folia Histochem Cytobiol.,* 2001; 39 (2): 127-8.

[83] Thomas P, De Lamballerie X, Garbe L, Castelnau O, Kleisbauer JP. [Detection of human papillomavirus by polymerase chain reaction in primary lung carcinoma] *Bull. Cancer,* 1996; 83 (10): 842-6.

[84] Yu Y, Yang A, Hu S, Yan H. Correlation of HPV-16/18 infection of human papillomavirus with lung squamous cell carcinomas in Western China. *Oncol. Rep.,* 2009; 21 (6): 1627-32.

[85] Kinoshita I, Dosaka-Akita H, Shindoh M, et al. Human papillomavirus type 18 DNA and E6-E7 mRNA are detected in squamous cell carcinoma and adenocarcinoma of the lung. *Br. J. Cancer,* 1995; 71 (2): 344-9.

[86] Baba M, Castillo A, Koriyama C, et al. Human papillomavirus is frequently detected in gefitinib-responsive lung adenocarcinomas. *Oncol. Rep.,* 2010; 23: 1085-92.

[87] Carpagnano GE, Koutelou A, Natalicchio MI, et al. HPV in exhaled breath condensate of lung cancer patients. *British journal of cancer,* 2011; 105 (8): 1183–90.

[88] Cheng YW, Chiou HL, Chen JT, et al. Gender difference in human papillomarvirus infection for non-small cell lung cancer in Taiwan. *Lung Cancer,* 2004; 46 (2): 165-70.

[89] Chiou HL, Wu MF, Liaw YC, Cheng YW, Wong RH, Chen CY, Lee H. The presence of human papillomavirus type 16/18 DNA in blood circulation may act as a risk marker of lung cancer in Taiwan. *Cancer,* 2003; 97 (6): 1558-63.

[90] Iwamasa T, Miyagi J, Tsuhako K, Kinjo T, Kamada Y, Hirayasu T, Genka K. Prognostic implication of human papillomavirus infection in squamous cell carcinoma of the lung. *Pathol. Res. Pract.,* 2000; 196 (4): 209-18.

[91] Cheng YW, Chiou HL, Sheu GT, et al. The association of human papillomavirus 16/18 infection with lung cancer among nonsmoking Taiwanese women. *Cancer Res.,* 2001; 61 (7): 2799-803.

[92] Kato T, Koriyama C, Khan N, et al. EGFR mutations and human papillomavirus in lung cancer. *Lung Cancer,* 2012; 78 (2): 144-7.

[93] Tung MC, Wu HH, Cheng YW, Wang L, et al. Association of epidermal growth factor receptor mutations with human papillomavirus 16/18 E6 oncoprotein expression in non-small cell lung cancer. *Cancer,* 2013; 119 (18): 3367-76.

[94] Cappuzzo F, Ligorio C, Jänne PA, et al. Prospective study of gefitinib in epidermal growth factor receptor fluorescence in situ hybridization-positive/phospho-Akt-positive or never smoker patients with advanced non-small-cell lung cancer: the ONCOBELL trial. *J. Clin. Oncol.,* 2007; 25 (16): 2248-55.

[95] Fukuoka M, Wu YL, Thongprasert S, et al. Biomarker analyses and final overall survival results from a phase III, randomized, open-label, first-line study of gefitinib

versus carboplatin/paclitaxel in clinically selected patients with advanced non-small-cell lung cancer in Asia (IPASS). *J. Clin. Oncol.*, 2011; 29 (21): 2866-74.

[96] Kim ES, Hirsh V, Mok T, et al. Gefitinib versus docetaxel in previously treated non-small-cell lung cancer (INTEREST): a randomised phase III trial. *Lancet,* 2008; 372 (9652): 1809-18.

[97] Arcilla ME, Chaft JE, Nafa K, et al. Prevalence, clinicopathologic associations, and molecular spectrum of ERBB2 (HER2) tyrosine kinase mutations in lung adenocarcinomas. *Clin. Cancer Res.*, 2012; 18: 4910-8.

[98] López-Malpartida AV, Ludeña MD, Varela G, García Pichel J. Differential ErbB receptor expression and intracellular signaling activity in lung adenocarcinomas and squamous cell carcinomas. *Lung Cancer,* 2009; 65 (1): 25-33.

[99] Casali C, Rossi G, Marchioni A, et al. A single institution-based retrospective study of surgically treated bronchioloalveolar adenocarcinoma of the lung: clinicopathologic analysis, molecular features, and possible pitfalls in routine practice. *J. Thorac. Oncol.,* 2010;5:830-6.

In: Fighting Lung Cancer through the HER Family ...
Editor: Diego Márquez-Medina
ISBN: 978-1-63321-092-9

Chapter 5

Laboratory I. Analysis of Human Epidermal Growth Factor Receptors: Conventional Analysis

Beatriz Bellosillo, Ph.D. and Luz Martínez-Avilés, B.S.
Pathology Department, Hospital del Mar University Hospital of Barcelona, Spain

Abstract

In the last 10 years development of tyrosine kinase inhibitors for the treatment of Non Small Cell Cancer (NSCLC) patients and the discovery that response to these treatments was dependent on the molecular status of the epidermal growth factor receptor (EGFR) gene has made the analysis of this human growth factor receptor mandatory prior to the initiation of any targeted therapy.

In this chapter we will review the considerations that must be taken into account when undergoing/undertaking EGFR analysis, as well as the role of other members of the EGFR family in NSCLC.

1. Introduction

As described in the previous chapters, the family of the human epidermal growth factor receptors (HER) or ErbB (erythroblastic leukaemia viral oncogene) receptors consists of four different members: HER1 (EGFR, ErbB1), HER2 (Neu, ErbB2), HER3 (ErbB3) and HER4 (ErbB4) which all have in their intracellular region a domain with tyrosine kinase (TK) activity. The formation of homodimers or heterodimers of the HER receptors following the binding of their ligands, results in the activation of a variety of signal transduction pathways that promote cell proliferation, angiogenesis, invasion of tumor cells and metastasis in various epithelial diseases.

2. EGFR in Non Small Cell Lung Cancer

The Epidermal Growth Factor Receptor (EGFR/HER1/ErbB1) is a 170 kDa transmembrane glycoprotein, containing an extracellular ligand binding domain, a transmembrane domain, a cytoplasmic region containing the TK domain and a carboxy-terminal region containing tyrosine residues of the receptor and regulatory elements. The binding of the ligand to the extracellular domain of the EGFR receptor produces its dimerization (homodimerization or heterodimerization with another HER receptor) which leads to its autophosphorylation and activation of the TK domain that, in turn, activates a cascade of mitogenic signals through two different signal transduction pathways. The first one is the KRAS -RAF- MEK- MAPK pathway responsible for the activation of gene transcription, entry into cell cycle and proliferation, and the second one is the PI3K/Akt/mTOR pathway involved in cell survival by inhibiting the process of apoptosis.

EGFR regulates essential cellular functions and has an oncogenic role in various tumors (head and neck, ovarian, endometrial, bladder, esophagus, stomach, brain, breast, colon and pancreas) by several activating mechanisms including overexpression, mutations and autocrine ligand production. EGFR alterations are associated with tumor proliferation, growth, invasion, metastatic capacity, inhibition of apoptosis and tumor angiogenesis [1].

The EGFR is overexpressed in 40-80% of many epithelial cancers including NSCLC [2] so inhibition of this receptor provided an effective alternative for the treatment of some neoplasms. Up to know, there are two major classes of molecules which act against the EGFR: monoclonal antibodies, which inhibit the receptor binding to its extracellular domain, and small-molecule TK inhibitors (EGFR-TKI), which inhibit the activation of the TK domain of the receptor.

EGFR-TKIs, such as gefitinib (Iressa) or erlotinib (Tarceva), are small molecules that can block the TK domain by competing with ATP for the binding to the TK domain. Initial studies with the EGFR-TKI gefinitib showed minimal adverse effects in NSCLC treated patients [3-5]. However, tumor responses were observed in only 10-19% of patients with advanced NSCLC refractory to chemotherapy [6, 7].

In 2004 several publications reported that the subgroup of patients who showed clinical responsiveness to EGFR-TKIs had specific activating mutations clustered around the ATP-binding pocket of the TK domain of the *EGFR* gene. These mutations cause a conformational change of the receptor that promotes an increase of the EGFR phosphorylation levels with independence of the binding of the ligand, leading to the constitutive activation of antiapoptotic pathways (Ras/MEK/ERK and Akt) [8-10]. The identification of these mutations in the *EGFR* gene represented the discovery of the first molecular marker of response to EGFR-TKIs treatment.

Responsiveness to EGFR-TKIs and the presence of *EGFR* mutations that confer sensitivity to these drugs is more frequently observed in several subgroups of patients: women, patients who have never smoked, patients with adenocarcinoma cell type and patients of East Asian origin [11, 12].

The *EGFR* gene is located at chromosome 7 (7p12.1-12.3) and it is constituted by 26 exons: exons 1-14 encode the extracellular domain, exon 15 encodes the transmembrane domain and exons 16-26 encode the intracellular portion of the receptor (Figure 1).

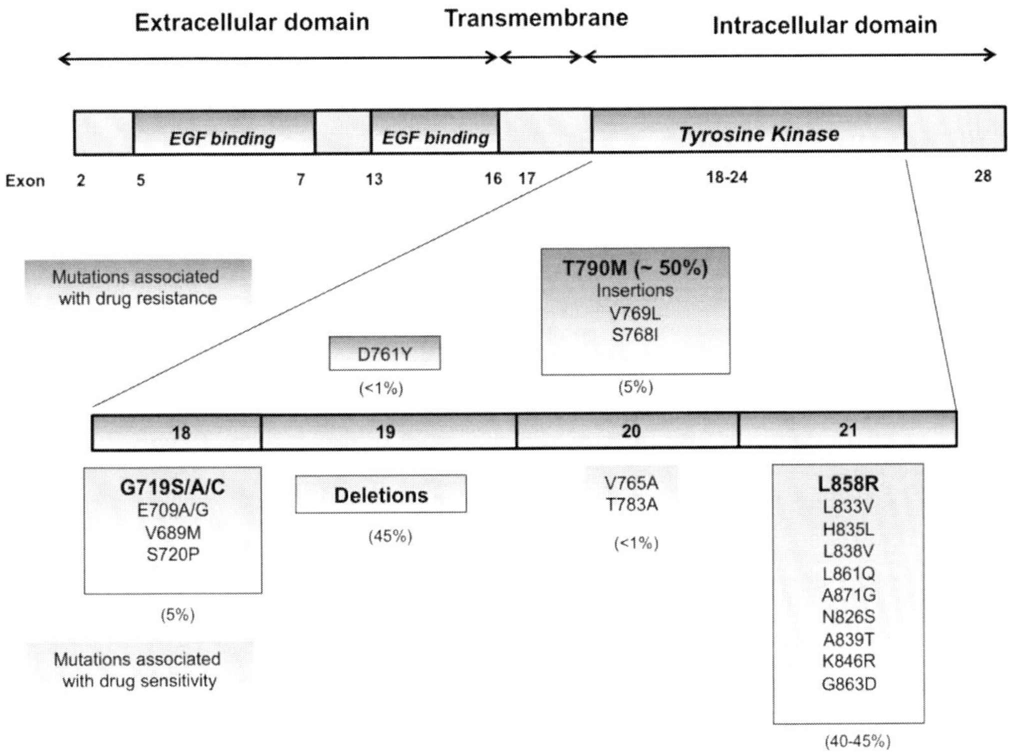

Figure 1. Distribution of the most frequent EGFR mutations affecting the EGFR tyrosine kinase domain.

Mutations in the *EGFR* gene related to the sensitivity of EGFR-TKIs in patients with NSCLC are mainly found in exons 18, 19, 20 and 21 of the gene. The most frequent mutations that confer sensitivity to EGFR-TKIs are several deletions that affect exon 19 of the *EGFR* gene (the most commonly affected region spans from codon 746 to codon 752) and a missense mutation resulting from the replacement of a leucine to an arginine at amino acid position 858 (p.L858R) which is located in exon 21. These mutations represent 85-90% of all *EGFR* mutated cases [13]. In addition, other uncommon mutations can also be detected in the *EGFR* gene. Among these infrequent mutations, the most commonly detected are various missense mutations that affect amino acid position glycine 719 at exon 18 (p.G719S/A, among others), or the p.L861Q missense mutation at exon 21, which have also been associated with a favorable effectiveness to EGFR-TKIs (Figure 1).

Finally, other *EGFR* mutations than can also be detected at diagnosis are in-frame deletion/insertions located at exon 20 or missense mutations at exon 19, but their clinical significance is still controversial (Figure 1) [14]. However, there is some evidence that these mutations might cause primary resistance to EGFR-TKIs [9, 10, 14-17] (Figure 1).

There are many other publications reporting rare and infrequent mutations affecting exons 18 to 21 of the *EGFR* gene. For example, recently two infrequent *EGFR* mutations located at exon 21 (p.R836C and p.T854S) have been reported; these mutations conferred low or no sensitivity to gefitinib, leading to a rapid progression of the disease [18]. Unfortunately, the predictive value of infrequent *EGFR* mutations is very often unknown, and thus their detection constitutes a challenge for treatment decision in routine clinical practice.

Most of the patients with *EGFR* mutations who initially respond to EGFR-TKIs finally relapse. In some cases, a second point mutation resulting in an amino acid substitution of threonine to methionine at amino acid position 790 (p.T790M) at exon 20 of the *EGFR* gene can also be observed. Structural modeling studies showed that the threonine at codon 790 appears to be critical for the binding of erlotinib to EGFR, and its substitution for methionine may interfere with the binding of the drug. Similar results were observed with gefitinib, suggesting that the presence of the p.T790M mutation confers resistance to EGFR-TKIs [19]. Regarding the origin of this resistance mutation, there are some studies that show that the p.T790M mutation can be a primary mutation [20, 21], present at the time of diagnosis that expands during the progression of the disease, whereas there are some other studies that show that it can also be a secondary mutation acquired after treatment with EGFR-TKIs [22, 23].

Table 1. Summary of four publications reporting on EGFR testing recommendations

	Shim et al.	Gómez et al.	Pirke et al.	Lindeman et al.
Patient Selection	1) Patients with NSCLC, especially adenocarcinoma 2) Other types if clinically indicated	1) Patients with advanced NSCLC: a) With non-squamous carcinoma and b) Non smokers with independence of the histological subtype	1) Patients with NSCLC: a) Adenocarcinoma and/or b) A negative smoking history	1) Lung adenocarcinoma 2) Mixed lung cancers with and adenocarcinoma component 3) Squamous or small cell histology in limited specimens where adenocarcinoma component cannot be completely excluded
Sample Source	1) Primary and metastatic sites 2) Biopsy and cytology specimens	1) Primary and metastatic sites 2) Biopsies and cytological specimens can be used if there are enough tumor cells	1) Primary and metastatic sites 2) Biopsy preferred over cytology	1) Primary and metastatic sites a) Formalin fixed paraffin-embedded specimens or fresh, frozen or alcohol-fixed specimens. b) Cytological samples are also suitable with cell blocks being preferred over smear preparations
Sample Processing	1) Routine preparation for tissue or cytology is suitable 2) Various methods can be used for mutation testing 3) The pathologist and oncologist should be aware of the pros and cons of each method	1) Routine preparation for tissue or cytology is suitable a) Determination of DNA quantity and quality is recommended. 2) Perform macrodissection or microdiseccion if needed 3) Various methods can be used for mutation testing: a) Sanger Sequencing and b) RT-PCR, are the most frequently used 3) Responsible should be aware of the pros and cons of each method	1) Determination of the ratio of malignant to normal cells within the sample is crucial for the detection of tumor-specific mutations a) 50% Tumor cells for DNA Sequencing b) Lower % acceptable for higher sensitivity techniques 2) Manual dissection or laser capture microdissection might be useful in certain cases 3) A variety of methods are used, but no consensus agreement on which was the best a) Direct sequencing b) ARMS c) Length analysis d) Denaturing high-performance liquid chromatography 4) Responsible should be aware of the pros and cons of each method	1) Pathologist should determine the adequacy of specimens by assessing cancer cell content and DNA quantity and quality (microdissection of tumor cells if needed) 2) Any validated EGFR testing method with sufficient performance characteristics can be used a) A test able to detect mutations in specimens with as little as 10% cancer cells is recommended b) A test able to detect individual mutations that have been reported at 1% of EGFR-mutated lung adenocarcinomas is recommended 3) Responsible should be aware of the pros and cons of each method

Table 1. (Continued)

	Shim et al.	Gómez et al.	Pirke et al.	Lindeman et al.
Turnaround Time	1) Pathologic diagnosis: 1-2 working days 2) Molecular diagnosis: 5-7 working days	1) Pathologic diagnosis: 2-3 working days 2) Molecular diagnosis: <7 working days	1)Pathologic diagnosis: 1-2 working days 2)Molecular diagnosis: 5-7 working days	1) *EGFR* and *ALK* analysis in 10 working days
Repeat examination	*Molecular testing should be repeated under the following situations:* 1) Poor sequence data 2) Cycle threshold too close to the defined cut-off limit (RT-PCR) 3) Sample with low tumor representation 4) Results are not matched with previously well-defined clinical-pathologic characteristics		*Molecular testing should be repeated under the following situations:* 1) A new (unreported) mutation is found because of the possibility of a false positive result. 2) Poor sequence data (with primary PCR and sequencing) 3) Cycle threshold is close to the defined cut-off limit (with the ARMS-based kits) 4) If other quality assessment criteria are not met	
Reporting format	1) Sample information 2) Type of method 3) Mutation status 4) Comments	1) Patient and doctor identification 2) Sample information (type of sample) 3) Type of method 4) Mutation status 5) Comments 6) Laboratory accreditation or participation in quality controls	1) Detail of biopsy sample and tissue extracted 2) Type of mutation analysis 3) Mutation present/absent 4) Interpretation	

ALK Anaplastic lymphoma kinase; **ARMS** Amplification refractory mutation systems; **DNA** Deoxyribonucleic acid; **EGFR** Epidermal growth factor receptor; **NSCLC** Non-small cell lung cancer; **PCR** Polymerase chain reaction; **RT-PCR** Real time polymerase chain reaction.

3. EGFR Mutational Testing

As mentioned above, it is mandatory to perform *EGFR* mutational analysis of tumor samples from NSCLC patients at the diagnostic routine to predict sensitivity to treatment with EGFR-TKIs such as gefitinib or erlotinib, which are drugs that target the EGFR ATP cleft. Main recommendations for EGFR analysis are summarized in Table 1 [24-27].

3.1. Candidate Patients

It is recommended to analyze *EGFR* mutation in patients with advanced NSCLC that have been diagnosed a non-squamous cell carcinoma, or do not smoke, regardless of histological subtype.

In the practical diagnostic routine, it is recommended to perform the mutational analysis of exons 18 to 21 of the *EGFR* gene, but if it is not possible to analyze all four exons, at least exons 19 and 21, where 90% of *EGFR* mutations are located, should be analyzed.

3.2. NSCLC Tumor Samples

In all cases determination of *EGFR* mutations should be made in a sample whose histology has been reviewed by a qualified person, usually the pathologist, to ensure that the sample contains tumor cells. The analysis of biomarkers in patients with lung cancer is typically performed in two types of samples, tissue samples and cytological samples.

Normally these samples have to be fixed to prevent their autolysis that could be produced by the presence of proteolytic enzymes or by the presence of microorganisms capable of degrading the cell. So fixation of the sample is done in order to maintain the tissue stability, the cells structure and to keep the original morphology.

For molecular biology studies it must take into account that sometimes one of the most commonly used fixatives such as formalin may lead to the modification and breakage of DNA molecules not allowing the performance of further molecular biology studies.

a) Tissue samples

- Bronchial biopsy: sample taken by bronchoscopy. Usually 3-6 tissue fragments are obtained (1 and 2 mm).
- Transbronchial biopsy: sample obtained during bronchoscopy, by puncture of the bronchial wall. Usually 2-3 tissue fragments are obtained (1-2 mm).
- Mediastinal lymph node biopsy: samples obtained from mediastinal lymphadenopathies. Usually 5-10 fragments are obtained (4-5 mm).
- Thoracentesis for pleural effusion: samples obtained from the parietal and visceral pleura, from variable size.
- CT-guided transthoracic fine-needle aspiration biopsy: one or various cylindrical fragments with a 0.5 mm diameter and 5 mm length might be obtained.
- Partial lung resection: in cases with peripheral tumors, resected lung fragments of medium or large size can be obtained.
- Pieces from surgical therapeutic resection: samples corresponding to individual lung lobes or pneumonectomies made with a therapeutic purpose.

b) Cytological samples

- Bronchoalveolar lavage: sample obtained after introducing, with the bronchoscope impacted in the segmental bronchus, around 10 ml of sterile saline solution that afterwards is sucked.
- Bronchial aspirate: bronchopulmonary secretions are collected in a tube interposed between a suction pump and the bronchoscope. Generally this material is used for microbiological study and the sample received by the pathologist usually corresponds to the aspirate after bronchoalveolar lavage.

- Bronchial brushing: Through the bronchoscope a brush can be passed to scrape the lesion. This process is usually done after the endoscopy when the biopsy has already been obtained.
- Endobronchial ultrasound-guided fine needle aspiration biopsy (EBUS): It is an ultrasound-guided transbronchial puncture of hilar lung tumors or paratracheal tumors without endoluminal affection or mediastinal lymph nodes.
- Lung puncture: It includes the transbronchial fine needle aspiration (FNA) and the peripheral pulmonary nodule FNA by CT guidance.
- Pleural fluid (thoracentesis): pleural fluid obtained by thoracentesis procedures.

Cytological samples collected in liquid media require no processing prior to staining, except for centrifugation if necessary, in order to concentrate cells and fix them into a slide before their staining. In some cases, when immunohistochemistry studies are required, samples obtained can be processed in a paraffin block.

c) Circulating free DNA

In some cases, there are difficulties in collecting sufficient tumor tissue for performing biomarkers analysis, especially in patients with advanced disease, in whom it would not be possible to perform a new biopsy or in cases in which the sample is insufficient to perform all diagnostic tests and another biopsy should be taken. In these situations, the detection of mutations in circulating free DNA in serum or plasma may be an alternative to determine the mutational status of *EGFR* or other biomarkers such as *KRAS*.

It must be taken into account, however, that in this sort of samples the amount of tumor DNA is very low, so very sensitive techniques have to be employed in order to be able to detect gene mutations.

4. Sample Processing

The ratio of tumor cells according to normal cells is crucial for adequate mutation testing. If the percentage of tumor cells in the sample is above 50%, no macrodissection is needed, especially if sensitive techniques are going to be used for the mutational analysis. In contrast, if the percentage of tumor cells is below 50% macrodissection or microdissection might be used to increase the ratio of tumor to normal tissue cells, and a more sensitive assay might be required.

After getting the sections of interests, the sample is deparaffinized using xylene and ethanol and the sample is incubated with proteinase K normally overnight. Afterwards, DNA can be extracted using commercial kits in a manual way or in an automated system.

Once the DNA is extracted, it would be recommendable to quantify the amount of DNA obtained as well as to perform a control PCR to ensure that the DNA is amplifiable. After that, *EGFR* testing could be performed using several methodologies (Figure 2).

4.1. Methodology

Different molecular techniques can be used to perform the *EGFR* mutational analysis as summarized in Table 2. These techniques have different sensitivities and limitations. Some assays can be used as screening tests, allowing the detection of most of the mutations that can occur in the region analyzed, as long as the mutant allele burden is above the limit of sensitivity of the technique, whereas other methodologies are targeted assays, usually allele-specific assays, with a very high sensitivity but where only a limited number of mutations can be detected.

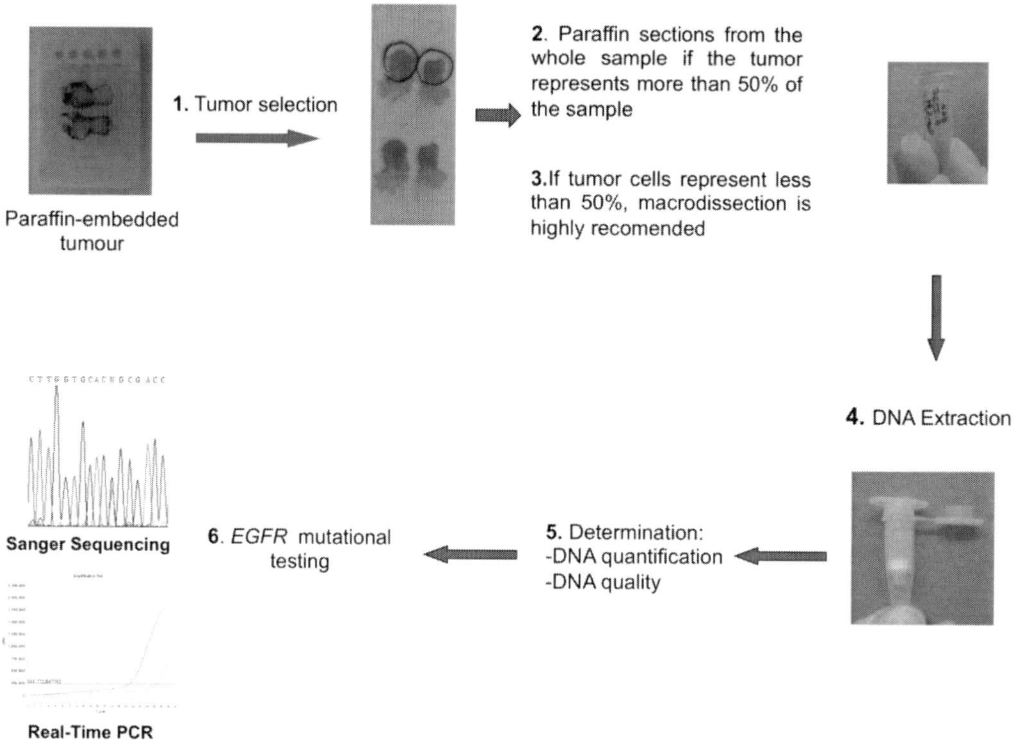

Figure 2. Workflow showing the main steps involved in *EGFR* mutational analysis.

Nevertheless, all assays are based on the amplification of the region of interest by the polymerase chain reaction (PCR). PCR amplification of the DNA from the region of interest is performed using a thermostable polymerase and primers (short DNA sequences of 15-25 nucleotides) that specifically hybridize to the two ends of the target region. The PCR reaction includes three steps: 1) denaturation (in which DNA is subjected to an elevated temperature of over 95°C so that the two strands are separated); 2) annealing (a stage of 1 to 2 minutes that is carried out between 50ºC and 65ºC; in this stage the primers bind specifically to the region studied); and 3) extension (a stage performed at 72°C and wherein the polymerase makes copies of the selected sequence). These three steps are cyclically repeated for 30-40 times and billions of copies of the region of interest are generated. The visualization of the PCR product can be performed by agarose gel electrophoresis or by capillary electrophoresis (the later has a higher capacity of separating DNA fragments of up to one-base pair resolution).

Table 2. Main molecular methodologies used for the detection of *EGFR* mutations. Sensitivity refers to the minimum percentage of mutant cells needed in the sample analyzed to be able to detect the mutation

		Sensitivity	Mutation
Screening assays	Sanger Sequencing	10-20%	Known and new
	Pyrosequencing	5%	Known and new
	Fragment size analysis	5%	Known and new
	CE-SSCP	1%	Known and new
Targeted assay	ARMS-PCR	3%	Known
	RT-PCR: a) Scorpions ARMS b) TaqMan	 1% 0.01%	 Known Known
Mutated allele enriched methods	PNA-PCR clamp	1%	Known
	COLD-PCR	1-10%	Known and new
	CAST-PCR	0.01%	Known

ARMS Amplification refractory mutation systems; **CAST-PCR**: Competitive Allele -Specific TaqMan® PCR; **COLD-PCR**: co-amplification at lower denaturation temperature-PCR; **CE-SSCP**: Capillary electrophoresis single-strand conformation analysis; **PNA-PCR clamp**: peptide nucleic acid locked polymerase chain reaction clamp.

The PCR technique has as main advantages that it is a fast technique that requires small starting material (allowing work with small biopsies or samples with low cellularity) and that it can be used to study partially degraded material (which is not uncommon among paraffin-embedded tissues) (Table 2).

4.2. Screening Assays

a) Sanger Sequencing

Direct DNA sequencing or Sanger sequencing is a method based on the selective incorporation of chain-terminating dideoxynucleotides (each nucleotide is fluorescently labeled with a different fluorochrome) by DNA polymerase during *in vitro* replication. PCR product is analyzed by capillary electrophoresis and the sequence determined from the detected fluorescence (Figure 3, upper panel).

Direct sequencing has been considered the gold standard for *EGFR* mutation analysis (as well as other mutational analysis). However, to apply this technology there must be a high ratio of mutated tissue with respect to non-mutated tissue (e.g., normal tissue) in the sample analyzed because if not, non-mutated DNA can mask the detection of mutations (especially when they are present in a low mutant allele burden), giving a false negative result.

b) Fragment size analysis

PCR amplification products are separated using an acrylamide gel, and the size of the PCR products will determine the presence of a mutation by comparison with a known size standard. If PCR is performed with fluorescent primers, PCR products can also be analyzed by capillary electrophoresis. This method is only useful when detecting deletions/insertions that alter the final length of the mutated PCR product in comparison with the wild type fragment (Figure 3, central panel).

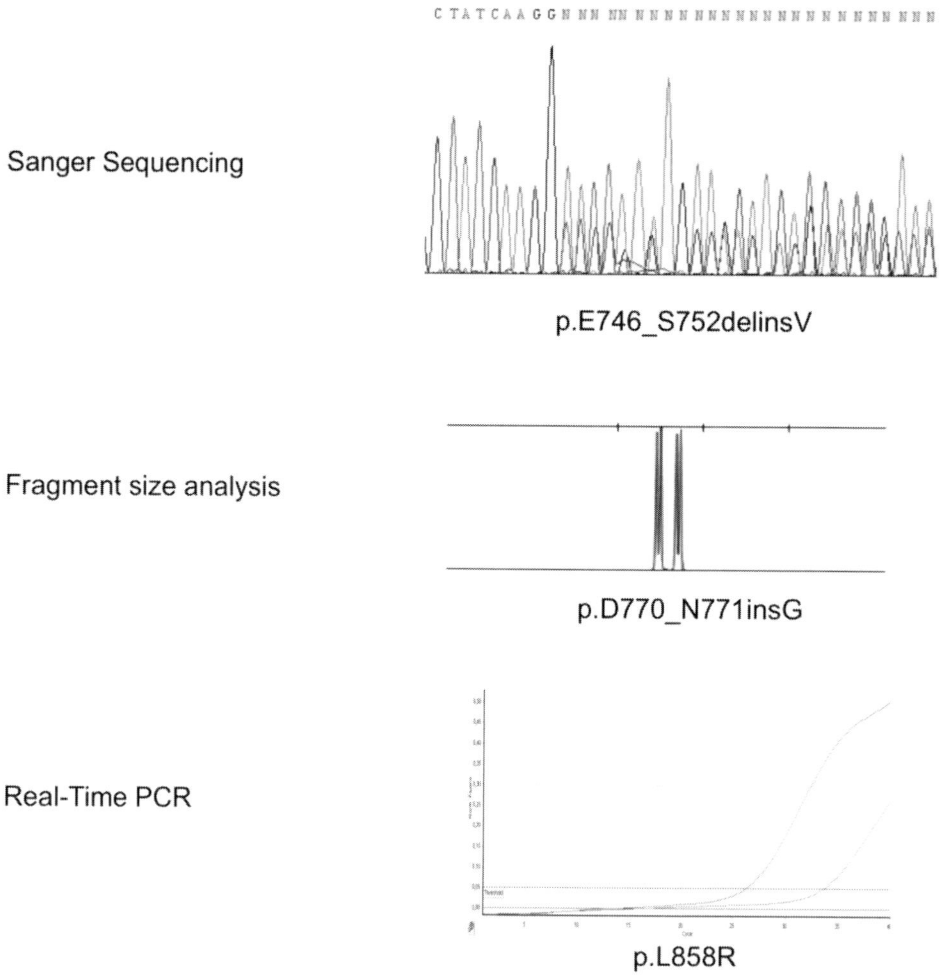

Figure 3. Detection of *EGFR* mutations by means of three different methodologies: Sanger sequencing (upper panel), PCR followed by capillary electrophoresis (central panel) and Real Time PCR (lower panel).

c) Pyrosequencing

Pyrosequencing is a *de novo* DNA sequencing method based on the sequencing-by-synthesis principle. This method measures the chemiluminiscent signal resulting from the pyrophosphate that is released during primer-directed DNA polymerase catalyzed nucleotide incorporation, during the sequencing reaction. Nucleotides are added and removed 1 at each time to avoid crossed signals. A chemiluminiscent signal is produced after the incorporation of each nucleotide and the sequence can be determined from the pyrogram interpretation.

d) Co-amplification at lower denaturation temperature-PCR *(COLD-PCR)*

COLD-PCR is a modified PCR method that utilizes the critical temperature at which mutation-containing DNA is preferentially melted over excess wild type alleles. This results in the preferential amplification of the mutant DNA increasing the sensitivity in order to detect the presence of low-level mutations. This PCR is used in combination with other methodologies for genotyping and detection of somatic mutations. These can include the use of PCR product for RFLP analysis, MALDI-TOF (matrix-assisted laser-desorption–time-of-flight) genotyping, or direct sequencing for detection of mutations by Sanger sequencing or pyrosequencing.

e) Capillary electrophoresis single-strand conformation analysis (CE-SSCP)

This is a screening method based on the principle of sequence-specific mobility of single-stranded DNA in a polymer. PCR product (PCR using fluorescent primers) is heat-denatured to separate the strands and subsequently cooled on ice to avoid reannealing. Finally, homoduplex/heteroduplex (with different electrophoretic mobility) will be analyzed by capillary electrophoresis and appropriate analysis software.

4.3. Targeted Assays

a) Amplification refractory mutation systems (ARMS)

Allele-specific PCR in which PCR primers are designed such that their 3' end nucleotides matches with the mutant or wild-type sequence. Under suitable conditions amplification will not take place if the 3' end has not perfectly paired and the two alleles (the wild type and the mutated) can therefore be distinguished. PCR products can be analyzed by electrophoresis in an agarose gel, although this technology has also been applied in real time PCR approaches.

b) Real Time PCR (quantitative PCR, qPCR)

Quantitative method in which the concentration of the PCR products are measured during the exponential phase using a fluorescence-detecting thermocycler machine (Figure 3, lower panel).

Commercial kits are mainly based in this methodology, although home-made assays can also be designed. In some cases the ARMS technology in combination with labeled probes are used for the detection of mutations with a high sensitivity. Real time PCR-based methods show a higher sensitivity than other previously described techniques, requiring a mutant DNA content of only 1%.

In order to increase the sensitivity of many of these assays as Sanger sequencing, fragment analysis or RT-PCR, addition of a blocker of the wild type allele to the reaction, can be used to enrich the mutant allele amplification and detection. The most commonly blocker used is the peptide nucleic acid locked polymerase chain reaction clamp (PNA-PCR Clamp).

In real-time PCR, this PNA can also be used, but there are also some commercial assays named CAST-PCR (Competitive Allele -Specific TaqMan® PCR), that combines allele-specific Taqman real time PCR with allele-specific MGB blockers to suppress amplification of the wild type allele, providing a better specificity and increasing the sensitivity of the assay.

5. EGFR Amplification

It has been reported that amplification of the *EGFR* gene might also be a predictor of response and survival in EGFR-TKI treated patients [28], although some studies show inconclusive information about the association between *EGFR* amplification and efficacy of EGFR-TKIs. *EGFR* amplification has been associated with a higher response rate and a benefit on survival from EGFR-TKIs, when compared to placebo [29, 30], although the benefit when EGFR-TKIs are compared head to head with conventional chemotherapy are more controversial [31, 32].

5.1. In Situ Hibridization

EGFR amplification is generally determined by *in situ* hybridization. *In Situ* Hibridization assays are based on the binding of probes to the region of interest, which is detected by chromogenic reagents. In the case of the chromogenic *in situ* hybridization (CISH) immunohistochemistry reactions with chromogen of alkaline phosphatase is used and in the silver stain *in situ* hybridization (SISH) the silver chromogen is used. The results of these techniques are interpreted using a normal microscope. Fluorescent microscopes are required to evaluate fluorescence *in situ* hybridations (FISH).

To study *EGFR* amplifications, two labeled probes are simultaneously used to detect the *EGFR* gene (7p12) and the chromosome 7 centromere (control probe). Probes are labeled with different fluorochromes (Figure 4). The stratification criteria for *EGFR* copy number gains, based on a retrospective study in advanced NSCLC patients treated with gefitinib [28, 33], are shown in Table 3.

Table 3. Stratification criteria of *EGFR* analysis by FISH in NSCLC patients

Categories	Cappuzzo et al. (2005)	Result
1	**Disomy** ≤2 copies in >90% of cells	NEGATIVE
2	**Low trisomy** ≤2 copies in ≥40% of cells 3 copies in 10-40% of cells ≥4 copies in <10% of cells	NEGATIVE
3	**High trisomy** ≤2 copies in ≥40% of cells 3 copies in ≥40% of cells ≥4 copies in <10% of cells	NEGATIVE
4	Low polysomy ≥4 copies in 10-40% of cells	NEGATIVE
5	High polysomy ≥4 copies in ≥40% of cells	POSITIVE
6	**Gene amplification** *EGFR* clusters Small clusters (4-10 copies) Ratio of *EGFR* gene to chromosome of ≥2 or ≥ 15 copies of *EGFR* per cell in ≥10% of analyzed cells	POSITIVE

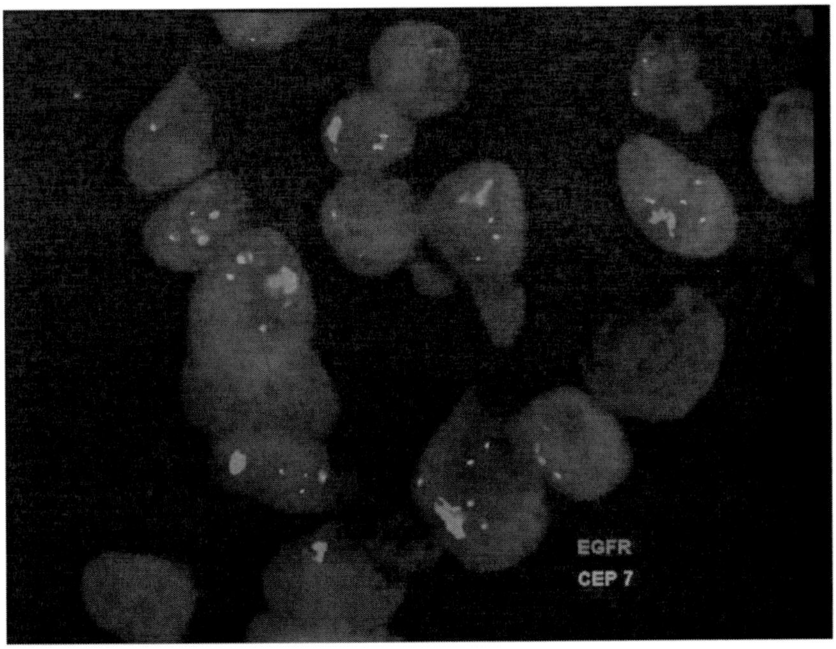

Figure 4. Detection of *EGFR* gene amplification by FISH analysis. *EGFR* signals (in red) show clusters of E*GFR* amplification.

6. EGFR Overexpression

The role of EGFR protein expression in predicting response to EGFR-TKIs is controversial, and therefore it is currently not considered at the decision of therapy.

EGFR protein expression is assessed by immunohistochemistry usually using methods and assessment criteria described in the publication of Hirsch et al. [34]. In this study, EGFR overexpression was assessed using the mouse anti-human EGFR, clone 31G7 monoclonal antibody [34]. According to this publication, only clear staining of the tumor cell membranes was considered positive. A semi quantitative approach was used to generate a score for each tissue as follows. The percentage of positive tumor cells per slide (0-100%) was multiplied by the dominant intensity pattern of staining: 1: negative; 2: weak; 3: moderate and 4: intense. Depending on the score obtained, samples were classified in negative or with low levels of expression (0-200), intermediate levels of expression (201-300) and high levels of expression (301-400).

There is no robust evidence about the predictive value of EGFR overexpression at the protein level with regard to TKIs. Some studies showed association between overexpression and benefit of TKIs in relation to response rate and decrease in the risk of progression or death [28, 29, 35] whereas some other studies did not observe this association [32, 34].

Nowadays neither *EGFR* amplification nor EGFR overexpression are accepted as criteria for selecting candidate patients for receiving therapy with TKIs. Only the *EGFR* mutational analysis is used as a predictive biomarker.

7. HER2 in NSCLC

HER2 (EGFR2, NEU, ERBB2) is a transmembrane receptor with TK activity, encoded by a gene located at chromosome 17q21. In comparison with other HER receptors, no specific ligand it is known for the HER2 receptor. HER2 activation can be independent of the binding of the ligand with the formation of homodimers or heterodimers in combination with EGFR, HER3 and HER4, and the binding of their specific ligands.

HER2 overexpression has been associated to many neoplasms such as breast cancer, gastric, ovary, prostatic and lung cancer and it might play an important role in the initiation of carcinogenesis, cancer progression and metastasis.

7.1. *HER2* Mutations in NSCLC

It has been mentioned that *EGFR* mutations can be found in a 15% of NSCLC patients. In some cases, mutations can be also found in the *HER2* gene with a lower incidence.

Several studies have reported mutations in the HER2 TK domain, showing frequencies of around 4-6% in NSCLC patients [36, 37]. As *EGFR* mutations, *HER2* mutations are preferentially detected in non-smoking females with lung adenocarcinoma, suggesting that these mutations have probably a role in the development of the lung cancer types that do not depend on tobacco smoke carcinogens, especially adenocarcinoma.

The most important mutations that affect the *HER2* gene are two different insertions of 12 pairs of bases located at exon 20, that alter the reading frame of the wild type HER2 sequence: the A775YVMA (represents 66% of all *HER2* mutations) and the M774AYVM insertion. These mutations result in excessive phosphorylation and activation of several proteins involved in cell signaling pathways than enhance neoplastic cells proliferation, resistance or decreased sensitivity to the action of reversible EGFR TKIs [36-41].

In a similar way to *EGFR* mutations, these alterations might also be a predictive marker for EGFR-TKI therapy considering that those patients carrying *HER2* exon 20 mutations will not respond to this treatment, and in the future it can become a target for new therapies.

In some studies, mutational analysis of the *HER2* exon 20 was performed with the use of a PCR assay flanking the potential mutated region of the gene. One of the primers was labeled with a fluorochrome so PCR products were analyzed by capillary electrophoresis in a genetic analyzer. Detection of PCR products with lengths different from the expected (if unmutated), determined the presence of *HER2* mutations [42]. Nevertheless, many other methodologies as the ones used for the *EGFR* mutational analysis can be applied in order to determine *HER2* exon 20 mutations.

7.2. *HER2* Amplification in NSCLC

HER2 gene amplification can be detected in NSCLC in a variable frequency (1-22%) depending on the analyzed series [43-46]. Recently, Takezawa et al. reported that *HER2* gene was amplified in 12% of tumors with acquired resistance to EGFR-TKIs versus only 1% of untreated lung adenocarcinoma. This study identified *HER2* amplification as a new mechanism of acquired resistance to EGFR-TKIs in EGFR-mutant NSCLC tumors, occurring independently of the *EGFR* p.T790M secondary mutation [43].

8. HER3 in NSCLC

HER3 is a transmembrane receptor encoded by a gene located at chromosome 12q13. It is the only member of the HER receptor family that lacks TK activity because of substitutions in crucial residues in the tyrosine kinase domain.

Up to now, HER3 has not been identified as a driving oncogene. Although HER3 does not have an oncogenic effect *per se*, it plays a critical role in HER2-mediated transformation and it is indispensable for continued tumor cell growth and proliferation driven by HER2 overexpression, and subsequent activation of the PI3K/Akt signaling. Indeed, high expression of HER3 can be observed in certain human cancers, so it has been suggested that it could be a novel therapeutic target [47].

Several studies have analyzed the role of HER3 in NSCLC. Several reports show overexpression of HER3 both at the mRNA and protein level [48], which, in turn, seems to be associated with a poor prognosis [49-51]. HER3 overexpression seems to play an important role in lung tumorigenesis as well as in the development of metastasis [51]. However, the signal transduction pathways involved in this effect remain to be elucidated.

HER3 expression could be associated to the presence of EGFR mutations [52]. In addition it may play a role in the responsiveness to EGFR-TKIs, as an association has been found between high levels of HER3 expression and gefitinib response or stabilization of disease [53].

No mutations in the HER3 gene have been detected in lung cancer [54], and regarding gene amplification, there are controversial results. Several publications have reported no gene amplifications affecting the *HER3* gene. However, one publication with a cohort of gefitinib-treated NSCLC reported up to 27% of *HER3* gene amplification by FISH. *HER3* amplification was associated to female gender and non-smoking patients, but not to tumor stage or histology, and it could be possible that gene amplification was due to the chemotherapy that patients had previously received [54].

On the other hand, HER3 might be also involved in EGFR-TKIs resistance. It is known that amplification of the MET receptor causes resistance to gefitinib in NSCLC with *EGFR* mutations. It seems that this resistance might be due to HER3-dependent activation of PI3K and AKT signaling, a pathway thought to be specific to EGFR/ERBB family receptor [55, 56].

In conclusion, further studies are needed to clarify the role of HER3 in NSCLC and its potential use as therapeutic target.

References

[1] Normanno N, Bianco C, Strizzi L, et al. The ErbB receptors and their ligands in cancer: an overview. *Curr Drug Targets*. 2005; 6 (3): 243–57.

[2] Arteaga CL. ErbB-targeted therapeutic approaches in human cancer. *Exp Cell Res*. 2003; 284 (1): 122–30.

[3] Ranson M, Hammond LA, Ferry D, et al. ZD1839, a selective oral epidermal growth factor receptor-tyrosine kinase inhibitor, is well tolerated and active in patients with solid, malignant tumors: results of a phase I trial. *Journal of clinical oncology: official journal of the American Society of Clinical Oncology*. 2002; 20 (9): 2240–50.

[4] Baselga J, Rischin D, Ranson M, et al. Phase I safety, pharmacokinetic, and pharmacodynamic trial of ZD1839, a selective oral epidermal growth factor receptor tyrosine kinase inhibitor, in patients with five selected solid tumor types. *J Clin Oncol*. 2002; 20 (21): 4292–302.

[5] Herbst RS, Maddox A-M, Rothenberg ML, et al. Selective oral epidermal growth factor receptor tyrosine kinase inhibitor ZD1839 is generally well-tolerated and has activity in non-small-cell lung cancer and other solid tumors: results of a phase I trial. *J Clin Oncol*. 2002; 20 (18): 3815–25.

[6] Kris MG, Natale RB, Herbst RS, et al. Efficacy of gefitinib, an inhibitor of the epidermal growth factor receptor tyrosine kinase, in symptomatic patients with non-small cell lung cancer: a randomized trial. *JAMA*. 2003; 290 (16): 2149–58.

[7] Fukuoka M, Yano S, Giaccone G, et al. Multi-institutional randomized phase II trial of gefitinib for previously treated patients with advanced non-small-cell lung cancer (The IDEAL 1 Trial). *J Clin Oncol*. 2003; 21 (12): 2237–46.

[8] Lynch TJ, Bell DW, Sordella R, et al. Activating mutations in the epidermal growth factor receptor underlying responsiveness of non-small-cell lung cancer to gefitinib. *N Engl J Med*. 2004; 350 (21): 2129–39.

[9] Pao W, Miller V, Zakowski M, et al. EGF receptor gene mutations are common in lung cancers from "never smokers" and are associated with sensitivity of tumors to gefitinib and erlotinib. *Proc Natl Acad Sci USA*. 2004; 101 (36): 13306–11.

[10] Paez JG, Jänne PA, Lee JC, et al. EGFR mutations in lung cancer: correlation with clinical response to gefitinib therapy. *Science*. 2004; 304 (5676): 1497–500.

[11] Miller VA, Kris MG, Shah N, et al. Bronchioloalveolar pathologic subtype and smoking history predict sensitivity to gefitinib in advanced non-small-cell lung cancer. *J Clin Oncol*. 2004; 22 (6): 1103–9.

[12] Miller VA, Riely GJ, Zakowski MF, Li AR, Patel JD, Heelan RT, et al. Molecular characteristics of bronchioloalveolar carcinoma and adenocarcinoma, bronchioloalveolar carcinoma subtype, predict response to erlotinib. *J Clin Oncol*. 2008; 26 (9): 1472–8.

[13] Rosell R, Moran T, Queralt C, et al. Spanish Lung Cancer Group. Screening for epidermal growth *N Engl J Med*. 2009; 361 (10): 958-67.

[14] Irmer D, Funk JO, Blaukat A. EGFR kinase domain mutations - functional impact and relevance for lung cancer therapy. *Oncogene*. 2007; 26 (39): 5693–701.

[15] Jänne PA, Engelman JA JB. Epidermal growth factor receptor mutations in non-small-cell lung cancer: implications for treatment and tumor biology. *J Clin Oncol.* 2005; 23 (14): 3227–34.

[16] Wu J-Y, Wu S-G, Yang C-H, et al. Lung cancer with epidermal growth factor receptor exon 20 mutations is associated with poor gefitinib treatment response. *Clin Cancer Res.* 2008; 14 (15): 4877–82.

[17] Greulich H, Chen T-H, Feng W, et al. Oncogenic transformation by inhibitor-sensitive and -resistant EGFR mutants. *PLoS Med.* 2005; 2 (11): e313.

[18] Mompradé E, Arriola E, Martínez-Avilés L. Two rare exon 21 EGFR mutations in patients treated with gefitinib. *J Thorac Oncol.* 2013; 8 (4): e36–7.

[19] Kobayashi S, Boggon TJ, Dayaram T, et al. EGFR mutation and resistance of non-small-cell lung cancer to gefitinib. *N Engl J Med.* 2005; 352 (8): 786–92.

[20] Pao W, Miller VA, Politi KA, et al. Acquired resistance of lung adenocarcinomas to gefitinib or erlotinib is associated with a second mutation in the EGFR kinase domain. *PLoS Med.* 2005; 2 (3): e73.

[21] Balak MN, Gong Y, Riely GJ, et al. Novel D761Y and common secondary T790M mutations in epidermal growth factor receptor-mutant lung adenocarcinomas with acquired resistance to kinase inhibitors. *Clin Cancer Res.* 2006; 12 (21): 6494–501.

[22] Maheswaran S, Sequist L V, Nagrath S, et al. Detection of mutations in EGFR in circulating lung-cancer cells. *N Engl J Med.* 2008; 359 (4): 366–77.

[23] Rosell R, Molina MA, Costa C, et al. Pretreatment EGFR T790M mutation and BRCA1 mRNA expression in erlotinib-treated advanced non-small-cell lung cancer patients with EGFR mutations. *Clin Cancer Res.* 2011; 17 (5): 1160–8.

[24] Pirker R, Herth FJF, Kerr KM, et al. Consensus for EGFR mutation testing in non-small cell lung cancer: results from a European workshop. *J Thorac Oncol.* 2010; 5 (10): 1706–13.

[25] Shim HS, Chung J-H, Kim L, et al. Guideline Recommendations for EGFR Mutation Testing in Lung Cancer: Proposal of the Korean Cardiopulmonary Pathology Study Group. *Korean J Pathol.* 2013; 47 (2): 100–6.

[26] Lindeman NI, Cagle PT, Beasley MB, et al. Molecular testing guideline for selection of lung cancer patients for EGFR and ALK tyrosine kinase inhibitors: guideline from the College of American Pathologists, International Association for the Study of Lung Cancer, and Association for Molecular Patho. *J Mol Diagn.* 2013; 15 (4): 415–53.

[27] Gómez JJ, de Castro J, Concha Á, et al. Recomendaciones para la determinación de biomarcadores en el carcinoma de pulmón no microcítico avanzado. Consenso nacional de la Sociedad Española de Anatomía Patológica y de la Sociedad Española de Oncología Médica. *Rev Esp Patol.* 2012; 45 (1): 14–28.

[28] Cappuzzo F, Hirsch FR, Rossi E, et al. Epidermal growth factor receptor gene and protein and gefitinib sensitivity in non-small-cell lung cancer. *J Natl Cancer Inst.* 2005; 97 (9): 643–55.

[29] Tsao M-S, Sakurada A, Cutz J-C, et al. Erlotinib in lung cancer - molecular and clinical predictors of outcome. *N Engl J Med.* 2005; 353 (2): 133–44.

[30] Hirsch FR, Varella-Garcia M, Bunn PA, et al. Molecular predictors of outcome with gefitinib in a phase III placebo-controlled study in advanced non-small-cell lung cancer. *J Clin Oncol.* 2006; 24 (31): 5034–42.

[31] Mok TS, Wu Y-L, Thongprasert S, et al. Gefitinib or carboplatin-paclitaxel in pulmonary adenocarcinoma. *N Engl J Med.* 2009; 361 (10): 947–57.
[32] Douillard J-Y, Shepherd FA, Hirsh V, et al. Molecular predictors of outcome with gefitinib and docetaxel in previously treated non-small-cell lung cancer: data from the randomized phase III INTEREST trial. *J Clin Oncol.* 2010; 28 (5): 744–52.
[33] Varella-Garcia M, Diebold J, Eberhard DA, et al. EGFR fluorescence in situ hybridisation assay: guidelines for application to non-small-cell lung cancer. *J Clin Patho*l. 2009; 62 (11): 970–7.
[34] Hirsch FR, Varella-Garcia M, Bunn PA, et al. Epidermal growth factor receptor in non-small-cell lung carcinomas: correlation between gene copy number and protein expression and impact on prognosis. *J Clin Oncol.* 2003; 21 (20): 3798–807.
[35] Cappuzzo F, Ciuleanu T, Stelmakh L, et al. Erlotinib as maintenance treatment in advanced non-small-cell lung cancer: a multicentre, randomised, placebo-controlled phase 3 study. *Lancet Oncol.* 2010; 11 (6): 521–9.
[36] Stephens P, Hunter C, Bignell G, et al. Lung cancer: intragenic ERBB2 kinase mutations in tumours. *Nature*. 2004; 431 (7008): 525–6.
[37] Li C, Fang R, Sun Y, et al. Spectrum of oncogenic driver mutations in lung adenocarcinomas from East Asian never smokers. *PloS one.* 2011; 6 (11): e28204.
[38] Pao W, Girard N. New driver mutations in non-small-cell lung cancer. *Lancet Oncol.* 2011; 12 (2): 175–80.
[39] Shigematsu H, Takahashi T, Nomura M, et al. Somatic mutations of the HER2 kinase domain in lung adenocarcinomas. *Cancer Res*. 2005; 65 (5): 1642–6.
[40] Buttitta F, Barassi F, Fresu G, et al. Mutational analysis of the HER2 gene in lung tumors from Caucasian patients: mutations are mainly present in adenocarcinomas with bronchioloalveolar features. International journal of cancer. *Int J Cancer.* 2006; 119 (11): 2586–91.
[41] Wang SE, Narasanna A, Perez-Torres M, et al. HER2 kinase domain mutation results in constitutive phosphorylation and activation of HER2 and EGFR and resistance to EGFR tyrosine kinase inhibitors. *Cancer cell.* 2006; 10 (1): 25–38.
[42] Nicoś M, Krawczyk P, Mlak R, et al. The presence of HER2 exon 20 insertion in patients with central nervous system metastases from non-small lung cancer--a potential application in classification for therapy. *Pneumonol Alergol Pol.* 2013; 81 (4): 294–7.
[43] Takezawa K, Pirazzoli V, Arcila ME, et al. HER2 amplification: a potential mechanism of acquired resistance to EGFR inhibition in EGFR-mutant lung cancers that lack the second-site EGFRT790M mutation. *Cancer Discov*. 2012; 2 (10): 922–33.
[44] Cappuzzo F, Varella-Garcia M, Shigematsu H, et al. Increased HER2 gene copy number is associated with response to gefitinib therapy in epidermal growth factor receptor-positive non-small-cell lung cancer patients. *J Clin Oncol.* 2005; 23 (22): 5007–18.
[45] Pugh TJ, Bebb G, Barclay L, et al. Correlations of EGFR mutations and increases in EGFR and HER2 copy number to gefitinib response in a retrospective analysis of lung cancer patients. *BMC Cancer.* 2007; 7: 128.
[46] Varella-Garcia M, Mitsudomi T, Yatabe Y, et al. EGFR and HER2 genomic gain in recurrent non-small cell lung cancer after surgery: impact on outcome to treatment with gefitinib and association with EGFR and KRAS mutations in a Japanese cohort. *J Thorac Oncol.* 2009; 4 (3): 318–25.

[47] Gullick WJ. The c-erbB3/HER3 receptor in human cancer. *Cancer Surv.* 1996; 27: 339–49.
[48] E. Felip, M. Salcedo, N. Murtra-Garrell, et al. Expression of ErbB2 and ErbB3 in resected non-small cell lung cancer (NSCLC) patients. *J Clin Oncol.* 2011; 29 (suppl; abstr 7037).
[49] Poller DN, Spendlove I, Baker C, et al. Production and characterization of a polyclonal antibody to the c-erbB-3 protein: examination of c-erbB-3 protein expression in adenocarcinomas. *J Pathol.* 1992; 168 (3): 275–80.
[50] Koumakpayi IH, Diallo J-S, Le Page C, et al. Low nuclear ErbB3 predicts biochemical recurrence in patients with prostate cancer. *BJU Int.* 2007; 100 (2): 303–9.
[51] Müller-Tidow C, Diederichs S, Bulk E, et al. Identification of metastasis-associated receptor tyrosine kinases in non-small cell lung cancer. *Cancer Res.* 2005; 65 (5): 1778–82.
[52] Kawano O, Sasaki H, Endo K, et al. ErbB3 mRNA expression correlated with specific clinicopathologic features of Japanese lung cancers. *J Surg Res.* 2008; 146 (1): 43–8.
[53] 53. and their ligands in lung adenocarcinomas that are sensitive to inhibition of epidermal growth factor receptor. *Cancer Res.* 2005; 65 (24): 11478–85.
[54] Sithanandam G, Anderson LM. The ERBB3 receptor in cancer and cancer gene therapy. *Cancer Gene Ther.* 2008; 15 (7): 413–48.
[55] Engelman JA, Zejnullahu K, Mitsudomi T, Song Y, Hyland C, Park JO, et al. MET amplification leads to gefitinib resistance in lung cancer by activating ERBB3 signaling. *Science.* 2007; 316 (5827): 1039–43.
[56] Arteaga CL. HER3 and mutant EGFR meet MET. *Nat Med.* 2007; 13 (6): 675–7.

In: Fighting Lung Cancer through the HER Family ...
Editor: Diego Márquez-Medina
ISBN: 978-1-63321-092-9

Chapter 6

Laboratory II. Experimental Analysis of Human Epidermal Growth Factor Receptors

Javier Hernández-Losa, Ph.D.
Molecular Biology Laboratory, Vall d'Hebron University Hospital of Barcelona, Spain

Abstract

The human epidermal growth factor (HER) family of tyrosine kinase receptors includes the epidermal growth factor (EGFR or HER1), the ErbB2 (HER2), ErbB3 (HER3), and ErbB4 (HER4) receptors. The HER family is implicated in the pathogenesis of many human malignancies including the non-small cell lung cancer (NSCLC). Different laboratory tests have been clinically validated to examine HER abnormalities with a prognostic and predictive value in NSCLC (*HER* amplifications, mRNA and protein overexpression, copy number aberrations, loss of heterozygosis, and methylation). The present chapter reviews novel and experimental technologies that are being developed to study the HER family and its signaling pathways in the "omic" era.

1. Introduction

Different clinically validated lab tests are available to detect abnormalities in the Human Epidermal Growth Factor (HER) family of cell receptors with a prognostic and predictive value in non-small cell lung cancer (NSCLC). Nevertheless, novel methodologies are being implemented in order to encompass new aberrations and to provide additional information of the HER family and its downstream pathways. The present chapter focuses on those emerging techniques.

2. Proteomic Analysis of HER Protein Expression in Non-Small Cell Lung Cancer

2.1. Electrophoresis-Based Techniques

Western blotting has been classically applied to detect HER proteins and their downstream effectors in both *in vitro* and *in vivo* models, and it is strongly recommended to be applied before the setting-up of any other molecular technique. The Western blot analysis quantifies the real amount of HER proteins, measures the protein size, and identifies variations in full-length isoforms. The existence of some predictive markers for targeted therapies such as the p95HER2 in breast cancer [1, 2], and the truncated HER2 [3], the sensitizing mutations of the Epidermal Growth Factor Receptor (EGFR) [4, 5], and *EGFR* amplifications [6] in NSCLC were initially reported by Western blotting.

The Kinetworks^{TM} Phospho-Site Screen 1.3 is an alternative electrophoresis-based method. The Phospo-Site provides a set of custom or preformed fluorochrome-tagged protein kinases that are compared with fluorochrome-tagged non-phosphorylated proteins by 2D fluorescence analysis. This method provides quantitative information of the HER amount, measures the ratio of phosphorylated (p-) proteins, and detects activated downstream pathways [7].

2.2. Spectrometric Methods

Some proteomic analyses based on 2D electrophoresis are being replaced by mass spectrometry. The SILAC (Stable Isotope Labeling by Amino acids in Cell culture) incorporates specific aminoacids (Normal Arg-O and Heavy Arg-6) into mammalian proteins *in vivo*, produces a mass shift of the corresponding peptides, and the relative protein abundance is detected by mass spectrometry. The Super-SILAC technology could be applied to distinguish lung adenocarcinomas from squamous cell carcinomas [8], and to explore the kinase network of NSCLC [9].

Spectrometry has been also applied to the Selected Reaction Monitoring multiplex quantification of EGFR, HER2, HER3, and Insulin Growth Factor receptor in formalin-fixed, paraffin-embedded (FFPE) samples. This technique provides an accurate measurement of native endogenous peptides in a soluble lysate using labeled, synthetic, internal standard peptides. The Selected Reaction Monitoring highly correlates with immunohistochemistry (IHC) and electrochemiluminiscense *in vitro* and breast cancer samples, and [10].

2.3. Immunohistochemistry

IHC applies a conventional antigen–antibody reaction to detect HER receptors in tumor sections. Several antibodies are available to detect EGFR in human FFPE NSCLC samples. However, an standard cutoff for IHC EGFR positivity has not been established, and the value of IHC EGFR-overexpression as a prognostic and predictive factor in NSCLC remains controversial. On contrary, the correlation between the IHC HER2-overexpression and the

HER-amplification detected by immunofluorescence *in situ* hybridization (FISH) is consistent in breast cancer [11-15]. In NSCLC, the *HER2*-amplification is rare and has been associated to a lower survival [16-20].

The IHC expression of HER3 and HER4 has been scarcely studied in NSCLC. HER3 is unable to be phosphorylated in response to NRG1 and NRG2. However, the HER3 basal activity allows the auto-phosphorylation and activates the PI3K-AKT downstream pathway in breast and lung cancer cells [21-23]. Different antibodies and antisense oligonucleotides are being developed to detect HER3 in NSCLC FFPE samples [24-26].

a) IHC analysis of phosphoproteins.

The presence of p-HER receptors and their kinase activity in NSCLC samples could be detected by IHC. Attempts to detect p-EGFR by IHC have been done. A high p-EGFR level has been associated with the presence of activating *EGFR*-mutations in NSCLC [27]. The phosphorylation of tyrosine 845 (pY845) and 1068 (pY1068) have been associated with *EGFR*-mutations in Asian patients with lung adenocarcinomas [28-32], and the phosphorylation of tyrosine 1173 (pY1173) has been associated with the presence of a lepidic pattern in lung adenocarcinomas [33]. Accordingly, p-EGFR could be eventually interpreted as an indirect marker of sensibility to tyrosine kinase inhibitors of the EGFR (EGFR-TKI).

b) Mutation analysis by IHC.

Monoclonal antibodies to detect *EGFR*-mutations in NSCLC small biopsies and surgical specimens are being developed. The correlation of IHC with the sequencing and real-time polymerase chain reaction (PCR) is high. The sensitivity and specificity of IHC to detect the E746_A750 deletion in exon 19, and the L858R point mutation in exon 21 is 60-70% and 80-95%, and 80% and 95-100%, respectively.

However, IHC does not detect all the *EGFR*-mutations, and a DNA confirmation of positive IHC is necessary. The IHC analysis of *EGFR*-mutations should be applied as a complementary method when DNA-based testing is unavailable, or when pathological procedures result in DNA degradation [34-41].

2.4. Protein Direct or Reverse Phase Assays

Protein chips can be combined with the phosphorylation analysis of protein lysates from cell lines, frozen tissues, FFPE samples [42], and laser micro-dissected samples [43], to quantify the presence of p-HER and p-EGFR.

The Direct Capture Technique derived from the Reverse Capture Protein Chips, and has been applied to detect prognostic and predictive signatures for anti-EGFR treatments in blood samples from NSCLC [44].

HER proteins can be quantified too using imaging techniques. HER receptors are labeled with different fluorochromes, and captured with a fluorescence-scanning camera. Then, an specific imaging software provides information about any single or dimer HER protein.

The Förster resonance energy transfer (FRET)-based assay also quantifies genuine protein-protein interactions. FRET could be used to calculate the amount of HER2 and HER3 dimers, and to suggest the status of HER signaling pathways in NSCLC samples. The TR-FRET, an antibody-based time-resolved assay, has been validated to analyze the EGFR and HER2-expression in breast cancer cryosections, and to quantify HER homo- or heterodimers [45]. This technique applies pairs of monoclonal antibodies against two distinct epitopes of the EGFR and HER. When the antibodies against the donor and the acceptor fluorophores are brought together, energy is released as fluorescence or transferred to the acceptor fluorophore, which re-emits it in a specific long-lived fluorescence at 665 nm that can be quantified.

The VeraTag is a proximity-based assay that quantifies proteins and protein complexes, and provides information about protein-protein interactions or about the activity of signaling pathways. The VeraTag provides a continuous, rather than semi-quantitative, measurement of HER1, HER2, and HER3-expression in FFPE samples [46], and has been validated in breast cancer samples and lung cancer cell lines [46, 47]. HER proteins and homodimers are detected through the release of fluorescent tags conjugated to specific HER antibodies, in the proximity of a second HER antibody. Over 14 different p-EGFR antibodies have been applied to quantify p-EGFR and to establish novel EGFR-AURKA interactions [48].

The Array 001 (R&D Systems) detects p-tyrosine receptors using capture antibodies against 42 custom or ready-to-use tyrosine kinase receptors in duplicate wells. Cell lysates are incubated overnight at 4ºC with the array in a specific buffer. HER receptors are linked to antibodies and p-receptors are detected by horseradish peroxidase-conjugated p-Tyr antibodies. This method avoids the western blotting and is useful to detect activated HER pathways and to establish the role of HER homo- and heterodimerization in *MET*-amplified cells [49].

The Bio-Plex Multiplex Immunoassay also analyzes pathway activations, and it has been validated in melanoma, breast, colon, lung, and pancreatic human cancers. This technique is based on the extraction of living cells from a tissue suspension taken from a solid tumor biopsy. Cells are distributed in different wells, and subsequently treated with drugs, growth factors, and/or other agents. Finally, a bead-based immunoassay enables different multiplexing to detect the unique signal to each antibody, even combining different antibodies in the same well. The PathMap profile focuses on the quantification of pathway alterations as biomarkers to predict the drug activity [50]. This technology was designed to detect tumor responses in fresh samples, and could be used to select live cells for further next-generation sequencing (NGS) with a SnapPath automatic platform.

The *Proseek Multiplex Oncology* I^{96x96} *Kit* quantifies proteins with the sensitivity of the so-called digital PCR. This technique uses a series of primers of selected flank proteins that are amplified by PCR when they are close together.

3. Transcriptomic Analysis

Transcriptomic analyzes the mRNA level of HER genes. The addition of dyes (e.g., SYBR Green, EvaGreen), or fluorochrome probes (e.g., Taqman, Bacon or Scorpion assays) increase the sensitivity and specificity of real time PCR, bypass the amplicon manipulation, and minimizes the risk of contamination. Some chip hybridization methods such as the Affymetrix U133 Gene Chip Microarray Hybridization have been designed to hybridize and to quantify the HER2 and EGFR mRNA in tumor samples, [51]. The NanoString system quantifies specific mRNA from FFPE samples [52], and detects those fusion genes such as KIF5B-RET and GOPC-ROS1 involved in the lung carcinogenesis. Some NGS applications such as RNA-Seq enable the amplification and sequencing of the entire transcriptome of the tumor cells [53].

The mRNA expression of HER3 and its main activator NRG1 should predict the prognosis and resistance to anti-EGFR treatments in lung cancer [45, 54, 55].

4. Genetic Analysis

4.1. Gene Amplification

Variations in the *EGFR* gene copy number are discussed to be a predictive marker to EGFR-TKI efficacy. The *EGFR*-amplification is present in 33-44% of lung adenocarcinomas, and could be partially associated with the presence of *EGFR*-mutation. However, it is not recommended as a predictive marker of EGFR-TKI benefit [56]. Dual probes such as Vysis (EGFR/CEP7), DAKO (EGFR/CEN7), Kreatech [HER1 (7p11)/SE7], Abnova (EGFR/CEN7q), and CytoTest (EGFR FISH probe) are available to analyze the *EGFR*-amplification.

HER2-amplification has been reported in 10% of lung adenocarcinomas, and it has been associated to EGFR-TKI acquired resistance in *EGFR*-mutant patients [57-58].

FISH has been rarely used to analyze HER3. One work reported that *HER3*-amplification predicted the sensitivity to gefitinib in advanced NSCLC [59]. The novel massive parallel sequencing techniques are able to detect copy number aberrations (CAN) and *HER*-amplifications in different human cancers, including NSCLC.

4.2. Mutation Analysis

Patients with specific *EGFR*-mutations in exons 18-21 are sensible to gefitinib, erlotinib or afatinib. On contrast, other specific mutations confer resistance to these treatments. A wide range of techniques is available to perform the mutational analysis, including the real-time PCR with probes (TaqMan and Scorpions) and dyes (SYBR Green and EvaGreen), the PCR plus hybridization, the melting curves, CAST PCR, COLD-PCR, and PNA-Clamp PCR. These methods increase the percentage of detected mutant alleles in comparison with the Sanger method. Mutations in the kinase domain of the *HER2* have been associated with a resistance to EGFR-TKIs.

HER3-mutations are found in 11% of colon and gastric tumors. However, they are rare in lung cancer [60, 61]. Nevertheless, the -256C/T HER3 polymorphism detected in some Korean patients has been associated with an increased risk of lung cancer in never smokers [62]. A NGS analysis of 188 Asian lung cancers revealed the uncommon presence of *HER4*-mutations [63].

Table 1. Main differences between sequencing methodologies

APPROACH	ADVANTAGES	DISADVANTAGES
Whole-genome sequencing	1. Comprehensive view of whole genome 2. Detection of all types of mutations 3. Standard procedure for all patients and tumor types	1. Expensive 2. Large datasets 3. Most findings are not clinically actionable
Whole-exome sequencing	1. 1-1.5% genome sequenced 2. Half the cost of whole-genome sequencing 3. Detects indels and SNPs	1. Smaller datasets (easier) 2. Miss fusion genes and many mutations 3. Most findings are not clinically actionable
Targeted gene sequencing	1. Cost-effective 2. Easy 3. Most findings clinically actionable	1. Many mutations missed 2. Requires the prior knowledge of genes 3. Benefits in a subset of patients

Table 2. Genome sequencers

	Genome Sequencer	HiSeq / MiSeq	5500W / SOLiD	Ion Torrent
Manufacturer (original / subsidiary)	Roche (454)	Illumina (Solexa)	Life Technologies (ABI)	Life Technologies (Ion Torrent)
Principle	Pyrosequencing	Reversible termination	Sequencing by ligation	Semiconductor sequencing
Run time	10 h	~27 h/4–39 h	6 days	2 h/1.5 h
High-throughput or genome line	GS FLX	HiSeq	5500W	Ion Proton
Targeted sequence or bench-top line	GS Junior	MiSeq	-	Ion PGM
Clonal amplification	Bridge PCR	Emulsion PCR	Emulsion PCR	Emulsion PCR
Sequencing enzyme	DNA polymerase	DNA polymerase	DNA ligase	DNA polymerase
Detected signal	Light	Fluorescence	Fluorescence	H^+ ion charge

A second series reported *HER4*-mutations in 5 out of 257 Asian lung tumor samples [64]. Nevertheless, these results were not reproduced in a third series analyzing 105 Japanese lung cancers with quantitative PCR and Sanger sequencing [65].

A wide range of high-throughput sequencing platforms is being developed, and they can be divided into three massive NGS parallel sequencing models: The whole-genome sequencing, the whole-exome sequencing, and the targeted gene sequencing (Table 1).

NGS is based on the combination of light detection and PCR. Each DNA nucleotide is marked in a different color, and an overlapping detection process is repeated 30–60 times to improve the resolution. Luminescence can be performed using the HiSeq or the MiSeq analyzer. The most relevant TruSeq method involves a cancer amplicon panel [66]. Roche developed the 454 FLX and the GS Junior Life Science, two genetic-based emulsion PCR and pyrosequencing analyzers.

The SOLiD sequencing performs a probe ligation-based mutational analysis. This sequencing platform combines the emulsion PCR and the ligation in color-space sequencing. The substitution of microbeads by nanobeads improves the sequence information (Table 2).

The Ion Torrent Applied Biosystems detects those pH changes caused by the release of protons in the nucleotide/base union. It included the Ion Ampliseq™ Cancer Panel with *EGFR*, *HER2*, and *HER4* genes that could be amplified in a multiplexed manner. Coming sequencers such as those from Pacific Biosciences or the GeneReader will include panels of gene-specific types of tumor.

4.3. Multiplexing Technologies

Several techniques have been implemented to detect relevant genes for the development and management of NSCLC. Sequenom combines the primer extension with the MALDI-TOF technology to obtain a gene mutational profile including the most common EGFR, HER2, HER4, and downstream pathways alterations in FFPE samples, [67]. Sequenom is used to screen patients for target phase I trials, and presents 5% sensitivity to detect mutant alleles in a wild-type background and a high concordance with specific real-time assays [68-69].

The SNaPshot analysis [70] combines the primer extension analysis with fluorochrome-labeled nucleotides, and provides the mutation analysis of selected single nucleotide polymorphisms (SNPs) after a gene-scanning analysis.

The mutation scanning (mutation multi-analyte panel or MUT-MAP) based on a TaqMan or allele-specific PCR (AS-PCR) assay pre-amplifies the DNAs using custom-designed primer sets before the TaqMan or the AS-PCR assays were performed. This technique provides the mutation profiling of EGFR, KRAS, PIK3CA, NRAS, BRAF, and AKT1 [71].

These methods are widely applied to analyze the tyrosine kinase profiling of different tumors, but fail to study pathway alterations from tumor suppressor genes such as TP53, PTEN, STK11, CDKN2A, ATM, which are altered in more than 70% of NSCLCs [72].

a) Experimental liquid biopsies

A new generation of liquid biopsies has been developed to obtain mutational information in NSCLCs. Some of them have been validated to monitor the patient response to target therapies, and they are becoming introduced in molecular laboratories.

The routine determination of *EGFR*-mutations in blood and serum provides easy access to biological samples, and the opportunity to monitor the response to EGFR-TKI. The main disadvantage of this method is its low sensitivity in comparison to the conventional analysis

[73, 74]. Novel technologies including the ARMS-Scorpions, the mutant-enriched liquidchip (ME-liquidchip), the digital PCR, and nanotechnologic platforms will detect *EGFR*-mutations in an infinitely low number of mutant copies [75, 76].

b) Single cells, circulating tumor cells, and cell-free DNA

Re-biopsy is difficult, invasive, and un-exact due to heterogeneity of lung cancer. The analysis of circulating cell-free tumor DNA released into plasma [77], circulating tumor cells (CTCs) [78] or Single Cells [79] represent a non-invasive liquid biopsy, and permit to observe evolution changes in the course of the disease. These techniques will help to discriminate the World Genome Amplification artifacts from the genuine genetic variants and the template genome [79].

5. Future Approaches in Epigenetics

New techniques are being developed to identify mechanisms of HER regulation, and they mainly focus on three epigenetic mechanisms: the DNA methylation, the histone tail modification, and the non-coding microRNA (miRNA) regulation.

5.1. DNA Methylation

The methylation of cytosine residues in CpG sites in the 5´region of genes has been extensively studied as an epigenetic mechanism of gene expression regulation. The hypermethylation (due to inactivation in tumor suppressor genes), and the hypomethylation (due to genomic instability and active transcription) are commonly described in human cancers. The sodium bisulfite treatment deaminates cytosine into uracil and does not interact with the t 5-methylcytosine. The PCRt of bisulfite-treated DNA amplifies uracil as thymine, and methylated cytosine as cytosine. The Methylation Specific Primers (MSP) has been used in *in vitro* and lung cancer [80]. Novel methodologies will be able to analyze *in vitro* sets of different gene promoters, and to quantify the methylation status of CpG islands by combining MSP and taqman assays in human samples [81-82].

5.2. Histone Tail Modifications

Lysine-rich tails of histones (H2A, H2B, H3, and H4) bulge from the nucleosome alter the chromatin structure and modulate the gene expression by methylation, acetylation, phosphorylation, sumoylation, and ubiquitination. The histone lysine acetylation /deacetylation by histone acetyltransferases, deacetylase enzimes HAT and HDAC, and the methylation/demethylation by histone methyltransferases (KMT) and histone dimethyltransferases (KDMT) have been extensively explores. The relationship between HDAC inhibitors and the EGFR and HER2 expression is being studied in lung cancer cell lines [83].

5.3. miRNAs

The miRNA is a small regulatory RNA (approximately 22 nucleotides long) that controls the gene expression binding the 3´untranslated region (UTR) of mRNA, and leading to either mRNA degradation or to the inhibition of the protein translation. The human genome includes more than 1000 mature miRNAs, and different miRNA signatures have been proposed to distinguish squamous carcinomas from adenocarcinomas, and to evaluate the risk of relapse in resected early lung cancers. The mir205 has been associated with HER3-expression in FFPE samples of breast cancer [84]. The miR-133b [85], miR-542-5p [86], miR-7 [87], and miR-21 [88], all of them down-modulators of the EGFR-expression, have been studied one by one or using miRNA *in vitro* and in FFPE samples.

References

[1] Anido J, Scaltriti M, Bech Serra JJ, Santiago Josefat B, Todo FR, Baselga J, Arribas J. Biosynthesis of tumorigenic HER2 C-terminal fragments by alternative initiation of translation. *EMBO J.*, 2006; 25 (13): 3234-44.

[2] Scaltriti M, Rojo F, Ocaña A, et al. Expression of p95HER2, a truncated form of the HER2 receptor, and response to anti-HER2 therapies in breast cancer. *J. Natl. Cancer Inst.*, 2007; 99 (8): 628-38.

[3] Cappuzzo F, Cho YG, Sacconi A, et al. p95HER2 truncated form in resected non-small cell lung cancer. *J. Thorac. Oncol.*, 2012; 7 (3): 520-7.

[4] Okamoto I, Kenyon LC, Emlet DR, et al. Expression of constitutively activated EGFRvIII in non-small cell lung cancer. *Cancer Sci.*, 2003; 94 (1): 50-6.

[5] Ji H, Zhao X, Yuza Y, et al. Epidermal growth factor receptor variant III mutations in lung tumorigenesis and sensitivity to tyrosine kinase inhibitors. *Proc. Natl. Acad. Sci. USA*, 2006; 103 (20): 7817-22.

[6] Sasaki H, Kawano O, Endo K, Yukiue H, Yano M, Fujii Y. EGFRvIII mutation in lung cancer correlates with increased EGFR copy number. *Oncol. Rep.*, 2007; 17 (2): 319-23.

[7] Oppermann FS, Klammer M, Bobe C, Cox J, Schaab C, Tebbe A, Daub H. Comparison of SILAC and mTRAQ quantification for phosphoproteomics on a quadrupole orbitrap mass spectrometer. *J. Proteome Res.*, 2013; 12 (9): 4089-100.

[8] Zhang W, Wei Y, Ignatchenko V, et al. Proteomic profiles of human lung adeno and squamous cell carcinoma using super-SILAC and label-free quantification approaches. Proteomics. 2014 Jan 22; doi: 10.1002/pmic.201300382. [Epub ahead of print].

[9] Ma PC, Tretiakova MS, Nallasura V, Jagadeeswaran R, Husain AN, Salgia R. Downstream signalling and specific inhibition of c-MET/HGF pathway in small cell lung cancer: implications for tumour invasion. *Br. J. Cancer,* 2007; 97 (3): 368-77.

[10] Hembrough T, Thyparambil S, Liao WL, et al. Application of selected reaction monitoring for multiplex quantification of clinically validated biomarkers in formalin-fixed, paraffin-embedded tumor tissue. *J. Mol. Diagn,* 2013; 15 (4): 454-65.

[11] Italiano A, Vandenbos FB, Otto J, et al. Comparison of the epidermal growth factor receptor gene and protein in primary non-small-cell-lung cancer and metastatic sites: implications for treatment with EGFR-inhibitors. *Ann. Oncol.,* 2006; 17 (6): 981-5.

[12] Pinter F, Papay J, Almasi A, et al. Epidermal growth factor receptor (EGFR) high gene copy number and activating mutations in lung adenocarcinomas are not consistently accompanied by positivity for EGFR protein by standard immunohistochemistry. *J. Mol. Diagn.,* 2008; 10 (2): 160-8.

[13] Gupta R, Dastane AM, Forozan F, Riley-Portuguez A, Chung F, Lopategui J, Marchevsky AM. Evaluation of EGFR abnormalities in patients with pulmonary adenocarcinoma: the need to test neoplasms with more than one method. *Mod. Pathol.,* 2009; 22 (1): 128-33.

[14] El-Zammar OA, Zhang S, Katzenstein AL. Comparison of FISH, PCR, and immunohistochemistry in assessing EGFR status in lung adenocarcinoma and correlation with clinicopathologic features. *Diagn. Mol. Pathol.,* 2009; 18 (3): 133-7.

[15] Liang Z, Zhang J, Zeng X, Gao J, Wu S, Liu T. Relationship between EGFR expression, copy number and mutation in lung adenocarcinomas. *BMC Cancer,* 2010; 10: 376.

[16] Al-Saad S, Al-Shibli K, Donnem T, Andersen S, Bremnes RM, Busund LT. Clinical significance of epidermal growth factor receptors in non-small cell lung cancer and a prognostic role for HER2 gene copy number in female patients. *J. Thorac. Oncol.,* 2010; 5 (10): 1536-43.

[17] Xia Q, Zhu Z, Wang J, Situ D, Zhou N, Jang W. Expression and association of HER2 with prognosis in early-stage (T1-T2N0M0) non-small cell lung cancer. *Tumour. Biol.,* 2012; 33 (5): 1719-25.

[18] Heinmöller P, Gross C, Beyser K, Schmidtgen C, Maass G, Pedrocchi M, Rüschoff J. HER2 status in non-small cell lung cancer: results from patient screening for enrollment to a phase II study of herceptin. *Clin. Cancer Res.,* 2003; 9 (14): 5238-43.

[19] Zinner RG, Glisson BS, Fossella FV, et al. Trastuzumab in combination with cisplatin and gemcitabine in patients with Her2-overexpressing, untreated, advanced non-small cell lung cancer: report of a phase II trial and findings regarding optimal identification of patients with Her2-overexpressing disease. *Lung Cancer,* 2004; 44 (1): 99-110.

[20] Ugocsai K, Mándoky L, Tiszlavicz L, Molnár J. Investigation of HER2 overexpression in non-small cell lung cancer. *Anticancer Res.,* 2005; 25 (4): 3061-6.

[21] Starr A, Greif J, Vexler A, et al. ErbB4 increases the proliferation potential of human lung cancer cells and its blockage can be used as a target for anti-cancer therapy. *Int. J. Cancer,* 2006; 119 (2): 269-74.

[22] Shi F, Telesco SE, Liu Y, Radhakrishnan R, Lemmon MA. ErbB3/HER3 intracellular domain is competent to bind ATP and catalyze autophosphorylation. *Proc. Natl. Acad. Sci. USA,* 2010; 107 (17): 7692-7.

[23] Holbro T, Beerli RR, Maurer F, Koziczak M, Barbas CF 3rd, Hynes NE. The ErbB2/ErbB3 heterodimer functions as an oncogenic unit: ErbB2 requires ErbB3 to drive breast tumor cell proliferation. *Proc. Natl. Acad. Sci. USA,* 2003; 100 (15): 8933-8.

[24] Bellezza G, Del Sordo R, Colella R, et al. Co-expression of receptors of the HER family correlates with clinical outcome in non-small cell lung cancer (NSCLC). *Virchows Arch.,* 2013; 463 (5): 663-71.

[25] Li C, Brand TM, Iida M, Huang S, Armstrong EA, van der Kogel A, Wheeler DL. Human epidermal growth factor receptor 3 (HER3) blockade with U3-1287/AMG888 enhances the efficacy of radiation therapy in lung and head and neck carcinoma. *Discov. Med.,* 2013; 16 (87): 79-92.

[26] Wu Y, Zhang Y, Wang M, et al. Downregulation of HER3 by a novel antisense oligonucleotide, EZN-3920, improves the antitumor activity of EGFR and HER2 tyrosine kinase inhibitors in animal models. *Mol. Cancer Ther.,* 2013; 12 (4): 427-37.

[27] Kawano D, Yano T, Shoji F, et al. The influence of intracellular epidermal growth factor receptor (EGFR) signal activation on the outcome of EGFR tyrosine kinase inhibitor treatment for pulmonary adenocarcinoma. *Surg. Today,* 2011; 41 (6): 818-23.

[28] Endoh H, Ishibashi Y, Yamaki E, et al. Immunohistochemical analysis of phosphorylated epidermal growth factor receptor might provide a surrogate marker of EGFR mutation. *Lung Cancer,* 2009; 63 (2): 241-6.

[29] McMillen E, Ye F, Li G, Wu Y, Yin G, Liu W. Epidermal growth factor receptor (EGFR) mutation and p-EGFR expression in resected non-small cell lung cancer. *Exp. Lung Res.,* 2010; 36 (9): 531-7.

[30] Felip E, Rojo F, Reck M, et al. A phase II pharmacodynamic study of erlotinib in patients with advanced non-small cell lung cancer previously treated with platinum-based chemotherapy. *Clin. Cancer Res.,* 2008; 14 (12): 3867-74.

[31] Kim SJ, Rabbani ZN, Dong F, et al. Phosphorylated epidermal growth factor receptor and cyclooxygenase-2 expression in localized non-small cell lung cancer. *Med. Oncol.,* 2010; 27 (1): 91-7.

[32] Li T, Ling YH, Perez-Soler R. Tumor dependence on the EGFR signaling pathway expressed by the p-EGFR:p-AKT ratio predicts erlotinib sensitivity in human non-small cell lung cancer (NSCLC) cells expressing wild-type EGFR gene. *J. Thorac. Oncol.,* 2008; 3 (6): 643-7

[33] Moldvay J, Barbai T, Bogos K, Piurko V, Fillinger J, Popper HH, Tímár J. EGFR autophosphorylation but not protein score correlates with histologic and molecular subtypes in lung adenocarcinoma. *Diagn. Mol. Pathol.,* 2013; 22 (4): 204-9.

[34] Brevet M, Arcila M, Ladanyi M. Assessment of EGFR mutation status in lung adenocarcinoma by immunohistochemistry using antibodies specific to the two major forms of mutant EGFR. *J. Mol Diagn.,* 2010; 12 (2): 169-76.

[35] Hasanovic A, Ang D, Moreira AL, Zakowski MF. Use of mutation specific antibodies to detect EGFR status in small biopsy and cytology specimens of lung adenocarcinoma. *Lung Cancer,* 2012; 77 (2): 299-305.

[36] Angulo B, Conde E, Suárez-Gauthier A, et al. A comparison of EGFR mutation testing methods in lung carcinoma: direct sequencing, real-time PCR and immunohisto chemistry. *PLoS One,* 2012; 7 (8): e43842.

[37] Xiong Y, Bai Y, Leong N, et al. Immunohistochemical detection of mutations in the epidermal growth factor receptor gene in lung adenocarcinomas using mutation-specific antibodies. *Diagn. Pathol.,* 2013; 8 (1): 27.

[38] Cooper WA, Yu B, Yip PY, et al. EGFR mutant-specific immunohistochemistry has high specificity and sensitivity for detecting targeted activating EGFR mutations in lung adenocarcinoma. *J. Clin. Pathol.,* 2013; 66 (9): 744-8.

[39] Liu X, Lu Y, Zhu G, et al. The diagnostic accuracy of pleural effusion and plasma samples versus tumour tissue for detection of EGFR mutation in patients with advanced

non-small cell lung cancer: comparison of methodologies. *J. Clin. Pathol.,* 2013; 66 (12): 1065-9.

[40] Seo AN, Park TI, Jin Y, Sun PL, Kim H, Chang H, Chung JH. Novel EGFR mutation-specific antibodies for lung adenocarcinoma: Highly specific but not sensitive detection of an E746_A750 deletion in exon 19 and an L858R mutation in exon 21 by immunohistochemistry. *Lung Cancer,* 2014; 83 (3): 316-23.

[41] Simonetti S, Molina MA, Queralt C, et al. Detection of EGFR mutations with mutation-specific antibodies in stage IV non-small-cell lung cancer. *J. Transl. Med.,* 2010; 8: 135.

[42] Assadi M, Lamerz J, Jarutat T, et al. Multiple protein analysis of formalin-fixed and paraffin-embedded tissue samples with reverse phase protein arrays. *Mol. Cell Proteomics,* 2013; 12 (9): 2615-22.

[43] VanMeter AJ, Rodriguez AS, Bowman ED, et al. Laser capture microdissection and protein microarray analysis of human non-small cell lung cancer: differential epidermal growth factor receptor (EGPR) phosphorylation events associated with mutated EGFR compared with wild type. *Mol. Cell Proteomics,* 2008; 7 (10): 1902-24.

[44] Farlow EC, Patel K, Basu S, et al. Development of a multiplexed tumor-associated autoantibody-based blood test for the detection of non-small cell lung cancer. *Clin. Cancer Res.,* 2010; 16 (13): 3452-62.

[45] Patel NV, Acarregui MJ, Snyder JM, Klein JM, Sliwkowski MX, Kern JA. Neuregulin-1 and human epidermal growth factor receptors 2 and 3 play a role in human lung development in vitro. *Am. J. Respir. Cell Mol. Biol.,* 2000; 22 (4): 432-40.

[46] Shi Y, Huang W, Tan Y, et al. A novel proximity assay for the detection of proteins and protein complexes: quantitation of HER1 and HER2 total protein expression and homodimerization in formalin-fixed, paraffin-embedded cell lines and breast cancer tissue. *Diagn. Mol. Pathol.,* 2009; 18 (1): 11-21.

[47] Larson JS, Goodman LJ, Tan Y, et al. Analytical Validation of a Highly Quantitative, Sensitive, Accurate, and Reproducible Assay (HERmark) for the Measurement of HER2 Total Protein and HER2 Homodimers in FFPE Breast Cancer Tumor Specimens. *Patholog. Res. Int.,* 2010; 2010: 814176.

[48] Chen TC, Liu YW, Huang YH, et al. Protein phosphorylation profiling using an in situ proximity ligation assay: phosphorylation of AURKA-elicited EGFR-Thr654 and EGFR-Ser1046 in lung cancer cells. *PLoS One,* 2013; 8 (3): e55657.

[49] Tanizaki J, Okamoto I, Sakai K, Nakagawa K. Differential roles of trans-phosphorylated EGFR, HER2, HER3, and RET as heterodimerisation partners of MET in lung cancer with MET amplification. *Br. J. Cancer,* 2011; 105 (6): 807-13.

[50] Krepler C, Vultur A, Xu W, Yu GH, Schuchter L, Clark DP. Functional profiling of live melanoma samples using a novel automated platform. *PLoS One,* 2012; 7 (12): e52760.

[51] Bhargava R, Gerald WL, Li AR, Pan Q, Lal P, Ladanyi M, Chen B. EGFR gene amplification in breast cancer: correlation with epidermal growth factor receptor mRNA and protein expression and HER-2 status and absence of EGFR-activating mutations. *Mod. Pathol.,* 2005; 18 (8): 1027-33.

[52] Suehara Y, Arcila M, Wang L, et al. Identification of KIF5B-RET and GOPC-ROS1 fusions in lung adenocarcinomas through a comprehensive mRNA-based screen for tyrosine kinase fusions. *Clin. Cancer Res.,* 2012; 18 (24): 6599-608.

[53] Kojima K, April C, Canasto-Chibuque C, et al. Transcriptome Profiling of Archived Sectioned Formalin-Fixed Paraffin-Embedded (AS-FFPE) Tissue for Disease Classification. *PLoS One,* 2014; 9 (1): e86961.

[54] Chen HY, Yu SL, Chen CH, et al. A five-gene signature and clinical outcome in non-small-cell lung cancer. *N. Engl. J. Med.,* 2007; 356 (1): 11-20.

[55] Tomizawa K, Suda K, Onozato R, Kuwano H, Yatabe Y, Mitsudomi T. Analysis of ERBB4 mutations and expression in japanese patients with lung cancer. *J. Thorac. Oncol.,* 2010; 5 (11): 1859-61.

[56] Dacic S, Yousem SA. Molecular testing in lung carcinoma: Quo vadis? *Am. J. Clin. Pathol.,* 2010; 134 (1): 7-9.

[57] Grob TJ, Kannengiesser I, Tsourlakis MC, et al. Heterogeneity of ERBB2 amplification in adenocarcinoma, squamous cell carcinoma and large cell undifferentiated carcinoma of the lung. *Mod. Pathol.,* 2012; 25 (12): 1566-73.

[58] Takezawa K, Pirazzoli V, Arcila ME, et al. HER2 amplification: a potential mechanism of acquired resistance to EGFR inhibition in EGFR-mutant lung cancers that lack the second-site EGFRT790M mutation. *Cancer Discov.,* 2012; 2 (10): 922-33.

[59] Cappuzzo F, Toschi L, Domenichini I, et al. HER3 genomic gain and sensitivity to gefitinib in advanced non-small-cell lung cancer patients. *Br. J. Cancer,* 2005; 93 (12): 1334-40.

[60] Jeong EG, Soung YH, Lee JW, et al. ERBB3 kinase domain mutations are rare in lung, breast and colon carcinomas. *Int. J. Cancer,* 2006; 119 (12): 2986-7.

[61] Jaiswal BS, Kljavin NM, Stawiski EW, et al. Oncogenic ERBB3 mutations in human cancers. *Cancer Cell,* 2013; 23 (5): 603-17.

[62] Sung JS, Jin L, Jo U, Park KH, Kim YH. Association between -276 C/T polymorphism of the ERBB3 gene and lung cancer risk in a Korean population. *Anticancer. Res.,* 2012; 32 (10): 4433-7.

[63] Ding L, Getz G, Wheeler DA, et al. Somatic mutations affect key pathways in lung adenocarcinoma. *Nature,* 2008; 455 (7216): 1069-75.

[64] Soung YH, Lee JW, Kim SY, et al. Somatic mutations of the ERBB4 kinase domain in human cancers. *Int. J. Cancer,* 2006; 118 (6): 1426-9.

[65] Sasaki H, Okuda K, Kawano O, et al. ErbB4 expression and mutation in Japanese patients with lung cancer. *Clin. Lung Cancer,* 2007; 8 (7): 429-33.

[66] Hubers AJ, Heideman DA, Yatabe Y, et al. EGFR mutation analysis in sputum of lung cancer patients: a multitechnique study. *Lung Cancer,* 2013; 82 (1): 38-43.

[67] Bar J, Damianovich M, Hout Siloni G, et al. Genetic Mutation Screen in Early Non-Small-Cell Lung Cancer (NSCLC) Specimens. *Clin. Lung Cancer,* 2014; 15 (2): 159-65.

[68] Dienstmann R, Serpico D, Rodon J, et al. Molecular profiling of patients with colorectal cancer and matched targeted therapy in phase I clinical trials. *Mol. Cancer Ther.,* 2012; 11 (9): 2062-71.

[69] Rodón J, Saura C, Dienstmann R, Vivancos A, Ramón y Cajal S, Baselga J, Tabernero J. Molecular prescreening to select patient population in early clinical trials. *Nat. Rev. Clin. Oncol.,* 2012; 9 (6): 359-66.

[70] Sequist LV, Heist RS, Shaw AT, et al. Implementing multiplexed genotyping of non-small-cell lung cancers into routine clinical practice. *Ann. Oncol.,* 2011; 22 (12): 2616-24.

[71] Patel R, Tsan A, Tam R, et al. Mutation scanning using MUT-MAP, a high-throughput, microfluidic chip-based, multi-analyte panel. *PLoS One,* 2012; 7 (12): e51153.
[72] Greulich H. The genomics of lung adenocarcinoma: opportunities for targeted therapies. *Genes Cancer,* 2010; 1 (12): 1200-10.
[73] Kim ST, Sung JS, Jo UH, Park KH, Shin SW, Kim YH. Can mutations of EGFR and KRAS in serum be predictive and prognostic markers in patients with advanced non-small cell lung cancer (NSCLC)? *Med. Oncol.,* 2013; 30 (1): 328.
[74] Rosell R, Moran T, Queralt C, et al. Screening for epidermal growth factor receptor mutations in lung cancer. *N. Engl. J. Med.,* 2009; 361 (10): 958-67.
[75] Xu F, Wu J, Xue C, et al. Comparison of different methods for detecting epidermal growth factor receptor mutations in peripheral blood and tumor tissue of non-small cell lung cancer as a predictor of response to gefitinib. *Onco. Targets Ther.,* 2012; 5: 439-47.
[76] Yung TK, Chan KC, Mok TS, Tong J, To KF, Lo YM. Single-molecule detection of epidermal growth factor receptor mutations in plasma by microfluidics digital PCR in non-small cell lung cancer patients. *Clin. Cancer Res.,* 2009; 15 (6): 2076-84.
[77] Murtaza M, Dawson SJ, Tsui DW, et al. Non-invasive analysis of acquired resistance to cancer therapy by sequencing of plasma DNA. *Nature,* 2013; 497 (7447): 108-12.
[78] Rosell R, Molina MA, Serrano MJ. EGFR mutations in circulating tumour DNA. *Lancet Oncol.,* 2012; 13 (10): 971-3.
[79] Macaulay IC, Voet T. Single cell genomics: advances and future perspectives. *PLoS Genet.,* 2014; 10 (1): e1004126.
[80] Zhao Y, Zhou H, Ma K, et al. Abnormal methylation of seven genes and their associations with clinical characteristics in early stage non-small cell lung cancer. *Oncol. Lett.,* 2013; 5 (4): 1211-8.
[81] Sano A, Kage H, Sugimoto K, et al. A second-generation profiling system for quantitative methylation analysis of multiple gene promoters: application to lung cancer. *Oncogene,* 2007; 26 (45): 6518-25.
[82] Hoque MO, Brait M, Rosenbaum E, et al. Genetic and epigenetic analysis of erbB signaling pathway genes in lung cancer. *J. Thorac. Oncol.,* 2010; 5 (12): 1887-93.
[83] Yu X, Guo ZS, Marcu MG, Neckers L, Nguyen DM, Chen GA, Schrump DS. Modulation of p53, ErbB1, ErbB2, and Raf-1 expression in lung cancer cells by depsipeptide FR901228. *J. Natl. Cancer Inst.,* 2002; 94 (7): 504-13.
[84] Markou A, Tsaroucha EG, Kaklamanis L, Fotinou M, Georgoulias V, Lianidou ES. Prognostic value of mature microRNA-21 and microRNA-205 overexpression in non-small cell lung cancer by quantitative real-time RT-PCR. *Clin. Chem.,* 2008; 54 (10): 1696-704.
[85] Liu L, Shao X, Gao W, et al. MicroRNA-133b inhibits the growth of non-small-cell lung cancer by targeting the epidermal growth factor receptor. *FEBS J.,* 2012; 279 (20): 3800-12.
[86] 86 Yamaguchi G, Takanashi M, Tanaka M, Fujita K, Ohira T, Kuroda M, Ikeda N. Isolation of miRNAs that target EGFR mRNA in human lung cancer. Biochem Biophys *Res. Commun.,* 2012; 420 (2): 411-6.

[87] Rai K, Takigawa N, Ito S, et al. Liposomal delivery of MicroRNA-7-expressing plasmid overcomes epidermal growth factor receptor tyrosine kinase inhibitor-resistance in lung cancer cells. *Mol. Cancer Ther.*, 2011; 10 (9): 1720-7.
[88] Seike M, Goto A, Okano T, et al. MiR-21 is an EGFR-regulated anti-apoptotic factor in lung cancer in never-smokers. *Proc. Natl. Acad. Sci. USA,* 2009; 106 (29):12085-90.

In: Fighting Lung Cancer through the HER Family …
Editor: Diego Márquez-Medina
ISBN: 978-1-63321-092-9

Chapter 7

Timing I: Dynamic Analysis of Human Epidermal Growth Factor Receptors. Role of Rebiopsy

Santiago Viteri, M.D. and Alejandro Martínez-Bueno, M.D.
Medical Oncology Department, Instituto Rosell de Oncología de Barcelona, Spain

Abstract

It is a well-established principle that precise diagnosis and accurate selection of treatment for Non-Small Cell Lung Cancer (NSCLC) patients relies on the information obtained in the basal tumor biopsy. It confirms the presence of neoplastic cells, identifies the histological subtype and provides tumor DNA and RNA to analyze molecular targets, as for instance the presence of sensitizing mutations of the epidermal growth factor receptor (*EGFR*), that can be specifically treated. However no systemic treatment has shown until now durable clinical responses due to the inevitable development of tumor resistance leading to treatment failure, disease progression and patient's death. During treatment tumor undergoes quick biological reprogramming and the molecular basis of these mechanisms of resistance remains incompletely characterized. New biopsies (rebiopsies) obtained in different moments of the evolution of the tumor stand as a unique tool to identify different mechanisms of resistance and allow the creation of new treatment strategies to prevent or overcome them. Some of these resistance mechanisms have been reported: the presence of additional resistant mutations like T790M in the kinase domain of the EGFR receptor; concomitant oncogenic alterations (like KRAS mutations, PIK3CA mutations or ALK translocations); co-activation of alternative growth factor receptors and others. This biological complexity explains why it is so challenging to design a successful therapeutic strategy and reinforces the incorporation of rebiopsies in the clinical management of NSCLC patients.

Another promising source of information of the molecular changes occurring in the tumor has been called "liquid biopsies", meaning the real possibility to detect and analyze tumor circulating fragments of cell free DNA or RNA in peripheral blood (serum or plasma), tumor cell free DNA o RNA stored in normal platelets and Circulating Tumor Cells. Liquid biopsies are very easy to obtain, completely safe for the patient and may provide a real time molecular snapshot of the tumor.

1. Background

As it has been fully described above, the Human Epidermal Growth Factor Receptors (HER) family plays a significant role in normal and cancerous cells. Specifically, these receptors are responsible for translating signals within the cells that have numerous effects such as growth, proliferation and survival [1].

While this cellular signaling is precisely regulated in normal cells, the aberrant activation of HER signaling pathways may result in uncontrolled growth and spread of cancer cells. The HER family consists in 4 structurally related cellular receptors: HER1, also known as the epidermal growth factor receptor (EGFR), HER2, HER3 and HER4, which interact in many ways [2]. In this chapter we will focus in the dynamic analyses of *HER1/EGFR* mutated tumors, as they harbor the main actionable mutations established to date for non-small cell lung cancer (NSCLC) patients.

HER1/EGFR deregulation has been described in multiple solid tumors including lung cancer, pancreatic cancer, glioblastoma and many others. Multiple mechanisms can cause the oncogenic hiperactivity of this signaling pathway including receptor over expression and the presence of activating mutations. The significant role of HER1/EGFR hyperactivity in cancer progression and the growing knowledge of this signaling pathway has allowed to develop a whole new cancer treatment strategy based on various classes of EGFR targeted agents.

One of the most remarkable achievements of this approach so far was the identification in 2004 of the presence of activating mutations in the intracellular tyrosine kinase domain of the EGFR. A relevant subset of NSCLC patients (between 10-15% of lung adenocarcinoma patients in Caucasian population) harbors *EGFR* mutations that act as oncogenic drivers. These mutations result in ligand-independent activation of the EGFR signaling cascade leading to cell proliferation, survival, migration and metastasis The survival and proliferation of this particular kind of tumors is fully dependent of the aberrant hyperactivity of this pathway to the point that its inactivation leads to cell death by apoptosis. This phenomenon has been named "oncogene addiction" and pinpoints a particularly interesting Achilles' heel to be targeted with specific agents.

The EGFR tyrosine kinase inhibitors (EGFR-TKI) are small molecules that bind to the intracellular domain of the EGFR in presence of activating mutations. This binding prevents the phosphorilation of the protein causing inactivation and avoiding downstream signaling. These drugs have proven to be far more active than conventional chemotherapy in the treatment of *EGFR* mutated advanced lung adenocarcinomas and represent the first steps into a precision medicine approach. Over 75% of patients harboring *EGFR* mutations have a clinical response to currently approved EGFR-TKI (gefinitb, erlotinib, afatinib) but disappointingly the duration of the response is short-lived and every patient eventually progresses and dies due to lethal drug resistance [3, 4]. This means that up to 25% of the *EGFR* mutated patients present primary innate resistance mechanisms that prevent EGFR-TKIs to effectively stop tumor growth.

Meanwhile, in the initially responding patients, treatment with EGFR-TKIs seems to activate early adaptive resistance mechanisms that ultimately overcome the action of the targeted treatment leading to clinical progression. The underlying biological basis of the evolution of EGFR targeted therapy resistance remains incompletely characterized, although some mechanisms have been described in various preclinical cellular and mouse models.

Very limited clinical studies have been published to date with a rebiopsy at the moment of progression to help to unveil the keystones of tumor anti-EGFR resistance. Some of these resistance mechanisms have been reported: the presence of additional resistant mutations like T790M in the kinase domain of the EGFR receptor; concomitant oncogenic alterations (like KRAS mutation, PIK3CA mutations or ALK translocation); co-activation of alternative growth factor receptors like MET amplification and histological transformations.

Thus, as the tumor biology suffers a quick reprogramming process during EGFR-TKI treatment, only dynamic analyses of the molecular changes that occur in the tumor cell can help us to understand adaptive resistance and develop strategies to overcome it. Serial rebiopsies of EGFR mutated patients offer a unique setting to adequately characterize this process.

2. Feasibility of Serial Rebiopsies in the Clinical Practice

Obtaining additional tumor biopsies is an invasive procedure and entails associated risks of perforation, bleeding or pneumothorax just to mention some of them. Although these are calculated risks a small but meaningful rate of severe complications may arise during the procedure. For that reason an adequate selection of rebiopsy candidate patients is mandatory, with a careful interrogation of comorbidities. It is also important to select the most suitable biopsy technique and the target lesion, because these aspects may be relevant to assure a successful biopsy. For instance, bone metastases should be avoided when considering a rebiopsy. The decalcification process necessary to preserve and analyze this kind of tissue usually destroys the tumor DNA and RNA therefore turning the material completely useless.

A recent publication prospectively examined the feasibility and safety of repeat biopsy for mutational analysis in patients with NSCLC who have a resistance history to previous chemotherapy [5]. In this trial 94 patients (31 men, 63 women; mean age ± standard deviation, 57 years ± 10.3) were selected for rebiopsy via percutaneous transthoracic lung biopsy under CT guidance. They reported a technical success rate for biopsy of 100%, meaning that all the procedures were able to obtain tumor tissue. In 75 (80%) of 94 patients, specimens were adequate for mutational analysis: 35 were tested for *EGFR* mutation, 34 for anaplastic lymphoma kinase gene (ALK) rearrangement, and six for both. Postprocedural complications occurred in 13 (14%) of 94 patients. 6 patients suffered pneumothorax (only 2 required chest tube) and 7 patients had non-fatal intrapulmonary hemorrhage.

New technologies as Endobronchial Ultrasound Bronchoscopy (EBUS) or Transbronchial Cryobiopsy are feasible and safe procedures for the patients and may yield enough tumor tissue to perform complete molecular assays including Whole Genome Sequencing (WGS) [6, 7].

One of the main caveats of rebiopsies is the concept of tumor heterogeneity. As it has been widely documented there can be different molecular profiles between the primary tumor and different metastatic localizations, even between different areas in the same tumor localization. This fact may cause the rebiopsy not to be fully representative of the main molecular changes active in the moment of tumor progression.

3. Detection and Understanding of Adaptive Resistance Mechanisms

The best-established mechanism of adaptive resistance in *EGFR* mutant patients is the detection of additional mutations in the same kinase domain in treament-resistant specimens. The most common *EGFR* mutation associated with adaptive treatment resistance involves a C-to-T change at nucleotide 2369 in exon 20, which results in threonine to methionine substitution at the amino acid position 790 (T790M) The T790M mutation was detected in 68% to 83% of rebiopsies of EGFR-mutant patients progressing to EGFR-TKIs [8, 9] and it is recognized as an acquired-resistance mutation in *EGFR*-mutant lung cancer [10, 11].

At least two molecular mechanisms explain how T790M confers drug resistance. First, the substitution of a bulky methionine at the place of threonine at position 790 leads to a steric hindrance that interferes with drug binding in the ATP pocket of EGFR [12]. This phenomenon, affecting the threonine gatekeeper residue in this protein, can also be found in other cases of secondary mutations leading to drug resistance, such as ABL (T315I) and KIT (T670I) that cause resistance to imatinib in chronic myeloid leukemia and gastrointestinal stromal tumors, respectively [13]. Second, the *EGFR* T790M mutation promotes the assembly of an active kinase conformation with high affinity for ATP binding [14]. As a proof of concept in preclinical models, the introduction of vectors carrying T790M to EGFR-TKIs sensitive cell lines caused resistance without substantially modifying EGFR tyrosine kinase activity [11].

It is hypothesized that *EGFR* T790M mutation is present in small fractions of tumor cells before treatment, and that this fraction of tumor cells could expand selectively with EGFR-TKIs treatment leading to progression [15].

Three other second-site mutations in *EGFR* have been associated with acquired resistance, including L747S (exon 19), D761Y (exon 19) and T854A (exon 21) [16-18]. Like the T790M, T854A is a drug contact residue and mutation to the smaller hydrophobic alanine residue may increase the size of the selectivity pocket, negatively impacting erlotinib binding [19]. L747S occurs at the start of the loop between the 3 strand and the -C helix and is thought to shift the equilibrium to- wards active conformation of the receptor. D761Y occurs in the -C helix and a salt bridge formed by D761Y may be disrupted by mutation to tyrosine, affecting the catalytic cleft of the receptor [19]. Consistent with the clinical data, D761Y, T790M and T854A were all identified in a comprehensive resistance mutation screen with erlotinib in vitro.

Two relevant studies have highlighted the treatment approach in patients with *EGFR* mutations at the time of clinical progression to erlotinib or gefitinib. The Massachusetts General Hospital experience found that 49% of patients acquired the T790M mutation [20]. Erlotinib was switched to chemotherapy at the time of clinical progression. Interestingly, after chemotherapy treatment, at the time of a second progression, the T790M mutation had disappeared in some cases and patients could be retreated with and respond to erlotinib.

PIK3CA mutations were found in 5% of patients, while MET amplification was detected in only 5% of the re-biopsied samples. In 14% of cases, there was a histological change in the re-biopsied material, the tumor was transformed to small-cell lung cancer and was sensitive to standard treatments [20].

The second experience is that of investigators from the Memorial Sloan Kettering Cancer Center in New York and from Vanderbilt University, as well as other hospitals. At the time of clinical progression to gefitinib or erlotinib, the addition of chemotherapy to the EGFR-TKI treatment provided optimal outcomes, with some patients even continuing EGFR-TKI treatment for more than six months after progression, with acceptable results [21].

New generation EGFR-TKIs have been developed in order to overcome resistance, particularly the coexistence of T790M mutation. Some of them bind irreversibly to the tyrosine kinase domain as afatinib. Others show panHer family activity as dacomitinib or neratinib. The most promising ones are specific T790M inhibitors like CO1686 (Clovis Oncology) and AZD9291 (AstraZeneca) that are being evaluated in ongoing clinical trials whose results are eagerly awaited.

4. New Perspectives

To our knowledge, the most ambitious project (submitted for publication at the moment of preparing this chapter) aimed to characterize the molecular landscape of EGFR-TKI therapy to contextualize and identify predictive response biomarkers and therapeutic targets to improve clinical outcomes has been conducted by the Cancer Therapeutics Innovation Group from San Francisco with the collaboration of our institution among others from different countries. In this project 32 matched, paired tumor biopsy samples obtained both before EGFR-TKI therapy and after the development of acquired clinical resistance from 16 patients with *EGFR*-mutant lung adenocarcinoma under informed consent were analyzed. Whole exome sequencing, targeted exome and whole transcriptome deep sequencing and data analysis was performed on nucleic acid extracted from the specimens and matched normal tissue, as described [22]. In this cohort the *EGFR* T790M resistance mutation was detected in 6 (37.5%) resistant cases. They also identified somatic mutations that have not previously been described in EGFR-TKI resistant NSCLC and that represent actionable therapeutic targets. These novel mutations include established activating mutations in KRAS (Q61K and A146T), PIK3CA (R108H), KIT (D579Y), and SMO (W535R), and an uncharacterized mutation within the kinase domain of PDGFRA (T894S). Notably, several of these mutations co-occurred with *EGFR* T790M in a single resistant specimen and many resistant tumors harbored multiple somatic alterations highlighting a previously unappreciated level of complexity and heterogeneity in the somatic mutation landscape in EGFR-TKI resistant clinical cases.

Consistent with prior studies [23], focal genomic amplification of MET was noted in 2 of the resistance specimens that also harbored T790M mutation. One of the cases was confirmed to have a canonical EML4-ALK fusion transcript in both the pre-treatment and therapy resistant tumor, with increased EML4-ALK expression in the resistant specimen. Although activating *EGFR* mutations and EML4-ALK fusions occur at low frequency prior to therapy [24], our findings indicate that these driver kinases can co-exist and evolve during EGFR-TKI clinical resistance.

In order to further delineate these molecular mechanisms, CTIG is sponsoring a new innovative protocol in cooperation with the Spanish Lung Cancer Group. The proposal consists in applying massively parallel sequencing technologies to patient samples obtained prior to the initiation of EGFR-TKI therapy, immediately following initiation (between 24h-120h after initiation) and at resistance (Figure 1). Given the molecular complexity and heterogeneity of every case of EGFR-driven NSCLC, obtaining comprehensive genomic and transcriptomic snapshots of tumor samples over the course of therapy represents the most sensitive strategy for delineating the evolution of each patient's disease.

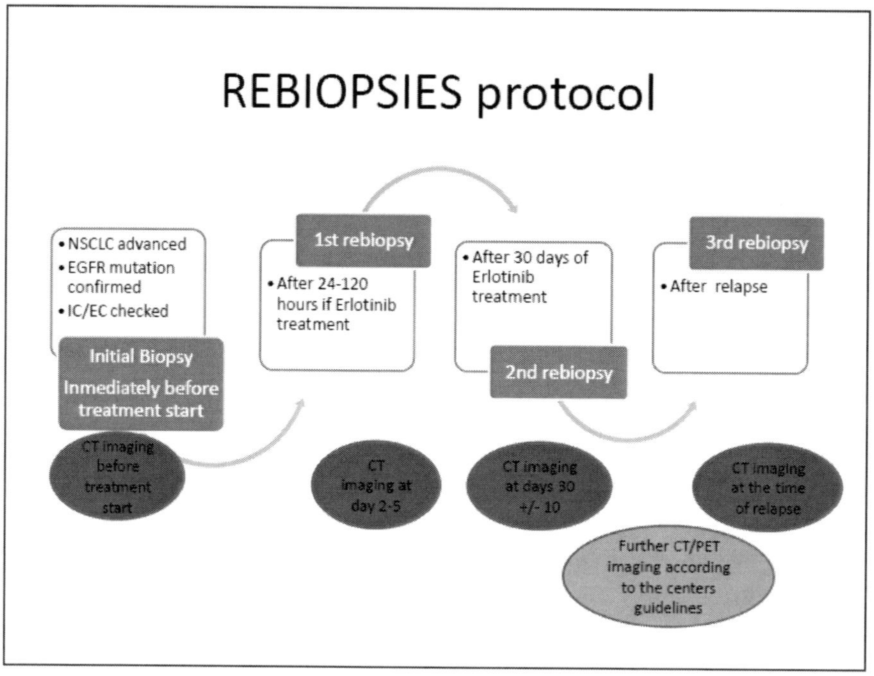

Figure 1. Rebiopsy protocol.

5. Liquid Biopsies and Treatment Real Time Monitorization

Another promising source of information of the molecular changes occurring in the tumor has been called "liquid biopsies", meaning the real possibility to detect and analyze tumor circulating fragments of cell free DNA or RNA in peripheral blood (serum or plasma) [25], tumor cell free DNA o RNA stored in normal platelets [26] and Circulating Tumor Cells (CTCs). Liquid biopsies are very easy to obtain, completely safe for the patient and may provide a real time molecular snapshot of the tumor. Liquid biopsies might be more representative of the relevant clone of cells leading disease progression, avoiding the risk of bias commented regarding tumor heterogeneity in solid tissue rebiopsies. For example, in a recent publication [27] it was reported that CTCs were detected (>1 CTC) at baseline in 78% of patients. Detected mutations in CTC were strongly concordant with mutation status in matched tumor. Higher baseline CTC counts were associated with response to treatment by Response Evaluation Criteria in Solid Tumors (RECIST) and decreased CTC counts upon treatment were associated with FDG-PET and RECIST response and longer progression-free survival.

However, due to the scarce amount of tumor genetic material obtained in liquid biopsies, newer and more sensitive techniques need to be validated in order to perform useful molecular determinations.

References

[1] Sliwkowski MX. *Diseases of the Breast.* 3rd ed. Harris JR, Lippman ME, Morrow M OC, editor. Lippincott Williams & Wilkins; 2004.

[2] Olayioye MA, Neve RM, Lane HA, Hynes NE. The ErbB signaling network: receptor heterodimerization in development and cancer. *EMBO J.* 2000; 19 (13): 3159-67.

[3] Mok TS, Wu Y-L, Thongprasert S, et al. Gefitinib or carboplatin-paclitaxel in pulmonary adenocarcinoma. *N Engl J Med.* 2009; 361 (10): 947-57.

[4] Rosell R, Carcereny E, Gervais R, et al. Erlotinib versus standard chemotherapy as first-line treatment for European patients with advanced EGFR mutation-positive non-small-cell lung cancer (EURTAC): a multicentre, open-label, randomised phase 3 trial. *Lancet Oncol.* 2012; 13 (3): 239-46.

[5] Yoon HJ, Lee HY, Lee KS, et al. Repeat biopsy for mutational analysis of non-small cell lung cancers resistant to previous chemotherapy: adequacy and complications. *Radiology.* 2012; 265 (3): 939-48.

[6] Sanz-Santos J, Cirauqui B, Sanchez E, et al. Endobronchial ultrasound-guided transbronchial needle aspiration in the diagnosis of intrathoracic lymph node metastases from extrathoracic malignancies. *Clin Exp Metastasis.* 2013; 30 (4): 521-8.

[7] Babiak A, Hetzel J, Krishna G, et al. Transbronchial cryobiopsy: a new tool for lung biopsies. *Respiration.* 2009; 78 (2): 203-8.

[8] Su K-Y, Chen H-Y, Li K-C, et al. Pretreatment epidermal growth factor receptor (EGFR) T790M mutation predicts shorter EGFR tyrosine kinase inhibitor response duration in patients with non-small-cell lung cancer. *J Clin Oncol.* 2012; 30 (4): 433-40.

[9] Arcila ME, Oxnard GR, Nafa K, et al. Rebiopsy of lung cancer patients with acquired resistance to EGFR inhibitors and enhanced detection of the T790M mutation using a locked nucleic acid-based assay. *Clin Cancer Res.* 2011; 17 (5): 1169-80.

[10] Pao W, Miller VA, Politi KA, et al. Acquired resistance of lung adenocarcinomas to gefitinib or erlotinib is associated with a second mutation in the EGFR kinase domain. *PLoS Med.* 2005; 2 (3): e73.

[11] Kobayashi S, Boggon TJ, Dayaram T, et al. EGFR mutation and resistance of non-small-cell lung cancer to gefitinib. *N Engl J Med.* 2005; 352 (8): 786-92.

[12] Yun C-H, Mengwasser KE, Toms A V, et al. The T790M mutation in EGFR kinase causes drug resistance by increasing the affinity for ATP. *Proc Natl Acad Sci USA.* 2008; 105 (6): 2070-5.

[13] Azam M, Seeliger MA, Gray NS, Kuriyan J, Daley GQ. Activation of tyrosine kinases by mutation of the gatekeeper threonine. Nat Struct Mol Biol. *Nature Publishing Group;* 2008; 15 (10): 1109-18.

[14] Nussinov R, Tsai C-J. Allostery in disease and in drug discovery. *Cell.* 2013; 153 (2): 293-305.

[15] Mumenthaler SM, Foo J, Leder K, Choi NC, Pao W, Mallick P, Michor F. Evolutionary Modeling of Combination Treatment Strategies To Overcome Resistance to Tyrosine Kinase Inhibitors in Non-Small Cell Lung Cancer. *Molecular Pharmaceutics.* 2011; 8 (6): 2069-79.

[16] Yamaguchi F, Fukuchi K, Yamazaki Y, et al. Acquired resistance L747S mutation in an epidermal growth factor receptor-tyrosine kinase inhibitor-naïve patient: A report of three cases. *Oncol Lett.* 2014; 7 (2): 357-60.

[17] Nguyen K-SH, Kobayashi S, Costa DB. Acquired resistance to epidermal growth factor receptor tyrosine kinase inhibitors in non-small-cell lung cancers dependent on the epidermal growth factor receptor pathway. *Clin Lung Cancer.* 2009; 10 (4): 281-9.

[18] Bean J, Riely GJ, Balak M, et al. Acquired resistance to epidermal growth factor receptor kinase inhibitors associated with a novel T854A mutation in a patient with EGFR-mutant lung adenocarcinoma. *Clin Cancer Res.* 2008; 14 (22): 7519-25.

[19] Pao W, Chmielecki J. Rational, biologically based treatment of EGFR-mutant non-small-cell lung cancer. *Nat Rev Cancer.* 2010; 10 (11): 760-74.

[20] Sequist LV, Waltman BA, Dias-Santagata D, et al. Genotypic and histological evolution of lung cancers acquiring resistance to EGFR inhibitors. *Sci Transl Med.* 2011; 3 (75): 75ra26.

[21] Goldberg SB, Oxnard GR, Digumarthy S, et al. Chemotherapy with Erlotinib or chemotherapy alone in advanced non-small cell lung cancer with acquired resistance to EGFR tyrosine kinase inhibitors. *Oncologist.* 2013; 18 (11): 1214-20.

[22] Gnirke A, Melnikov A, Maguire J, et al. Solution hybrid selection with ultra-long oligonucleotides for massively parallel targeted sequencing. *Nat Biotechnol.* 2009; 27 (2): 182-9.

[23] Engelman JA, Zejnullahu K, Mitsudomi T, et al. MET amplification leads to gefitinib resistance in lung cancer by activating ERBB3 signaling. *Science.* 2007; 316 (5827): 1039-43.

[24] Miyanaga A, Shimizu K, Noro R, et al. Activity of EGFR-tyrosine kinase and ALK inhibitors for EML4-ALK-rearranged non-small-cell lung cancer harbored coexisting EGFR mutation. *BMC Cancer.* 2013; 13: 262.

[25] Kim H-R, Lee SY, Hyun D-S, et al. Detection of EGFR mutations in circulating free DNA by PNA-mediated PCR clamping. J Exp Clin Cancer Res. J*ournal of Experimental & Clinical Cancer Research.* 2013; 32 (1): 50.

[26] Nilsson RJA, Balaj L, Hulleman E, et al. Blood platelets contain tumor-derived RNA biomarkers. *Blood.* 2011; 118 (13): 3680-3.

[27] Punnoose E a, Atwal S, Liu W, et al. Evaluation of circulating tumor cells and circulating tumor DNA in non-small cell lung cancer: association with clinical endpoints in a phase II clinical trial of pertuzumab and erlotinib. *Clin Cancer Res.* 2012; 18 (8): 2391-401.

In: Fighting Lung Cancer through the HER Family ...
Editor: Diego Márquez-Medina
ISBN: 978-1-63321-092-9

Chapter 8

Timing II. Appropriate Time to Determine the Presence of *EGFR* Mutation and Sequence of Treatment

Teresa Morán, M.D.*[1]*, Enric Carcereny, M.D.*[1]*,
María de los Llanos Gil, M.D.*[1]*, Laia Vilà, M.D.*[1]*, Alberto Indacochea*[1]
***and Jordi Remón, M.D.*[2]**
[1]Medical Oncology Department, Catalan Institut of Oncology,
Germans Trias i Pujol University Hospital of Badalona, Spain
[2]Medical Oncology Department, Hospital of Mataró, Spain

Abstract

The discovery of the *epidermal growth factor receptor* (*EGFR*) mutations in Non-Small Cell lung cancer opened a new understanding in lung tumor biology and has changed the way we approach the care of our patients. Currently, there is general consensus about the importance of having this piece of molecular information, so as to offer a targeted therapy with tyrosine kinase inhibitors against *EGFR* (EGFR-TKI) in those patients whose result is positive for *EGFR* mutations. Moreover, the cumulative clinical experience directs the clinic care towards the EGFR-TKI as upfront treatment in *EGFR*-mutant patients.

In this chapter, we will review the evidence for using EGFR-TKI in first line. There is room for debate in the sequence of treatment when the *EGFR* positive result returns positive once the chemotherapy has been started; for which EGFR-TKI should be used or for other potential strategies in this setting.

1. Introduction

The landscape of cancer therapy has undergone far-reaching changes since the advent of tyrosine kinase inhibitors against the epidermal growth factor receptor (EGFR-TKI).

Effective agents against different types of tumors are now available in the clinical setting, including inhibitors of the C-Kit kinase in gastrointestinal stromal tumors and of the BCR-ABL kinase in chronic myeloid leukemia [1-3]. The discovery of *EGFR* mutations in 2004 lead to a change in the paradigm of how lung cancer patients are classified and treated [4-7]. The EGFR model is just one example of oncogene-addicted biology in lung cancer. Currently, mutations and chromosomal rearrangements affecting different oncogenes, such as ALK, BRAF, RET and ROS1, have been well established as oncogenic driver mutations in lung cancer [8-17].

EGFR is a transmembrane receptor frequently overexpressed in lung cancer that plays a central role in tumor development [4]. The presence of *EGFR* mutations produces oncogene-addiction meaning that tumors harboring *EGFR* mutations are selectively controlled by the exclusive signal that comes down from the EGFR, without being affected by signals that come from other receptors. Thus, with an appropriate drug, this selective and exclusive signal could be shut down leading to the cell growth arrest and apoptosis [18, 19]. Deletions in exon 19 affecting the LREA fragment and point mutations in exon 21 (L858R) are the most frequent mutations, accounting for an 85% of *EGFR* mutations. These mutations are highly responsive to EGFR-TKI [20, 21]. G719X (3%) and L861Q (2%) are other EGFR-TKI sensitive mutations [22]. More recently, other minority mutations, such as exon 19 insertions (1%) have been reported, which are also responsive to EGFR-TKI [23]. Mutations affecting exon 20 of the *EGFR* have been associated to resistance to EGFR-TKI [24-27] (Figure 1).

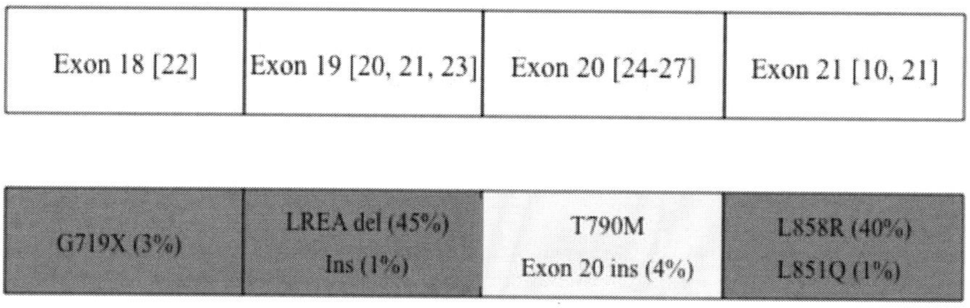

Figure 1. Distribution of EGFR mutations. Dark grey represents TKI-sensitive mutations. Light grey represents TKI-resistant mutations.

Several studies have suggested that EGFR-TKIs are highly active in NSCLC patients harboring *EGFR* mutations. Single arm prospective studies testing both gefitinib and erlotinib in *EGFR*-mutant population demonstrated a high rate of response (75%) and median progression-free survival (PFS) times ranging from 9 to 12 months, a significantly better results when considering the results in unselected NSCLC patient treated with chemotherapy [28-30]. Additional clinical trials comparing EGFR-TKI versus chemotherapy in NSCLC patients harboring *EGFR* mutations have demonstrated the superiority of erlotinib, gefitinib and afatinib over different chemotherapy schedules when administered as first-line therapy. These trials demonstrated consistent results in terms of response rate, PFS, tolerability and quality of life [31-38]. Moreover, other groups have reported favorable results when *EGFR*-mutant patients receive EGFR-TKI as second or subsequent line of therapy [39-42].

Although EGFR determination to establish a genotype-directed therapy is very appealing, some practical considerations can jeopardize it. The timeline when obtaining the *EGFR* mutation result and the type of sample to evaluate the presence of *EGFR* mutation can both be challenging. Different groups have achieved turnaround times from one to two weeks [43, 44] The European *EGFR* Workshop Group considered 7 working days as an optimal timeline [45]. Generally, the amount of diagnostic tissue is scarce in lung cancer, a fact that can limit the evaluation of *EGFR* mutations or other biomarkers. Different groups have developed optimal techniques to obtain sufficient amount of tissue using minimal invasive sampling [eg. endobronchial ultrasound with transbronchial needle aspiration] or by optimizing *EGFR* detection in a cytology sample [46-49].

Table 1. Summary of relevant facts regarding EGFR mutations

Key points: *EGFR* mutations
•NSCLC harboring *EGFR* mutations defines a distinct subgroup of lung cancer.
•Deletions in exon 19 and point mutations are the most frequent mutations and confer sensitivity to TKI [20,21].
•Insertions in exon 19 and other mutations such as G719X and L816Q are potential drug-sensitive mutations [22,23].
•Mutations affecting exon 20 have been related to resistance to TKI [24-27].
•EGFR mutational status can be evaluated in surgical specimens, small biopsies and even cytology samples [46-49].

2. EGFR-TKI as First-Line Therapy in Patients Harboring *EGFR* Mutations: A Review on the Literature

Several clinical trials comparing EGFR-TKI and chemotherapy have been carried out in recent years [31-38]. Consistently, all these trial demonstrated a superiority of EGFR-TKI over chemotherapy in terms of response and PFS. This superiority of the EGFR-TKI is irrespective of the TKI that has been compared (erlotinib, gefitinib or more recently afatinib), and the benefit is extensive in all *EGFR*-mutant patients, irrespective of their ethnic background. Most of the trials included quality of life evaluation and revealed a positive impact of the EGFR-TKI when compared to chemotherapy. None of these trials have demonstrated superiority of the EGFR-TKI over the chemotherapy in overall survival (OS). The effect of the cross-over, by which patients assigned to receive chemotherapy as upfront therapy received EGFR-TKI as second line, is the responsible for the lack of differences in survival. However, there is available data that suggests higher survival rates for patients with *EGFR* mutations treated with EGFR-TKI [50, 51]. A retrospective analysis, carried out in two historical cohorts of Japanese population, demonstrated that *EGFR*-mutant patients treated with the sequence EGFR-TKI followed by chemotherapy, once gefitinib was approved in Japan, lived longer than those patients treated with chemotherapy followed by EGFR-TKI during the years before gefitinib was approved (27.2 months versus 13.6 months; $p< 0.01$) [50]. Also, although gefitinib is a drug no longer available in the US since 2005, 250 patients with *EGFR*-mutations who were receiving gefitinib in an Expanded Access Program were still alive in the evaluation performed in 2011 [51]. These two experiences have methodological limitations; but the data suggest the long-term survival of *EGFR*-mutant patients treated with EGFR-TKI.

The IRESSA Pan-Asian Study (IPASS) was the first randomized clinical trial that confirmed the superiority of EGFR-TKI over chemotherapy in first line in NSCLC patients harboring *EGFR* mutations [31]. Patients were included according to clinical characteristics (adenocarcinoma, never or light smokers) and not to a molecular selection. Since the trial was performed in Asian population where *EGFR* mutations are two to three times more prevalent that in Western population, the rate of patients harboring *EGFR* mutations was high (21.4% confirmed *EGFR*-mutant patients). The study included 1,217 patients who were randomly assigned to receive either gefitinib or paclitaxel and carboplatin. Gefitinib was superior to chemotherapy in the entire population in terms of PFS, the primary endpoint of the trial, with a Hazard Ratio (HR) of 0.74 (95% CI 0.65-0.85; p< 0.001). This difference was more striking in the population tested positive for *EGFR* mutations that accounted for a total of 261 patients. The HR for PFS in this group of patients was 0.48 (95% CI 0.36-0.64; p< 0.001). Response rate was significantly higher in the gefitinib arm (71% versus 47%; p< 0.001) when compared to chemotherapy arm. Quality of life was evaluated and patients treated in the gefitinib arm exhibited the higher scores and the higher benefit when compared to patients assigned to chemotherapy. No differences in OS were found. Patients assigned to receive chemotherapy were treated with EGFR-TKI as second-line; this is the reason for the lack of difference in OS, 21.6 versus 21.9 months in gefitinib and chemotherapy group, respectively. Although patients were selected using clinical features in the IPASS trial, and these clinical characteristics were associated to a higher likelihood of the presence of *EGFR* mutations, those patients who received EGFR-TKI as first line and were *EGFR* wild type did poorly (HR 2.58, 95% CI 2.05-3.98; p< 0.001). This is one of the main contributions of this trial. Genotyping and confirmation of the presence of *EGFR* mutations should always be the basis to select EGFR-TKI therapy rather than clinical characteristics to avoid the harmful effect of the EGFR-TKI in non-mutant *EGFR* patients.

Two additional clinical trials performed in Asian population have compared gefitinib versus chemotherapy in first line in *EGFR*-mutant population: the North-East Japan Study group 002 trial (NEJ002) and the West Japan Thoracic Oncology Group 3405 trial (WJTOG3405) [32-34]. The NEJ002 randomized 227 patients harboring *EGFR* mutations to receive gefitinib versus carboplatin and paclitaxel. RR was 74% versus 31%, respectively (p< 0.001) [32]. PFS were 10.8 versus 5.4 months, respectively (HR 0.30, 95% CI 0.22-0.41; p< 0.001). No differences in OS were found (30.5 months versus 23.6 months, respectively). In an updated analysis, OS remained without differences (27.7 months versus 26.6 months, respectively; HR 0.884, 95% CI 0.634–1.241; p= 0.483) [33]. The WJTOG-3405 compared gefitinib versus cisplatin and docetaxel [34]. One hundred and seventy-five patients were randomly assigned to either treatment. RR was 62% versus 32%, respectively (p< 0.001). PFS was 9.2 versus 6.3 months, respectively (HR 0.48, 95% CI 0.33-0.71; p< 0.001). Again, the effect of the crossover therapy at the time of progression did not demonstrate differences in OS.

The OPTIMAL and the European Tarceva versus Chemotherapy trial (EURTAC) compared erlotinib and chemotherapy as upfront therapy in *EGFR*-mutant population [35, 36]. The OPTIMAL trial included 175 *EGFR*-mutant patients who were randomly assigned to receive erlotinib or carboplatin and gemcitabine [35]. RR was 83% and 36%, respectively. PFS was 13.1 versus 4.6 months (p< 0.001), respectively (HR 0.16, 95% CI 0.10-0.26; p<

0.001). No differences in OS were reported. In comparison to previous trials that were performed in Asian population, the EURTAC trial was the first one that compared the TKI erlotinib versus different chemotherapy schedules in Caucasian *EGFR* population (N= 173) [36]. RR was 63 versus 18% (p< 0.001) in each arm, respectively. PFS was 9.4 versus 5.2 months (HR 0.37, 95% CI 0.25-0.54; p< 0.001). OS did not differ in both groups (19.3 months versus 19.5 months, respectively; HR 1, 95% CI 0.65-1.7; p non-significant). One of the main contributions of the EURTAC trial was that treatment selection success depends on the molecular selection rather than on the ethnic background.

More recently, the results of the LUX –Lung 3 trial have been published [37, 38]. This phase III trial investigated the efficacy of afatinib, a panHER inhibitor that blocks EGFR, HER2 and HER4 with a wide preclinical activity against *EGFR* mutations, in comparison to one of the most efficacious chemotherapy schedules: cisplatin and pemetrexed [37]. This study was performed globally, so Asian and non-Asian patients were included. A total of 1,269 patients were screened, and 345 were finally treated. Afatinib was associated with a prolongation of PFS (11.1 months for afatinib and 6.9 months for chemotherapy; HR 0.58, 95% CI 0.43-0.78; p= 0.001). Median PFS for patients with common sensitizing mutations (deletion in exon 19 and L858R in exon 21 that accounted for 308 patients) was 13.6 months for afatinib and 6.9 months for chemotherapy (HR, 0.47, 95% CI 0.34-0.65; p= 0.001). Significantly higher RR was observed with afatinib compared with chemotherapy according to both independent (56% and 23%, respectively) and investigator (69% and 44%, respectively) assessments (both p< 0.001). Median OS has not yet been reached for any group; however, OS did not differ between afatinib and chemotherapy in the overall study population (16.6 months versus 14.8 months, respectively; HR 1.12, 95% CI 0.73-1.73; p< 0.6). Quality of life results were reported separately [38]. Afatinib was associated with better control of cough and dyspnea when compared with chemotherapy. Diarrhea, dysphagia, and sore mouth were higherin the afatinib group. Global health status and quality of life was also improved over time with afatinib compared with chemotherapy.

Afatinib has also been compared to chemotherapy (cisplatin and gemcitabine) in the LUX-Lung 6 trial carried out in Asian population. Three hundred and sixty-four patients were randomly assigned to each arm (242 to afatinib, 122 to gemcitabine and cisplatin). Median PFS was significantly longer in the afatinib group versus the chemotherapy group (11 months versus 5.6 months; HR 0.28, 95% CI 0.20-0.39; p< 0.0001). RR was 66.9% versus 23%, respectively (p< 0.0001). OS data were immature with 42.6% of deaths at the time of the analysis. Median OS was 22.1 versus 22.2 months (HR 0.95, 95% CI 0.68−1.33; p= 0.76).

The rate of patients not receiving the EGFR-TKI as second line treatment when assigned to chemotherapy arm in the previous studies reinforces the importance of an early therapy with TKI in this population. According to IPASS, NEJ002, WJTOG3405, EURTAC and LUX-Lung-3, the proportion of patients who were crossovered to EGFR-TKI ranged from 58% to 95%, meaning that up to 42% of patients who harbored an *EGFR* mutation missed the opportunity of receiving EGFR-TKI treatment [31, 32, 34-37].

Once the role of EGFR-TKI over chemotherapy as the first choice for the *EGFR*-mutant population has been extensively set and accepted by the medical community, there is an additional question that arises in this setting. The CALGB 30406 trial sought to evaluate the role of combining a EGFR-TKI (erlotinib) plus chemotherapy [52]. This study was aimed to patients with NSCLC who had adenocarcinoma, were never or limited former smokers, or had *EGFR* mutant tumors. Patients were assigned to receive erlotinib alone (N= 81) or a combination of erlotinib, carboplatin and paclitaxel (ECP) (N= 100). PFS was similar in both groups (5 months versus 6.6 months, respectively; p= 0.1988). RR did not differ in both groups (35% versus 46%, respectively). OS was similar in both groups (24.6 months versus 19.8 months, respectively). *EGFR* mutation analysis was possible in 91% (164 of 181) of patients. *EGFR* mutations were detected in 40% (51 of 128) of never smokers and in 42% (15 of 36) of light former smokers. In the erlotinib group, RR (70% versus 9%), PFS (14.1 months versus 2.6 months), and OS (31.3 months versus 18.1 month) favored *EGFR*-mutant patients. In the ECP group, RR (73% versus 30%), PFS (17.2 months versus 4.8 months), and OS (38.1 months versus 14.4 months) favored *EGFR*-mutant patients, as well. However, the incidence of grades 3 to 4 hematologic (2% versus 49%; p< 0.001) and non-hematologic (24% versus 52%; p< 0.001) toxicity was greater in patients treated with ECP. Therefore, similar efficacy results and an excess of toxicity makes unnecessary to expose a patient to an EGFR-TKI plus chemotherapy as upfront therapy.

Table 2. Summary of relevant facts regarding treatment approach in patients harboring EGFR mutations

Key points: Therapy in *EGFR*-mutant NSCLC patients
•Retrospective studies demonstrate impressive response rates, progression-free survival times when *EGFR*-mutant patients are treated with TKI [6, 7, 39-42].
•Single arm studies reproduced similar results when TKI was administered as first-line therapy [28-30].
•TKI in first line in this population is superior to chemotherapy, in terms of response and progression-free survival [31,32,34-37].
•No differences in overall survival have been documented, due to the cross-over effect [3-33, 34-37].
•TKI in first line in this population has demonstrated a significant improvement in quality of life when compared to chemotherapy [31-35, 37].
•Currently available TKI are erlotinib, gefitinib and afatinib.
•If chemotherapy has been started before the EGFR mutational status is known, TKI can be potentially included in the therapeutic scheme as follows •Switch chemotherapy to TKI (not recommended) •Delaying the initiation of TKI once the progression to chemotherapy occurs (not recommended) •Using the TKI in a maintenance fashion after completing the chemotherapy (preferable option)

3. Chosing the TKI

Erlotinib, gefitinib and afatinib have demonstrated superior results to different chemotherapy schedules, including the most efficacious scheme (cisplatin and pemetrexed) [31-38]. However, as of today, no head-to-head comparison has been carried out with different EGFR-TKI. On a practical basis, we assume a similar activity of the three drugs, even though preclinical data have shown that similar but not equal chemical structures are recognized; erlotinib plasma concentrations are above the necessary dose to inhibit EGFR at a standard dose; gefitinib at a standard dose does not inhibit the *EGFR* wild type and erlotinib is a more potent inhibitor of *EGFR*-mutant forms than gefitinib [53-56]. Recently, a meta-nalysis that included data of the phase III trials that have compared EGFR-TKI versus chemotherapy in first-line in *EGFR*-mutant patients has been reported [57]. Overall, patients treated with erlotinib and gefitinib did better than patients treated with chemotherapy in terms of PFS, RR and disease control rate (HR 0.25, OR 1.05 and OR 2.7, respectively for erlotinib; and HR 0.43, OR 1.06 and OR 2.6, respectively for gefitinib). Patients treated with afatinib attained better outcomes compared to patients treated with chemotherapy in terms of OS (HR 0.95). Although no comparisons among erlotinib, gefitinib and afatinib achieved statistical significance, there was a trend for erlotinib in terms of PFS and RR when compared to gefitinib and afatinib (HR 0.58 and OR 2, respectively for gefitinib; and 0.57 and OR 1.5, respectively for afatinib). Currently, two clinical trials are ongoing with the goal of comparing two different TKI in *EGFR*-mutant population: the LUX-lung 7 (NCT01466660), a randomised phase IIb comparing afatinib versus gefitinib and the ARCHER 1050 comparing gefitinib vs dacomitinib, an irreversible pan-HER EGFR-TKI [58-59].

Table 3. Summary of phase III trials comparing first-line EGFR-TKI versus chemotherapy in patients with EGFR mutations

					PFS				**OS**		**COR (%)**
Trial	N	RR%	OR%	p	mo	HR	p	mo	HR	p	
IPASS* [31]											
gefitinib	132	71	2.8	<0.001	9.6	0.48	<0.001	21.6	1.0	NS	75
Chemotherapy	129	47			6.3			21.9			64
NEJ002 [32,33]											
gefitinib	114	74	6.3	<0.001	10.8	0.3	<0.001	27.7	0.884	0.483	68
chemotherapy	113	31			5.4			26.6			95
WJTOG3405 [34]		62	3.4	<0.001	9.2	0.48	<0.001	35.5	NR	NS	19
gefitinib	87	32			6.3			38.8			58
chemotherapy	88										
OPTIMAL [35]		83	NR	<0.001	13.1	0.16	<0.001	NR	NR	NR	NR
erlotinib	82	36			4.6			NR			NR
chemotherapy	72										
EURTAC [36]											37
erlotinib	86	83	NR	<0.001	9.4	0.37	<0.001	19.3	1.0	NS	76
chemotherapy	87	36			5.2			19.5			
LUX-Lung 3 [37]											
afatinib	230	56	NR	<0.001	11.1	0.58	0.001	16.6	1.12	0.6	62
chemotherapy	115	23			6.9			14.8			65
LUX-Lung 6 [38]											
afatinib	242	66.9	NR	<0.0001	11	0.28	<0.0001	22.1	0.95	0.76	
chemotherapy	122	23			5.6			22.2			

COR Cross-over rate to Chemotherapy or TKI

4. Timing for the EGFR-TKI

The ideal scenario of starting EGFR-TKI treatment in *EGFR*-mutant patients is sometimes limited when the clinical situation demands to start treatment before *EGFR* genotype is known. The question in these cases is how to proceed with the treatment once the result turns positive for an *EGFR* mutation and the patient has started chemotherapy. Different alternatives could be hypothesized in this situation. First, to stop the chemotherapy and to start EGFR-TKI immediately; second, to delay the initiation of EGFR-TKI until the progression to chemotherapy occurs; third, to administer the EGFR-TKI once four to six courses of chemotherapy have been completed, in a maintenance fashion.

4.1. Switch Chemotherapy to EGFR-TKI

We can hypothesize that since patient with EGFR mutations do better with EGFR-TKI, chemotherapy should be immediately suspended in order to start the EGFR-TKI as soon as possible. However, a hasty decision could be detrimental for the patient, loosing the option of an active treatment.

The IPASS study, that included a clinically selected population, showed a high RR in *EGFR*-mutant patient treated with a carboplatin chemotherapy regimen. RR was 47.3% in the subgroup of patients with *EGFR* mutations treated with chemotherapy versus 23.5% for those EGFR wild type patients treated with the same chemotherapy scheme [31]. The Spanish Lung Cancer Group experience demonstrated, in a non-comparative study, that patients who received the EGFR-TKI as first-line compared to second or third-line after chemotherapy attained similar results in terms of PFS and OS [43]. PFS for patients receiving first-line therapy was 14 months (95% CI 9.7-18.3) and second-line therapy was 13 months (95% CI 9.7-16.3; p= 0.62), respectively. OS for patients receiving first-line therapy was 28 months (95% CI 22.7-33), and 27 months (95% CI 19.9-34.1; p= 0.67) for those receiving second-line therapy, respectively. RR was not associated with the fact of receiving the EGFR-TKI in first-line or subsequent lines. However, other phase III trials comparing EGFR-TKI and chemotherapy have reported lower RR, ranging from 15 to 36%, when *EGFR*-mutant patients receive chemotherapy as first line therapy [32, 34-37].

Some groups have reported a high association of *EGFR* mutations and ERCC1 expression when compared with EGFR wild type NSCLC specimens. However, as the authors stated in their conclusions whether those findings could be translated into enhanced clinical efficacy of *EGFR*-mutant forms to platinum-containing chemotherapy is still unclear [60]. If a patient is tolerating chemotherapy well, it could be effective in some patients with *EGFR* mutations, so the interruption of the chemotherapy should not be recommended unless there are problems with tolerance.

4.2. Initiation of the EGFR-TKI When Progression Occurs

Another possible approach consists on waiting until disease progression is documented and starting the EGFR-TKI as a second-line therapy. This approach associates the risk that some *EGFR*-mutant patients will miss the most efficacious therapy. According to data from the phase III trials comparing TKI versus chemotherapy in first line, a significant proportion of patients ranging from 5% to 42% did not receive EGFR-TKI treatment once progression occurred [31, 32, 34-37]. Although these clinical trials were not designed to test the effect of the cross-over, these data suggest that even though *EGFR*-mutant patients were followed very closely, the possibility of missing the EGFR-TKI treatment is real. Based on these results, we could not recommend this approach.

4.3. EGFR-TKI as Maintenance Once the First-Line Chemotherapy Is Completed

The role of maintenance therapy with a EGFR-TKI after chemotherapy in patients with *EGFR* mutations has not been formally evaluated. Maintenance erlotinib versus placebo after upfront chemotherapy was studied in the Sequential Tarceva in unresected NSCLC (SATURN) trial [61]. PFS was longer in the erlotinib arm (HR 0.71, 95% CI 0.62-0.82; p< 0.001). OS was also longer in the erlotinib arm (HR 0.81, 95% CI 0.7-0.95; p< 0.0088). The PFS benefit was strikingly greater in patients with *EGFR* mutations, with a median PFS of 44 and 14 weeks for erlotinib and placebo, respectively (HR 0.1, 95% CI 0.04-0.25; p< 0.001). No OS advantage was found in the *EGFR*-mutant subgroup, likely as a result of a high rate of crossover from placebo to erlotinib in this group. According to these results, we can justify the use of erlotinib after chemotherapy in *EGFR*-mutant population. Again, the potential rate of patients with a likelihood of not receiving a EGFR-TKI reinforces this approach [31, 32, 34-37].

5. Final Recommendations

5.1. What Treatment Should We Select as the First Option for *EGFR*-Mutant Patients?

Currently, there is cumulative evidence demonstrating that EGFR-TKI should be the treatment of for this population as upfront therapy. [31-38].

5.2. A patient of Mine Has All the Clinical Features Related to the Presence of *EGFR* Mutations. Can I Start the Patient on EGFR-TKI Treatment and Suspend It If the Result Turns Negative?

There is evidence of the detrimental effect of administering EGFR-TKI as first line in patients not harboring *EGFR* mutations [31].

5.3. How Much Time Should the Patients and Physicians Wait for the *EGFR* Results?

This waiting time may vary depending on the performance status of the patient and the willingness to remain out of therapy until the definitive result is available. We consider acceptable a timeline from 7 to 14 days [43-45].

5.4. How Should We Proceed When We Obtain a Non-Conclusive Result for *EGFR* Analysis?

According to the detection method available in each center, we strongly recommend to repeat a biopsy or to obtain a cytology sample to repeat the analysis. This material could also be crucial to screen for other mutations in case of a definitive *EGFR* negative result.

5.5. How Should We Proceed Once Chemotherapy Has Been Started and the *EGFR* Mutation Result Turns Positive?

If tolerance to chemotherapy is correct, we can consider the administration of four cycles of chemotherapy and start the EGFR-TKI immediately after the last cycle of chemotherapy. If a patient presents side effects related to chemotherapy, chemotherapy should be stopped and we could switch to EGFR-TKI. In this situation, completing the chemotherapy and waiting for the progression to star the EGFR-TKI could take away the patient for receiving the best therapy for their *EGFR*-mutant disease [31-38, 62].

5.6. Is There Any Role for Combining an EGFR-TKI and Chemotherapy as First Line Therapy in *EGFR* Patients?

On the basis of the CALGB 30406 trial results, there is no evidence of a clinical benefit of this approach. Moreover, there is an increase of toxicity when both treatments are combined [52].

5.7. Which TKI Should I Choose?

To date there has not been a direct comparison between erlotinib and gefitinib. According to the data derived from the different trials we have assumed that, in the clinical setting, both gefitinib and erlotinib are equally efficacious. Currently, two clinical trials are ongoing and may shed some light in this question. However, the pharmaceutical policies at each center may direct the availability of the different EGFR-TKI [53-59].

References

[1] Hayden EC. Personalized cancer therapy gets closer. *Nature*. 2009; 458: 131-2.

[2] Demetri GD, von Mehren M, Blanke CD, et al. Efficacy and safety of imatinib mesylate in advanced gastrointestinal stromal tumors. *N. Engl. J. Med.* 2002; 347: 472-80.

[3] Druker BJ, Sawyers CL, Kantarjian H, et al. Activity of a specific inhibitor of the BCRABL tyrosine kinase in the blast crisis of chronic myeloid leukemia and acute lymphoblastic leukemia with the Philadelphia chromosome. *N. Engl. J. Med.* 2001; 344: 1038-42.

[4] Yarden Y, Sliwkowski MX. Untangling the ErbB signalling network. *Nat. Rev. Mol. Cell Biol.* 2001; 2:127-37.

[5] Sequist LV, Bell DW, Lynch TJ, Haber DA. Molecular predictors of response to epidermal growth factor receptor antagonists in non-small-cell lung cancer. *J. Clin. Oncol.* 2007; 25: 587-95.

[6] Lynch TJ, Bell DW, Sordella R, et al. Activating mutations in the epidermal growth factor receptor underlying responsiveness of non-small-cell lung cancer to gefitinib. *N. Engl. J. Med.* 2004; 350: 2129-39.

[7] Paez JG, Jänne PA, Lee JC, et al. EGFR mutations in lung cancer: correlation with clinical response to gefitinib therapy. *Science.* 2004; 304: 1497-500.

[8] Soda M, Choi YL, Enomoto M, et al. Identification of the transforming EML4-ALK fusion gene in non-small-cell lung cancer. *Nature*. 2007; 448: 561–6.

[9] Shaw AT, Yeap BY, Mino-Kenudson M, et al. Clinical Features and Outcome of Patients With Non Small-Cell Lung Cancer Who Harbor EML4-ALK. *J. Clin. Oncol.* 2009; 26: 4247-53.

[10] Kwak EL, Bang YJ, Camidge DR, et al. Anaplastic lymphoma kinase inhibition in non small-cell lung cancer. *N. Engl. J. Med.* 2010; 363: 1693–703.

[11] Paik PK, Arcila ME, Fara M, et al. Clinical characteristics of patients with lung adenocarcinomas harboring BRAF mutations. *J. Clin. Oncol.* 2011; 29 (15): 2046-51.

[12] Marchetti A, Felicioni L, Malatesta S, et al. Clinical features and outcome of patients with non-small-cell lung cancer harboring BRAF mutations. *J. Clin. Oncol.* 2011; 29 (26): 3574-9.

[13] Lipson D, Capelletti M, Yelensky R, et al. Identification of new ALK and RET gene fusions from colorectal and lung cancer biopsies. *P J.Nat. Med.* 2012; 18 (3): 382-4.

[14] Takeuchi K, Soda M, Togashi Y, Suzuki R, et al. RET, ROS1 and ALK fusions in lung cancer. *Nat. Med.* 2012; 18 (3): 378-81.

[15] Kohno T, Ichikawa H, Totoki Y, et al. KIF5B-RET fusions in lung adenocarcinoma. *Nat. Med.* 2012; 18 (3): 375-7.

[16] Li C, Fang R, Sun Y, et al. Spectrum of oncogenic driver mutations in lung adenocarcinomas from East Asian never smokers. *PLoS One*. 2011; 6 (11): e28204.

[17] Bergethon K, Shaw AT, Ou SH, et al. ROS1 rearrangements define a unique molecular class of lung cancers. *J. Clin. Oncol.* 2012; 30 (8): 863-70.

[18] Sordella R, Bell DW, Haber DA, Settleman J. Gefitinib-sensitizing EGFR mutations in lung cancer activate anti-apoptotic pathways. *Science.* 2004 Aug 20;305(5687):1163-7.

[19] Sharma SV, Bell DW, Settleman J, Haber DA. Epidermal growth factor receptor mutations in lung cancer. *Nat Rev Cancer.* 2007; 7 (3): 169-81.

[20] Greulich H, Chen TH, Feng W, et al. Oncogenic transformation by inhibitor-sensitive and -resistant EGFR mutants. *PLoS Med.* 2005; 2 (11): e313.

[21] Politi K, Zakowski MF, Fan PD, Schonfeld EA, Pao W, Varmus HE. Lung adenocarcinomas induced in mice by mutant EGF receptors found in human lung cancers respond to a tyrosine kinase inhibitor or to down-regulation of the receptors. *Genes Dev.* 2006; 20 (11): 1496-510.

[22] Horn L, Chen H, Lovly CM, Andrews J, Yeh P, Levy MA, Pao W. DIRECT: DNA-mutation Inventory to Refine and Enhance Cancer Treatment--A catalogue of clinically relevant somatic mutations in lung cancer. *J. Clin. Oncol.* 2011; 29: 494s (suppl; abstr 7575).

[23] He M, Capelletti M, Nafa K, et al. EGFR exon 19 insertions: a new family of sensitizing EGFR mutations in lung adenocarcinoma. *Clin. Cancer Res.* 2012; 18 (6): 1790-7.

[24] Nguyen KS, Kobayashi S, Costa DB. Acquired resistance to epidermal growth factor receptor tyrosine kinase inhibitors in non-small-cell lung cancers dependent on the epidermal growth factor receptor pathway. *Clin. Lung Cancer.* 2009; 10 (4): 281-9.

[25] Yu HA, Arcila ME, Hellmann MD, Kris MG, Ladanyi M, Riely GJ. Poor response to erlotinib in patients with tumors containing baseline EGFR T790M mutations found by routine clinical molecular testing. *Ann. Oncol.* 2014; 25 (2): 423-8.

[26] Pan Y, Zhang Y, Li Y, et al. Prevalence, Clinicopathologic Characteristics, and Molecular Associations of EGFR Exon 20 Insertion Mutations in East Asian Patients with Lung Adenocarcinoma. *Ann. Surg. Oncol.* 2014 doi 10.1245/s10434-013-3452-1 [Epub ahead of print].

[27] Yasuda H, Park E, Yun CH, et al. Structural, Biochemical, and Clinical Characterization of Epidermal Growth Factor Receptor (EGFR) Exon 20 Insertion Mutations in Lung Cancer. *Sci. Transl. Med.* 2013; 5 (216): 216ra177.

[28] Sequist LV, Martins RG, Spigel D, et al. First-line gefitinib in patients with advanced non-small-cell lung cancer harboring somatic EGFR mutations. *J. Clin. Oncol.* 2008; 26 (15): 2442-9.

[29] Inoue A, Suzuki T, Fukuhara T, et al. Prospective phase II study of gefitinib for chemotherapy-naive patients with advanced non-small-cell lung cancer with epidermal growth factor receptor gene mutations. *J. Clin. Oncol.* 2006; 24 (21): 3340-6.

[30] Asahina H, Yamazaki K, Kinoshita I, et al. A phase II trial of gefitinib as first-line therapy for advanced non-small cell lung cancer with epidermal growth factor receptor mutations. *Br. J. Cancer.* 2006; 95 (8): 998-1004.

[31] Mok TS, Wu YL, Thongprasert S, et al. Gefitinib or carboplatin-paclitaxel in pulmonary adenocarcinoma. *N. Engl. J. Med.* 2009; 361 (10): 947-57.

[32] Maemondo M, Inoue A, Kobayashi K, et al. Gefitinib or chemotherapy for non-small-cell lung cancer with mutated EGFR. *N. Engl. J. Med.* 2010; 362 (25): 2380-8.

[33] Inoue A, Kobayashi K, Maemondo M, et al. Updated overall survival results from a randomized phase III trial comparing gefitinib with carboplatin-paclitaxel for chemo-naïve non-small cell lung cancer with sensitive EGFR gene mutations (NEJ002). *Ann. Oncol.* 2013; 24 (1): 54-9.

[34] Mitsudomi T, Morita S, Yatabe Y, et al. Gefitinib versus cisplatin plus docetaxel in patients with non-small-cell lung cancer harbouring mutations of the epidermal growth factor receptor (WJTOG3405): an open label, randomised phase 3 trial. *Lancet Oncol.* 2010; 11 (2): 121-8.
[35] Zhou C, Wu YL, Chen G, et al. Erlotinib versus chemotherapy as first-line treatment for patients with advanced EGFR mutation-positive non-small-cell lung cancer (OPTIMAL, CTONG-0802): a multicentre, open-label, randomised, phase 3 study. *Lancet Oncol.* 2011; 12 (8): 735-42.
[36] Rosell R, Carcereny E, Gervais R, et al. Erlotinib versus standard chemotherapy as first-line treatment for European patients with advanced EGFR mutation-positive non-small-cell lung cancer (EURTAC): a multicentre, open-label, randomised phase 3 trial. *Lancet Oncol.* 2012; 13 (3): 239-46.
[37] Sequist LV, Yang JC, Yamamoto N, et al. Phase III study of afatinib or cisplatin plus pemetrexed in patients with metastatic lung adenocarcinoma with EGFR mutations. *J. Clin. Oncol.* 2013; 31 (27): 3327-34.
[38] Wu YL, Zhou C, Hu CP, et al. Afatinib versus cisplatin plus gemcitabine for first-line treatment of Asian patients with advanced non-small-cell lung cancer harbouring EGFR mutations (LUX-Lung 6): an open-label, randomised phase 3 trial. *Lancet Oncol.* 2014; 15 (2): 213-22.
[39] Jackman DM, Yeap BY, Sequist LV, et al. Exon 19 deletion mutations of epidermal growth factor receptor are associated with prolonged survival in non-small cell lung cancer patients treated with gefitinib or erlotinib. *Clin. Cancer Res.* 2006; 12 (13): 3908-14.
[40] Taron M, Ichinose Y, Rosell R, et al. Activating mutations in the tyrosine kinase domain of the epidermal growth factor receptor are associated with improved survival in gefitinib-treated chemorefractory lung adenocarcinomas. *Clin. Cancer Res.* 2005; 11 (16): 5878-85.
[41] Cortes-Funes H, Gomez C, Rosell R, et al. Epidermal growth factor receptor activating mutations in Spanish gefitinib-treated non-small-cell lung cancer patients. *Ann. Oncol.* 2005; 16 (7): 1081-6.
[42] Han SW, Kim TY, Hwang PG, et al. Predictive and prognostic impact of epidermal growth factor receptor mutation in non-small-cell lung cancer patients treated with gefitinib. *J. Clin. Oncol.* 2005; 23 (11): 2493-501.
[43] Rosell R, Moran T, Queralt C, et al. Screening for epidermal growth factor receptor mutations in lung cancer. *N. Engl. J. Med.* 2009; 361 (10): 958-67.
[44] Sequist LV, Heist RS, Shaw AT, et al. Implementing multiplexed genotyping of non-small-cell lung cancers into routine clinical practice. *Ann. Oncol.* 2011; 22 (12): 2616-24.
[45] Pirker R, Herth FJ, Kerr KM, et al. Consensus for EGFR mutation testing in non-small cell lung cancer: results from a European workshop. *J. Thorac. Oncol.* 2010; 5 (10): 1706-13.
[46] Garcia-Olivé I, Monsó E, Andreo F, et al. Endobronchial ultrasound-guided transbronchial needle aspiration for identifying EGFR mutations. *Eur. Respir. J.* 2010; 35 (2): 391-5.

[47] Molina-Vila MA, Bertran-Alamillo J, Reguart N, et al. A sensitive method for detecting EGFR mutations in non-small cell lung cancer samples with few tumor cells. *J. Thorac. Oncol.* 2008; 3 (11): 1224-35.
[48] Navani N, Lawrence DR, Kolvekar S, et al. Endobronchial ultrasound-guided transbronchial needle aspiration prevents mediastinoscopies in the diagnosis of isolated mediastinal lymphadenopathy: a prospective trial. *Am. J. Respir. Crit. Care Med.* 2012; 186 (3): 255-60.
[49] Billah S, Stewart J, Staerkel G, Chen S, Gong Y, Guo M. EGFR and KRAS mutations in lung carcinoma: molecular testing by using cytology specimens. *Cancer Cytopathol.* 2011; 119 (2): 111-7.
[50] Takano T, Fukui T, Ohe Y, et al. EGFR mutations predict survival benefit from gefitinib in patients with advanced lung adenocarcinoma: a historical comparison of patients treated before and after gefitinib approval in Japan. *J. Clin. Oncol.* 2008; 26 (34): 5589-95.
[51] Woodcock J: AstraZeneca Pharmaceuticals LP. Withdrawal of approval of a new drug Application for IRESSA. *Federal Register* 2012; 77; 2423-4.
[52] Jänne PA, Wang X, Socinski MA, et al. Randomized phase II trial of erlotinib alone or with carboplatin and paclitaxel in patients who were never or light former smokers with advanced lung adenocarcinoma: CALGB 30406 trial. *J. Clin. Oncol.* 2012; 30 (17): 2063-9.
[53] Costa DB, Schumer ST, Tenen DG, Kobayashi S. Differential responses to erlotinib in epidermal growth factor receptor (EGFR)-mutated lung cancers with acquired resistance to gefitinib carrying the L747S or T790M secondary mutations. *J. Clin. Oncol.* 2008; 26 (7): 1182-4.
[54] Hidalgo M, Bloedow D. Pharmacokinetics and pharmacodynamics: maximizing the clinical potential of Erlotinib (Tarceva). *Semin. Oncol.* 2003; 30 (3 Suppl 7): 25-33.
[55] Carey KD, Garton AJ, Romero MS, et al. Kinetic analysis of epidermal growth factor receptor somatic mutant proteins shows increased sensitivity to the epidermal growth factor receptor tyrosine kinase inhibitor, erlotinib. *Cancer Res.* 2006; 66 (16): 8163-71.
[56] Li J, Karlsson MO, Brahmer J, Spitz A, Zhao M, Hidalgo M, Baker SD. CYP3A phenotyping approach to predict systemic exposure to EGFR tyrosine kinase inhibitors. *J. Natl. Cancer Inst.* 2006; 98 (23): 1714-23.
[57] Lopes G, Haaland B. Comparative effectiveness of gefitinib, erlotinib, afatinib and chemotherapy in the first line treatment of patients with advanced non small cell lung cancer (NSCLC) and epidermal growth factor receptor (EGFR) mutations. *J. Thorac. Oncol.* 2013; 8 (suppl): 2: S895. Abst P2.11-015.
[58] LUX-Lung 7: A Phase IIb Trial of Afatinib(BIBW2992) Versus Gefitinib for the Treatment of 1st Line EGFR Mutation Positive Adenocarcinoma of the Lung. *ClinicalTrials.gov Identifier*: NCT01466660.
[59] ARCHER-1050: A Study of Dacomitinib vs. Gefitinib in 1st-Line Treatment Of Advanced NSCLC. *ClinicalTrials.gov Identifier*: NCT01774721.
[60] Gandara DR, Grimminger P, Mack PC, Lara PN Jr, Li T, Danenberg PV, Danenberg KD. Association of epidermal growth factor receptor activating mutations with low ERCC1 gene expression in non-small cell lung cancer. *J. Thorac. Oncol.* 2010; 5 (12): 1933-8.

[61] Cappuzzo F, Ciuleanu T, Stelmakh L, et al. Erlotinib as maintenance treatment in advanced non-small-cell lung cancer: a multicentre, randomised, placebo-controlled phase 3 study. *Lancet Oncol.* 2010; 11 (6): 521-9.

In: Fighting Lung Cancer through the HER Family ...
Editor: Diego Márquez-Medina
ISBN: 978-1-63321-092-9

Chapter 9

Treatment I - Treatment of Unselected Patients with Epidermal Growth Factor Tyrosine Kinase Inhibitors

Edurne Arriola, M.D. Ph.D., Álvaro Taus, M.D. and David Casadevall, M.D.
Oncology Department, Hospital del Mar University Hospital of Barcelona, Spain

Abstract

EGFR-tyrosine kinase inhibitors (EGFR-TKI) have proven effective in Non-small-cell lung cancer (NSCLC). With implementation of molecular analysis in clinical practice, it is now common knowledge that patients with certain mutations in the tyrosine kinase domain, which result in increased downstream *EGFR* signalling, show greater benefit with these therapies when compared with mutation-negative patients. However, several studies have consistently reported that a benefit also exists in patients with *EGFR* unknown or wild type status. In this chapter we present an overview of the current clinical evidence for EGFR-TKI use in patients with locally advanced or metastatic NSCLC, focusing on patients with no known *EGFR* mutation. The mechanism by which a subgroup of patients benefits from these treatments remains unclear, and thus, adequate patient selection is yet not possible. The second part of this chapter will focus on the different efforts so far made to elucidate the molecular networks implicated in tumor susceptibility to EGFR-TKI treatment. Finally, several studies with the aim of developing new patient selection strategies based on biomarkers and gene expression patterns will be presented.

1. Introduction

Since the discovery of oncogene driver mutations, activation of the Epidermal Growth Factor Receptor (*EGFR*) pathway has been one of the most thoroughly studied oncogenic phenomenons of the last decade. Up to 60% of Non-small-cell Lung Cancer (NSCLC) patients in clinically selected populations may present with a constitutively increased signaling through *EGFR*, which in turn activates downstream cell signaling cascades implicated in cell survival and tumorigenesis [1].

Activating somatic mutations of the *EGFR* tyrosine-kinase domain, which lead to increased *EGFR* downstream signaling, confer susceptibility to molecularly targeted inhibition of the tyrosine kinase domain [2]. Inhibition of this pathway with specific tyrosine-kinase inhibitors in these patients has shown a clear benefit in terms of progression-free survival when compared to chemotherapy [3]. gefitinib (AstraZeneca) and erlotinib (Roche/Genentech) are the most widely used *EGFR* Tyrosine-kinase inhibitors (EGFR-TKI). Both agents are approved as first-line treatment of advanced NSCLC with known activating mutations of the *EGFR* tyrosine-kinase domain.

First-line treatment of unselected patients with advanced NSCLC consists of platinum-based doublets. In the second-line setting, docetaxel and pemetrexed have shown similar results in terms of benefit in progression-free survival (PFS) and overall survival (OS) when compared to single agent chemotherapy and best supportive care [4-6].

In the year 2005, there was no clear evidence of benefit from third-line chemotherapy in NSCLC patients. It was in that context that Shepherd et al. [7] conducted the randomized BR.21 trial, comparing Erlotinib to Placebo in patients with advanced NSCLC who had received at least one previous chemotherapy regimen and were ineligible for further treatment with chemotherapy (PS 0-3). The benefit in PFS, OS and quality of life observed in the Erlotinib group lead to its approval in second and third-line therapy in patients with unknown or wild-type *EGFR*.

In this and many other early studies with *EGFR*-TKIs, molecular analysis of tumor samples was not required, and benefit from *EGFR*-TKIs would be associated to certain clinic and histological characteristics (see below). In unselected patients with previously treated NSCLC, treatment with *EGFR*-TKIs showed responses in 4 to 28% of cases [8] and disease stabilization in approximately 45% [7].

Patients with *EGF*R-mutant NSCLC show larger benefit from *EGFR-TKI* treatment than from chemotherapy [3, 9, 10]. Even though benefits have been reported in unselected and/or *EGFR* wild-type patients, the role of *EGFR*-TKI in this population remains controversial. In a recent meta-analysis of 23 trials using *EGFR-TKIs*, mutational status was only known in 31% of the patients, limiting the statistical power to detect differences between mutation-positive and –negative patients [11].

In this chapter, we will review the current clinical evidence for the use of *EGFR-TKI* in unselected NSCLC, assuming that the majority of these patients are wild-type. We will also analise the scientific evidence underlying the potential benefit observed with these treatments in this unselected population.

2. Addition of EGFR-TKIs to First-Line Chemotherapy

Erlotinib in combination with a platinum-based doublet was evaluated in two large randomized phase III trials. In the TALENT trial, Gatzemeier and colleagues [12] evaluated the combination of cisplatin and gemcitabine plus erlotinib or placebo in 1,172 unselected patients with advanced NSCLC. The TRIBUTE trial [13] compared the addition of erlotinib/placebo to the combination of carboplatin and paclitaxel in the same setting as the TALENT trial. Two equivalent studies were conducted with gefitinib, INTACT1 (cisplatin-gemcitabine + gefitinib/placebo) and INTACT 2 (carboplatin-paclitaxel + gefitinib/placebo) in cohorts comparable to the ones participating in the erlotinib trials [14, 15]. *EGFR* mutational status was not reported in the aforementioned studies and no survival benefit was observed with the addition of erlotinib or gefitinib to platinum-based chemotherapy. Subgroup analysis did not reveal any differences in efficacy according to histology. In a retrospective analysis of *EGFR* mutational status of the pacients participating in the TRIBUTE trial [16], Eberhard et al. observed a higher response rate in *EGFR*-mutant patients in both chemotherapy and chemotherapy plus erlotinib groups. Interestingly, however, *EGFR* mutations were not significantly associated with a benefit in OS or PFS. These findings suggest that there is no benefit in the addition of EGFR-TKI to standard first-line chemotherapy.

3. EGFR-TKI as First Line Treatment

Initially, probability of response to *EGFR-TKI*s was thought to be associated with certain clinical characteristics (Adenocarcinoma histology, Asian race, female gender and never-smokers). In the IPASS trial [9], a selected population according to these characteristics was randomized to receive gefitinib monotherapy versus a combination of carboplatin and paclitaxel as first line treatment. Mutation analysis was possible in approximately 36% of the patients included in the study, and 60% of these harbored activating *EGFR* mutations. This study reached its primary endpoint, showing non-inferiority of gefitinib compared to carboplatin-paclitaxel in terms of PFS in clinically selected patients. As expected, in the subgroup analysis, gefitinib was superior in patients with known *EGFR* mutations (HR for progression or death 0.48; $p<0.001$) and provided a better quality of life for the general population. Also, non-mutated patients treated with gefitinib presented worse outcome. Interestingly, however, the objective response rate was significantly superior in the gefitinib group when compared to the chemotherapy group (43% versus 32%, respectively; $p< 0.001$) and this difference was greater in the mutation-positive group. Notably, one patient in the gefitinib group with wild-type *EGFR* showed a partial response. Another study with similar design to the IPASS trial but with a smaller Korean population conducted by Han and colleagues [17] (First-SIGNAL) evaluated the administration of gefitinib compared with a combination of gemcitabine and cisplatin in Asian, never-smoking patients with advanced Lung Adenocarcinoma. Although molecular analysis was only available in 30% of the patients, the objective response rate in the mutation-negative subgroup was almost 26%. This study failed to meet its primary endpoint, since gefitinib was not superior to cisplatin-gemcitabine in terms of overall survival.

A third first-line trial (TORCH) evaluating the role of *EGFR-TKI*s in unselected population was conducted between Canada and Italy including a vast majority of non-asian patients. Out of 760 clinically unselected patients, twenty percent were never-smokers and 44.5% non-adenocarcinomas. This trial evaluated the non-inferiority of erlotinib followed by cisplatin-gemcitabine at progression versus the reverse strategy [18]. Mutation analysis was available in 36% of the patients, of which only 39 had an activating *EGFR* mutation. In the general population, erlotinib preceeding chemotherapy was associated with a worse outcome, and therefore this strategy was not further recommended.

Other trials have evaluated the clinical efficacy of *EGFR-TKI*s in molecularly unselected patients usually unfit for clinical trials. One hundred and three patients with advanced NSCLC and PS 2 were randomized to receive either erlotinib or a combination of carboplatin-paclitaxel in a study conducted by Lilenbaum et al. [19]. Ninety two percent had a smoking history, 63% were adenocarcinoma and the proportion of Asian patients was less than 15%. Only five patients in the overall population had an *EGFR* mutation, and all of them were in the chemotherapy group. The primary endpoint in this study was PFS, which was inferior in the erlotinib group, although not statistically significant (1.9 months vs 3.5 months; HR1.45; p= 0.063).

In another phase II study with predominantly Western patients with poor PS (2 or 3), comparing gefitinib to placebo, there were no statistically significant differences compared to placebo in terms of PFS, OS or the overall response ratio (ORR) [20].

Crino et al. [21] conducted a phase II trial in chemotherapy-naïve patients with locally advanced or metastatic NSCLC who were 70 years of age or more and were not candidates to platinum based chemotherapy. Patients were randomly assigned to receive either gefitinib or vinorelbine in monotherapy. Of the 196 patients, the vast majority (89%) had a smoking history, 55% had non-adenocarcinoma histology and 14% were Asian. Evaluation of results according to *EGFR* mutation was not possible due to small numbers (only 7 mutations detected in 65 samples available for study). Gefitinib failed to show superiority against vinorelbine in terms of PFS.

A more recent Asian open-label randomized trial compared erlotinib versus vinorelbine in elderly Taiwanese patients with similar characteristics (79% smokers, 63% adenocarcinomas). Primary endpoint was to detect differences in response rate between groups. Tissue sample availability for molecular studies was 53%. In the overall population, erlotinib was superior to vinorelbine in terms of response rate (22.8% had a partial response with erlotinib versus 8.9% patients with vinorelbine, respectively; p= 0.04) and progression-free survival (4.57 vs 2.53 months, respectively; p= 0.03). No differences in response rate were observed in subgroup analyses. Interestingly, *EGFR*-mutant patients in both arms had longer PFS compared to their non-mutated counterparts. In the EGFR-unknown subgroup, PFS was longer for patients in the erlotinib group (5.07 versus 2.17 months; p= 0.07). [22].

4. EGFR-TKI As Maintenance Therapy

A double blind randomized phase III (SATURN) trial evaluated switch maintenance treatment with erlotinib or placebo in patients with advanced NSCLC that had not shown progression after 4 cycles of a platinum-doublet [23]. The primary endpoint of this study was PFS. Although tissue collection for analysis was required, 43% of the samples were unavailable for mutational analysis. Patients were predominantly Caucasians (15% Asians), 80% had a smoking history and 44% were adenocarcinomas. Six percent of *EGFR* activating mutations were detected. In the overall population, erlotinib improved PFS compared to placebo (12.3 vs 11.1 weeks, respectively; HR0.71; p< 0.01) and OS (12 months vs 11 months, respectively. HR0.81; p= 0.009).

Table 1. Phase III trials evaluating first-line and maintenance with EGFR-TKI

Trial (Ref.)	Year	N	Regimens	Mutational status (%)	PE	Efficacy in OP	Subgroup analysis
INTACT 1 [14]	2004	1,093	C+Gem+G vs. C+Gem+P	Not reported	OS	9.9mo vs. 10.9mo *p=0.46*	
INTACT 2 [15]	2004	1,037	Cb+T+G vs. Cb+T+P	Not reported	OS	9.8mo vs. 9.9mo *p=0.64*	
TRIBUTE [13]	2005	1,059	Cb+T+E vs. Cb+T+P	29 of 228 avl. (12.8%)	OS	10.6mo vs. 10.5mo *p=0.95*	
TALENT [12]	2007	1,172	C+Gem+E vs. C+Gem+P	Not reported	OS	10.7mo vs. 11mo *p=0.486*	
IPASS [9]	2009	1,217	G vs. Cb+T	261 of 437 avl. (59.7%)	PFS	5.7mo vs. 5.8mo *p<0.001*	EGFR mutated: PFS HR, 0.83; EGFR wt: PFS HR, 2.85; interaction p<0.001
SATURN [23]*	2010	889	E vs. P	49 of 446 avl. (10.9%)	PFS	3mo vs. 2.77mo *p<0.001*	EGFR mutated: PFS HR, 0.10; EGFR wt: PFS HR, 0.78; interaction p<0.001; EGFR mutated: OS HR, NR; EGFR wt: OS HR, 0.77
First-SIGNAL [17]	2012	313	G vs. C+Gem	42 of 96 avl. (43.8%)	OS	22.3mo vs. 22.9mo *p= 0.604*	EGFR mutated: PFS HR, 0.54; EGFR wt: PFS HR, 1.41

Ref., reference in text; OP, overall study population; PE, Primary endpoint; ADC, adenocarcinoma; C, cisplatin; Cb, carboplatin; D, docetaxel; E, erlotinib; EGFR, epidermal growth factor receptor; G, gefitinib; Gem, gemcitabine; HR, hazard ratio; NR, not reported; OS, median overall survival; P, placebo; Pem, pemetrexed; PFS, median progression free survival; T, paclitaxel; wt, wild type; avl, available.

Efficacy in OP: only primary endpoints reported.

* All of the above presented studies evaluate first-line treatment except the SATURN Trial, which evaluated maintenance therapy after platinum-doublet (see text).

The benefit from erlotinib was greater in the *EGFR*-mutant subgroup. However, this benefit persisted in the *EGFR* wild-type subgroup in terms of PFS (HR0.78; p= 0.02) as well as OS (HR0.77; p= 0.02). A similar phase III trial published by Gaafar et al. [24] compared maintenance therapy with gefitinib versus placebo after 2-6 cycles of a platinum-doublet. 76% of the study population were males, 46% had adenocarcinoma and 74% had a smoking history. PFS was longer in the gefitinib group compared to the placebo group (4.1 versus 2.9 months, respectively. HR0.61; p= 0.002) with no significant differences observed in terms of OS. The ATLAS study [25], a randomized phase III trial comparing addition of erlotinib/placebo to maintenance with bevacizumab after 4 cicles of bevacizumab-containing first-line chemotherapy, was recently published. No mutational analysis was performed. Significant improvement in PFS was observed with the combination of erlotinib + bevacizumab compared with erlotinib + placebo (4.8 versus 3.7 months, respectively. HR0.71; p< 0.001) but no statistically significant differences were observed in terms of OS.

5. EGFR-TKI Role at Progression from First- or Second-Line Therapies

As mentioned previously in this chapter, the BR.21 trial compared the administration of erlotinib versus placebo in unselected population after progression to one or two previous chemotherapy regimens. Patients that received erlotinib had longer OS than those who received placebo (6.7 months versus 4.7, respectively; HR 0.70; p< 0.001) despite an objective response rate of only 8% observed in the erlotinib group. Zhu et al. [26] conducted a retrospective analysis of the patients in the erlotinib group with available tissue, detecting an ORR of 7% in the subgroup of *EGFR* wild-type patients.

The ISEL study [27] evaluated the efficacy of gefitinib compared to placebo in the same context as in the BR.21 trial. No statistical differences in terms of PFS or OS were detected in the overall population. However, preplanned subgroup analysis revealed improved survival with gefitinib in never-smokers and in patients of Asian origin (HR 0.67; p= 0.012 and HR 0.66; p= 0.01, respectively). Fifteen percent of the participating patients had available tissue for analysis, and a response rate of 2.8% was reported with gefitinib in *EGFR* wild-type patients [28]. The INTEREST trial [29] was an open-label randomized phase III trial designed to detect non-inferiority of gefitinib when compared with docetaxel after treatment with one or more platinum-based regimens. The study met its primary endpoint (median OS with gefitinib 7.6 months compared to 8 months with docetaxel (HR 1.02 meeting the predefined non-inferiority criterion). This effect was maintained when analysing non-adenocarcinoma and non-Asian patients. In a retrospective analysis of the cases with available tumor samples (25,5%), a benefit in terms of ORR and PFS was observed in *EGFR*-mutated patients compared to those with wild-type *EGFR*, but no differences in terms of OS were observed [30]. Patients participating in the SATURN trial (see above) who progressed during first-line chemotherapy were offered enrolment in the TITAN study [31]. Patients were randomized to receive erlotinib or chemotherapy (docetaxel or pemetrexed, at investigator's discretion). Although the trial was insufficiently powered to detect non-inferiority, no statistically significant differences in terms of survival were detected between the two arms. *EGFR* mutational analysis was possible in 44% of patients, and only 5% harboured activating *EGFR* mutations. No statistical differences in survival between arms were detected in the *EGFR* wild-type population. A trial conducted by the Hellenic Oncology Research Group (HORG trial) [32] was designed to detect superiority of pemetrexed compared to erlotinib in the second- or third-line treatment setting. Primary endpoint was time-to-progression, and no statistically significant differences were detected between the two arms. Tumor samples were available for mutational analysis in 34% of the patients, and 9% of these patients harboured an activating mutation. Consistent with previous findings, in the subset of *EGFR* wild-type patients, response and disease control rates with erlotinib were 7.3% and 21.8%, respectively.

The recently published Tarceva Italian Lung Optimization Trial (TAILOR) [33] compared second-line administration of erlotinib versus docetaxel in a Western population (1% Asians) with confirmed wild-type *EGFR*. The trial demonstrates superiority in terms of PFS and a non statistically significant trend to better OS of docetaxel compared to erlotinib in second line in EGFR wt NSCLC patients (OS 8.2 months in the docetaxel group versus 5.4 months in the erlotinib group. HR0.73; p= 0.05). Again, response and disease control rates in the erlotinib group were 3 and 23%, respectively. A similar study conducted in Japan (DELTA) [34] failed to show superiority in terms of PFS of erlotinib compared to docetaxel in a second- or third-line setting. In the subgroup of *EGFR* wild-type patients, PFS was longer for those patients receiving docetaxel (PFS 2.9 vs 1.3 months for those receiving erlotinib, respectively. HR1.452; p= 0.01).

Table 2. Relevant second and third-line phase III trials

Trial (Ref.)	Year	N	Regimens	Mutational status (%)	PE	Efficacy in OP	Subgroup analysis
BR.21 [7]	2005	731	E vs. P	34 of 204 avl. (16.7%)	OS	6.7mo vs. 4.7mo p<0.001	EGFR mutated: OS HR, 0.55; EGFR wt OS HR, 0.74; interaction p=0.47
ISEL [27]	2005	1,692	G vs. P	26 of 215 avl. (12.1%)	OS	5.6mo vs. 5.1mo p=0.089	NR
INTERES T [29]	2008	1,433	G vs. D	44 of 297 avl. (14.8%)	OS	7.6mo vs. 8mo *	EGFR mutated: OS HR, 0.83; EGFR wt: OS HR, 1.02; interaction p=0.59
TITAN [31]	2012	424	E vs. D/Pem	18 of 167 avl. (10.8%)	OS	5.3mo vs. 5.5mo p=0.073	EGFR mutated: OS HR, 1.19; EGFR wt: OS HR 0.85
HORG [32]	2013	368	E vs. Pem	11 of 123 avl. (8.9%)	TTP	3.9mo vs. 3mo *p=0.195*	NR

Ref., reference in text; ADC, adenocarcinoma; C, cisplatin; Cb, carboplatin; D, docetaxel; E, erlotinib; EGFR, epidermal growth factor receptor; G, gefitinib; Gem, gemcitabine; HR, hazard ratio; NR, not reported; OS, median overall survival; TTP: time to tumor progression; P, placebo; Pem, pemetrexed; PFS, median progression free survival; T, paclitaxel; wt, wild type; avl., Available.
*Study designed to detect non-inferiority in both arms. The results met the non-inferiority criteria.

A Chinese randomized phase II trial in wild-type *EGFR* patients previously treated with platinum-based chemotherapy compared the administration of gefitinib with that of pemetrexed. PFS was significantly longer in the pemetrexed group compared to the gefitinib group (4.8 vs 1.6 months, respectively. HR 0.54 $p < 0.001$) [35]. Like in the previous study, some benefit was observed in the gefitinib group (ORR of 2.4% and disease stabilization of 12.2%). In most situations, treatment in the second- and third-line setting in patients with advanced NSCLC provides limited benefit. The main interest in using *EGFR*-TKI in this context is route of administration, manageable toxicity and benefit in quality of life in comparison with chemotherapy in patients that may present poor PS. As presented above, chemotherapy is clearly superior in first line for *EGFR* wild-type patients and marginally superior in second-line. However, there is consistent data of a clinically significant benefit from *EGFR-TKI*s observed in unselected or *EGFR* wild-type patients, with response rates reaching 8% in some studies and disease control rates around 25%. It is clear that further studies are needed to better determine which patients, *EGFR*-mutants aside, will benefit from *EGFR* inhibition.

In the next section, the possible mechanisms related to *EGFR*-TKI treatment benefit in *EGFR* wild-type NSCLC patients will be reviewed.

6. Biological Evidence for *EGFR* Inhibition in EGFR Wild-Type NSCLC

The EGFR (HER1) belongs to a family of receptors with a common architecture (HER2, 3 and 4). These receptors have an extracellular ligand binding portion, a single transmembrane helix and an intracellular tyrosin kinase domain and C-terminal tail that serve as a scaffold for adapter molecules. A variety of EGFR ligands, mainly amphyregulin, TGFalpha and EGF, upon binding, drive the formation of homo- or heterodimers that activate the receptors and amplify their signal. In cancer cells, the phosphorylation of the tyrosine kinase domain eventually results in the recruitment of intracellular substrates and binding of adaptor molecules that activate downstream signalling pathways. One of the major signalling pathways downstream *EGFR* is the Ras- Raf-MAP kinase route. Another important target of the *EGFR* signalling is the PI3K-Akt pathway. Finally, *EGFR* activation also recruits PKC and Jak/Stat. The activation of these pathways induces transcriptional programs that result in increased proliferation, survival, motility, and invasion [36].

Several mechanisms have been postulated as alternative ways of activation of the EGFR pathway.

6.1. Overexpression of EGFR Ligands

Eleven ligands have been reported to bind to the HER/ErbB receptor family including EGF, transforming growth factor alpha (TGFa), amphiregulin, betacellulin, heparin-binding EGF and epiregulin. These are synthesized as membrane-anchored precursor forms that are then cleaved to generate soluble ligands. In some cases, these membrane-anchored isoforms can also act as biologically active ligands. Moreover, stromal cells have been described to release amphiregulin and TGFa. Thus activation of *EGFR* by its ligands can happen through paracrine, autocrine and juxtacrine mechanisms. Upon binding, they induce a conformational change in the receptor and activate several signalling pathways (see above) [36].

Various preclinical studies in NSCLC cell lines have been conducted to investigate the status of these ligands and their relationship to *EGFR*-TKI resonse. Fujimoto et al. detected high expression of HER/ErbB family members and their ligands in gefitinib sensitive cells [37]. Yonesaka et al. found an association between high levels of amphiregulin (Areg) and response to gefitinib. High levels of Areg, acting through autocrine signalling and thus increasing *EGFR* dimerization and activation, were predictors of sensitivity to gefitinib. Treatment with this agent induced cell cycle arrest in these cells, preferentially by inhibition of Extracellular signal-reculated kinases (ERK) 1 and 2, but not by Akt phosphorylation. In the same study, immunohistochemical analysis of tumor specimens from erlotinib and/or gefitinib treated patients revealed a significant association between high Areg staining and stable disease after *EGFR-TKI* treatment (p= 0.028) [38].

Conversely, several studies reached the opposite conclusion, and found that high Areg levels could be associated with resistance to gefitinib [39-41]. Areg expression was found to prevent activation of the proapoptotic protein BAX in the presence of gefitinib, thus interfering with its apoptotic effect. Transfection of recombinant Areg to a gefitinib-sensitive cell line (H322) rendered it resistant to gefitinib treatment. Furthermore, Areg inhibition through anti-Areg siRNA restored gefitinib sensitivity in a previously resistant cell line (H358) in vitro and in vivo [39]. Another study by the same authors [40] revealed the ability of Areg to reduce acetylation of ku70, thus allowing this protein to sequester and inactivate BAX. Moreover, efficacy of the combination of gefitinib with vorinostat (a histone deacetylase inhibitor) was shown in an in vivo murine model.

In a retrospective analysis of tumor samples from *EGFR* wild-type patients treated with *EGFR-TKI*s (erlotinib or gefitinib), Chang et al. [42] studied the differences in Areg expression determined by immunohistochemistry, using a previously described H-score method [43] and a cut-off value established in the study by Yonesaka et al. [38]. Patients with an Areg expression H-score of more than 100 (Areg positive) had longer OS than those Areg negative patients (p= 0.012).

Other studies have focused on detecting serum levels of circulating EGFR ligands, as they may be valid surrogate markers of intratumor ligand-EGFR interaction intensity.

Two Japanese studies found that low serum Areg and/or low serum TGF-alfa were favourable prognostic factors in patients receiving gefitinib [44, 45]. Interestingly however, these results were not reproduced in a Dutch study, where high levels of serum Areg were found to be predictive of benefit with *EGFR*-TKI treatment [46]. An additional study of tumor samples from the BR.21 trial identified high circulating Areg levels as an independent unfavourable prognostic factor (HR1.88; p= 0.0002), although not predictive of response to erlotinib. Conversely, high TGF-alfa levels predicted lack of benefit from erlotinib (p= 0.04), but had no prognostic value [47].

6.2. Other Members of the HER/ErbB Family

Upon ligand stimulation, *EGFR* forms homodimers or heterodimers with the other HER family members [48]. Several studies have been published demonstrating the importance of the status of other EGFR family members in response to *EGFR-TKI*s. HER2 is overexpressed in various cancers through gene amplification that constitutively activates the protein. As briefly exposed above, HER3 expression has also been associated with sensitivity to *EGFR-TKI*s. HER3 is unique among the HER/ErbB family members because it lacks significant tyrosin kinase activity. However, it heterodimerizes with others members of the family and couples to the PI3K/Akt pathway, initiating intracellular signalling pathway. *HER2* amplification and overexpression has been reported in NSCLC, although their prognostic significance remains unclear [49, 50]. *HER2* mutations have been reported in 1.7-9.8% of NSCLC patients. Mutations consist of in-frame insertions in exon 20, leading to constituve activation of the kinase domain. They are usually not associated with gene amplification, protein overexpression or *EGFR* mutations. In a retrospective analysis of HER2-mutant NSCLC patients reported by Mazières et al. four patients were treated with Afatinib, all of them reaching disease control [51, 52].

In preclinical cell models, *HER2* activating mutations have been reported to be predictive of resistance to gefitinib, while rendering the cell sensitive to HER2 inhibition to agents such as lapatinib or trastuzumab. Sensitivity to *EGFR*-TKI was regained through knockdown of mutant *HER2* in H1781 lung cancer cells [53].

Conversely, *HER2* gene copy number gain has been reported to predict sensitivity to *EGFR*-TKI in a large panel of NSCLC cell lines [54]. Furthermore, in *EGFR*-positive (determined by immunohistochemistry and FISH) NSCLC patients, *HER2* high copy number was associated with better ORR and higher disease control rate with gefitinib compared to those with low or no gain [55].

Ise et al. have reported the antiproliferative effects of gefitinib and erlotinib cell lines overexpressing *HER2* but not *EGFR*, through decrease in Akt phosphorylation [56]. Transfection of HER2 cDNA to NSCLC cell lines augmented their sensitivity to gefitinib in a study by Hirata and colleagues [57], diminishing Akt phosphorylation through inhibition of HER2/HER3 dimer formation and HER3 phosphorylation. In a study by Amman et al. cell lines that overexpressed HER2 and were sensitive to both erlotinib and gefitinib, presented also high HER3 expression [58]. Thus, the role of HER3 expression in mediating *EGFR*-TKI sensitivity of HER2-overexpressing NSCLC remains to be elucidated.

Downregulation of PI3K/Akt pathway through HER3 inhibition has been described as a growth inhibitory mechanism of gefitinib in wild-type NSCLC cell lines [59], and HER3 expression seems to mediate erlotinib sensitivity in pancreatic and colorectal cancer cell lines [60, 61]. In the clinical setting, a study by Cappuzzo et al. reported a higher benefit from gefitinib treatment in terms of PFS in patients whose tumors had HER3 overexpression. This benefit was more important in patients that had also *EGFR* overexpression ("*HER3*-positive" and "*EGFR*-positive" as defined by FISH criteria) [62].

Mutations in the receptor ligand binding and the tyrosine kinase domains of HER4 have been detected in lung adenocarcinoma cells [63], as well as protein overexpression, which can be found alone or co-expressed with other receptors of the *EGFR*-family [64]. In a panel of lung cancer cell lines, a somatic mutation in *HER4* was detected in a gefitinib-resistant cell line with squamous histology [54]. There is still insufficient data to establish a link between *HER4* mutation and/or overexpression and sensitivity to *EGFR*-TKIs.

Globally, it seems that HER family receptors' status has an impact in the response of wild-type *EGFR* lung cancer to *EGFR-TKI*s. Although clinical data are not mature it seems that combination of *EGFR-TKI*s with other receptor inhibitors or the use of panHER inhibitors could be a promising strategy for the treatment of patients with activation of the HER family members.

6.3. Epithelial to Mesenchymal Transition (EMT)

Epithelial-to-mesenchymal transition (EMT) is a cellular process that enables cells to migrate and invade surrounding tissues. This phenomenon is essential for a normal embryogenesis [65]. However, it has also been observed in carcinogenesis, providing cancer cells the ability to be locally invasive and to generate distant metastases [66]. For the loss of cell polarity and acquisition of an invasive phenotype, epithelial cells must abandon their attachment to the surrounding tissue and cells. Therefore, one of the initial features observed in EMT is loss of protein E-cadherin, which is a major constituent in adhesive cell-to-cell junctions [65, 66].

This transition is initiated a the transcriptional level by Snail1, a transcriptional factor that is key for the induction of EMT, which will be later maintained by other transcriptional factors such as Zeb1 and 2 [67]. Expression of markers such as vimentin, fibronectin or N-cadherin is characteristic of a mesenchymal phenotype, while expression of E-cadherin and/or proteins of the catenin family (α, β, γ, and/or δ) usually appertain to cells with an epithelial phenotype [65, 68]. Several studies in different tumor models have identified EMT as an unfavourable prognostic factor, as predictor of chemoresistance and sensitivity to EGFR-TKI [69-74].

In a panel of NSCLC cell lines, Yauch and colleagues detected that the concentrations of erlotinib necessary to inhibit growth were lower in those cell lines expressing an epithelial phenotype compared to those that had a mesenchymal phenotype [69]. Consistent with the previous findings, Thomson et al. found an association between overexpression of fibronectin and/or vimentin and resistance to erlotinib in vitro and in vivo. Moreover, erlotinib-sensitive cell lines expressed no or little of these proteins and, interestingly, showed high expression of E-cadherin [70].

Two studies with similar design that included cells of different lineages (NSCLC, Head and Neck Squamous Cell Carcinoma and Hepatoma cell lines) reached equivalent conclusions using gefitinib [72, 73]. Interestingly, gefitinib sensitivity was more strongly related to cellular phenotype (epithelial or mesenchymal) than to tumor origin [72]. In the gene expression analysis, gefitinib-sensitive NSCLC and Head and Neck Squamous Cell Carcinoma cell lines clustered together, as did the insensitive counterparts.

In the previously mentioned study by Yauch et al. [69], an immunohistochemical analysis of tumor specimens from a subset of patients participating in the TRIBUTE trial (see above) [13] was performed, evaluating levels of cellular E-cadherin staining and dividing patients in E-cadherin positive and –negative. No statistically significant differences between the two groups were found in terms of ORR and OS. Interestingly however, in E-cadherin-positive patients, receiving the combination of erlotinib plus chemotherapy was associated with a statistically significant difference in time to progression compared to receiving chemotherapy alone (34 vs 19.3 weeks, respectively; p= 0.003) [69]. A similar retrospective analysis performed onm the participants of the BATTLE trial. Of twenty patients with wild-type *EGFR* and *KRAS* who received erlotinib, those who reached disease control at 8 weeks of treatment (the primary endpoint of the study) presented with a more epithelial phenotype (defined by a 76-gene signature) compared to those that without disease control, although this difference was of borderline significance [75].

Several studies have attempted to explore the interrelation of EMT and the *EGFR* pathway. Cells sensitive to *EGFR*-TKIs with an epithelial phenotype have been reported to show *EGFR* and HER3 overexpression [70]. In contrast, expression and phosphorylation of *EGFR* family members is decreased in cell lines with a mesenchymal phenotype. Thus, mesenchymal-like cells are capable to maintain their proliferative potential independently of *EGFR*-pathway signalling [74]. Indeed, an EMT-like state reached through TGF-beta stimulation in the H358 NSCLC cell line showed *EGFR*-independent activation of the Mek-Erk pathway through acquired platelet-derived growth factor receptor (PDGFR) and fibroblast growth factor receptor (FGFR) expression and signalling. These cells were resistant to *EGFR* inhibition, but responded to pharmacological inhibition of *PDGFR* and *FGFR* [74].

Integrin-linked kinase (ILK) is a serine/threonine protein kinase localized at the focal adhesion that is stimulated by growth factor and extracellular matrices and interacts with the cytoplasmic domains of beta1 and beta3 integrins, mediating many signalling pathways between the cell and its environment [76]. It is essential in for embryonic development and its overexpression inhibits E-cadherin expression, thus inducing an epithelial-to-mesenchymal transition [77]. Increased expression of ILK has been reported in hepatoma cell lines that presented a mesenchymal-like phenotype. Moreover, inactivation of ILK in these cells induced a transition to a more epithelial-like phenotype and increased their sensitivity to *EGFR* inhibition in vivo [73]. In a retrospective study of 134 Japanese patients with Stage IA-IIIA resected NSCLC, ILK expression was a prognostic factor for survival (p=0.02) [78].

Acquisition of *PDGFR* and *FGFR* has been described as another way for mesenchymal-like NSCLC cells to maintain survival independent of *EGFR* activity. In a study with 14 NSCLC cell lines, both epithelial and mesenchymal-like cells showed expression of PDGF ligands. However, expression of *PDGFR*-alfa and -beta was only detected in mesenchymal-like cells. In this study, *EGFR* blockade by erlotinib showed increased *PDGFR* autophosphorylation and downstream activation in mesenchymal-like cells. Similar findings were detected in regard to *FGFR* and FGF-ligands expression and activity. Interestingly, in a cell line that underwent an epithelial-to-mesenchymal-like transition induced by TGF-beta stimulation, increased levels of *PDGFR*, PDGF-ligands, *FGFR*, FGF-ligands and transcription factors such as Snail, Zeb1 and Zeb2 were detected, along with a significant decrease in erlotinib-sensitivity. Treatment of this cell line with a TGF-beta receptor inhibitor reversed this process and re-sensitized the cells to erlotinib [73].

Hystone deacetylases (HDAC) are key participants of the epigenetic changes that lead to gene expression or repression. This family of enzimes is specialized in catalysing the removal of acetyl groups from lysine residues in histones, which ultimately leads to chromatin condensation and gene silencing. Through this mechanism they have been described as inducers of differentiation or apoptosis in tumor cells [79], and have been recognized as promising targets in cancer therapeutics [80]. Snail mediates E-cadherin repression through HDAC recruitment, and treatment with Trychostatin A (a known HDAC inhibitor) restored E-cadherin expression in preclinical studies [81].

E-cadherin expression and its association with *EGFR*-TKI sensitivity is mentioned above. In an elegant study, Witta et al. demonstrated increased antitumoral activity of gefitinib in previously resistant NSCLC cell lines after transfection of E-cadherin. Furthermore, resistant cells that were subject to treatment with the histone deacetylase inhibitor MS-275 (Entinostat) showed an increase in *EGFR* expression, and 4 previously resistant NSCLC cell lines showed increased sensitivity to gefitinib after pretreatment with MS-275. Remarkably, in one cell line, inhibitory effect of MS-275 plus gefitinib was similar to gefitinib alone in a cell line with known *EGFR* exon 21 L858R mutation [71]. On the basis of these findings, a recent phase II randomized study in unselected previously treated patients with advanced NSCLC compared administration of erlonib + entinostat versus erlotinib + placebo. In the overall study population, no benefit in PFS was observed between groups. However, a planned subgroup analysis in those patients harbouring E-cadherin-positive tumors (defined by immunohistochemistry), showed higher OS for those who had received the combination (median OS 9.4 months vs. 5.4 months, respectively; HR 0.35; p= 0.03) [82]. Thus, it seems that addition of an histone deacetylase inhibitor to an anti-*EGFR* would only be beneficial before cells have acquired a mesenchymal phenotype, being more effective in preventing *EGFR* resistance rather than reversing it.

6.4. Gene Signatures

In an effort to improve the ability to select patients who will potentially benefit from *EGFR-TKI* treatment, several studies set out to identify different gene expression profiles that would correlate with susceptibility to *EGFR* inhibition. In this direction, Kakiuchi et al. described a 12 gene signature obtained from NSCLC biopsy samples of patients treated with gefitinib.

Based on this, the investigators designed a scoring system capable to discriminate between responders and non-responders to gefitinib and validated it by semi-quantitative PCR and immunohistochemistry. Also in this study, serum Areg levels from an independent cohort of NSCLC patients were obtained and analysed. Non-responders to gefitinib showed higher serum Areg levels. These findings were validated in an in Vitro model, concluding that Areg high levels might inhibit apoptosis induced by gefitinib [83]. In a cohort of previously treated NSCLC patients, Tan et al. failed to identifying a gene expression profile that would predict clinical benefit from erlotinib [84].

Using a different approach, Balko et al. [85] obtained a gene expression pattern form NSCLC cell lines based on more than 150 genes, which correctly predicted erlotinib sensitivity. These findings were further validated in NSCLC tumor samples. Coldren et al. [86] conducted a similar study with gefitinib.

In both studies, genes included in the signature were representative of increased *EGFR* downstream signalling activation. Hence, cell lines harbouring the T790M mutation were classified as "sensitive" using this method, although further experiments confirmed their resistance. Therefore, until more accurate techniques step forward, screening of *EGFR* mutations remains capital in determining EGFR-TKI sensitivity.

The clear advantage of this approach is that the look at the complexity of the tumour can be addressed evaluating multiple genes simultaneously that may be involved in the behaviour of a particular tumour.

However, in the intent to limit the number of genes to be used in a platform we are probably leaving out genes that are more relevant that the ones we include. Further validation in human samples of patients treated with these drugs is warranted to take this approach further.

6.5. MicroRNAs

MicroRNAs are regulatory RNAs that are responsible for posttranscriptional gene silencing by degrading the mRNA or preventing its translation. Studies on expression of these miRNA signatures have revealed interesting data regarding association of miRNAs to sensitivity to *EGFR*-TKIs.

Using a panel of cell lines derived from different histologic subtipes (pancreatic, lung and colorectal cancer), Bryant et al. [87] identified a miRNA expression pattern that correlated with erlotinib sensitivity. Furthermore, expression of miRNAs represented in this signature was implicated with epithelial-to-mesenchymal transition (EMT, see above). Different individual miRNAs have been related to *EGFR*-TKI sensitivity. Overexpression of miR-146a [88], miR-7 [89], and miR-200c[90] have been described as predictors of *EGFR*-TKI sensitivity in cell line models, and have been proposed as prognostic biomarkers. In the World Conference on Lung Cancer 2013, Li et al. presented a study that demonstrated a relation between loss of miR-200c, consequent loss of epithelial phenotype and lack of response to *EGFR*-TKI in *EGFR* wild type cells. In this study, these findings were validated in tumor samples from NSCLC patients [91].

Recently, a study by the Catalan Institute of Oncology [92] reported the effects of silibinin, a compound isolated from a plant extract (*Sylibum marianum*), in reversing EMT-mediated resistance to erlotinib through alteration of miR-200c levels. Orally administered single-agent Silibinin showed growth inhibitory activity in erlotinib-resistant tumor xenografts. Furthermore, silibinin induced a mesenchymal-to-epithelial transition through increase in miR-200c expression and decrease of transcription factors such as Zeb1 and proteins such as N-Cadherin. Growth inhibitory effect of erlotinib + sibilinin was higher than that of each treatment alone.

6.6. Proteomics

Attempts have been made to develop blood tests that would predict response to EGFR-TKI treatment. Development of a serum-based method used in mass spectrometry and based on soft ionization techniques, usually used in biochemistry and with applications in clinical microbiology, led to commercialization of VeriStrat®. Briefly, VeriStrat® is a test that uses matrix-assisted laser desorption ionization on a time-of-flight mass spectrometer (MALDI-TOF) to detect and analyse proteins present in patients plasma or serum. Using serum samples from patients who would later be treated with gefitinib, a MALDI-TOF analysis was used to differentiate patients with different outcomes, with the intention to identify a valid and non-invasive predictive marker for EGFR-TKI benefit. The result was a binary classification of the patients (VeriStrat Good vs VeriStrat Poor) based on an 8-peak protein signature that was further validated in independent cohorts retrospectively. Reproducibility of the method was confirmed by performance of the technique at two different institutions, with an observed concordance of 97.1% between results [93]. In two independent cohorts treated with erlotinib and gefitinib classified, patients classified as VeriStrat Good had better outcomes than patients classified as VeriStrat Poor (HR of death 0.47, p= 0.009 and HR of death 0.33, p= 0.0007). This classification did not predict outcome of patients that were not treated with EGFR-TKIs [93]. More recently, in a study using pre-treatment plasma samples of patients participating in the BR.21 trial (explained above), patients classified as Good had a significantly higher response rate than Poor patients (11.5% vs. 1.1%, p= 0.002), and Good classification remained significantly associated with response after adjusting for possible confounding factors. However, regarding PFS and OS, the classification had prognostic, but failed to show predictive value for benefit from erlotinib [94]. Finally, preliminary data from a prosective study (PROSE) using Veristrat classification have been recently presented, showing that VeriStrat Poor patients who receive erlotinib have worse outcomes than tose that receive chemotherapy [95].

Conclusion

In current literature, there is clear evidence of a moderate but significant benefit from EGFR-TKI treatment in a subset of clinically and molecularly unselected patients, including EGFR wild-type patients. Data are still insufficient as to draw definitive conclusions, but many of the studies presented above offer different approaches to elucidate the biologic mechanisms that might explain the results observed in the clinic. Independently of the method used, these findings seem to converge in that an alteration of tumor dependence on EGFR signaling for growth and proliferation (beyond those who harbor an activating mutation) plays an important role in the susceptibility to these treatments. Interestingly, different ways for tumors to overcome EGFR dependence, based on epigenetic changes and resulting in altered transcription programs (e.g., EMT), are implicated in invasion and metastasis, and thus become potential targets for future treatment development. Further advance in this research will surely contribute to the understanding of carcinogenesis and will undoubtedly be a step forward to personalized cancer medicine.

References

[1] Wheeler DL, Dunn EF, Harari PM. Understanding resistance to EGFR inhibitors-impact on future treatment strategies. *Nat. Rev. Clin. Oncol.* 2010; 7 (9): 493-507.

[2] Lynch TJ, Bell DW, Sordella R, et al. Activating mutations in the epidermal growth factor receptor underlying responsiveness of non-small-cell lung cancer to gefitinib. *N. Engl. J. Med.* 2004; 350 (21): 2129-39.

[3] Maemondo M, Inoue A, Kobayashi K, et al. Gefitinib or chemotherapy for non-small-cell lung cancer with mutated EGFR. *N. Engl. J. Med.* 2010; 362 (25): 2380-8.

[4] Fossella FV, DeVore R, Kerr RN, et al. Randomized phase III trial of docetaxel versus vinorelbine or ifosfamide in patients with advanced non-small-cell lung cancer previously treated with platinum-containing chemotherapy regimens. The TAX 320 Non-Small Cell Lung Cancer Study Group. *J. Clin. Oncol.* 2000; 18 (12): 2354-62.

[5] Shepherd FA, Dancey J, Ramlau R, et al. Prospective randomized trial of docetaxel versus best supportive care in patients with non-small-cell lung cancer previously treated with platinum-based chemotherapy. *J. Clin. Oncol.* 2000; 18 (10): 2095-103.

[6] Hanna N, Shepherd FA, Fossella FV, et al. Randomized phase III trial of pemetrexed versus docetaxel in patients with non-small-cell lung cancer previously treated with chemotherapy. *J. Clin. Oncol.* 2004; 22 (9): 1589-97.

[7] Shepherd FA, Rodrigues Pereira J, Ciuleanu T, et al. Erlotinib in previously treated non-small-cell lung cancer. *N. Engl. J. Med.* 2005; 353 (2): 123-32.

[8] Fukuoka M, Yano S, Giaccone G, et al. Multi-institutional randomized phase II trial of gefitinib for previously treated patients with advanced non-small-cell lung cancer (The IDEAL 1 Trial) [corrected]. *J. Clin. Oncol.* 2003; 21 (12): 2237-46.

[9] Mok TS, Wu YL, Thongprasert S, Yang CH, Chu DT, Saijo N, et al. Gefitinib or carboplatin-paclitaxel in pulmonary adenocarcinoma. *N. Engl. J. Med.* 2009; 361 (10): 947-57.

[10] Rosell R, Carcereny E, Gervais R, et al. Erlotinib versus standard chemotherapy as first-line treatment for European patients with advanced EGFR mutation-positive non-small-cell lung cancer (EURTAC): a multicentre, open-label, randomised phase 3 trial. *Lancet Oncol.* 2012; 13 (3): 239-46.

[11] Lee CK, Brown C, Gralla RJ, et al. Impact of EGFR inhibitor in non-small cell lung cancer on progression-free and overall survival: a meta-analysis. *J. Natl. Cancer Inst.* 2013; 105 (9): 595-605.

[12] Gatzemeier U, Pluzanska A, Szczesna A, et al. Phase III study of erlotinib in combination with cisplatin and gemcitabine in advanced non-small-cell lung cancer: the Tarceva Lung Cancer Investigation Trial. *J. Clin. Oncol.* 2007; 25 (12): 1545-52.

[13] Herbst RS, Prager D, Hermann R, et al. TRIBUTE: a phase III trial of erlotinib hydrochloride (OSI-774) combined with carboplatin and paclitaxel chemotherapy in advanced non-small-cell lung cancer. *J. Clin. Oncol.* 2005; 23 (25): 5892-9.

[14] Giaccone G, Herbst RS, Manegold C, et al. Gefitinib in combination with gemcitabine and cisplatin in advanced non-small-cell lung cancer: a phase III trial--INTACT 1. *J. Clin. Oncol.* 2004; 22 (5): 777-84.

[15] Herbst RS, Giaccone G, Schiller JH, et al. Gefitinib in combination with paclitaxel and carboplatin in advanced non-small-cell lung cancer: a phase III trial--INTACT 2. *J. Clin. Oncol.* 2004; 22 (5): 785-94.

[16] Eberhard DA, Johnson BE, Amler LC, et al. Mutations in the epidermal growth factor receptor and in KRAS are predictive and prognostic indicators in patients with non-small-cell lung cancer treated with chemotherapy alone and in combination with erlotinib. *J. Clin. Oncol.* 2005; 23 (25): 5900-9.

[17] Han JY, Park K, Kim SW, et al. First-SIGNAL: first-line single-agent iressa versus gemcitabine and cisplatin trial in never-smokers with adenocarcinoma of the lung. *J. Clin. Oncol.* 2012; 30 (10): 1122-8.

[18] Gridelli C, Ciardiello F, Gallo C, et al. First-line erlotinib followed by second-line cisplatin-gemcitabine chemotherapy in advanced non-small-cell lung cancer: the TORCH randomized trial. *J. Clin. Oncol.* 2012; 30 (24): 3002-11.

[19] Lilenbaum R, Axelrod R, Thomas S, et al. Randomized phase II trial of erlotinib or standard chemotherapy in patients with advanced non-small-cell lung cancer and a performance status of 2. *J. Clin. Oncol.* 2008; 26 (6): 863-9.

[20] Goss G, Ferry D, Wierzbicki R, et al. Randomized phase II study of gefitinib compared with placebo in chemotherapy-naive patients with advanced non-small-cell lung cancer and poor performance status. *J. Clin. Oncol.* 2009; 27 (13): 2253-60.

[21] Crino L, Cappuzzo F, Zatloukal P, et al. Gefitinib versus vinorelbine in chemotherapy-naive elderly patients with advanced non-small-cell lung cancer (INVITE): a randomized, phase II study. *J. Clin. Oncol.* 2008; 26 (26): 4253-60.

[22] Chen YM, Tsai CM, Fan WC, et al. Phase II randomized trial of erlotinib or vinorelbine in chemonaive, advanced, non-small cell lung cancer patients aged 70 years or older. *J. Thorac. Oncol.* 2012; 7 (2): 412-8.

[23] Cappuzzo F, Ciuleanu T, Stelmakh L, et al. Erlotinib as maintenance treatment in advanced non-small-cell lung cancer: a multicentre, randomised, placebo-controlled phase 3 study. *Lancet Oncol.* 2010; 11 (6): 521-9.

[24] Gaafar RM, Surmont VF, Scagliotti GV, et al. A double-blind, randomised, placebo-controlled phase III intergroup study of gefitinib in patients with advanced NSCLC, non-progressing after first line platinum-based chemotherapy (EORTC 08021/ILCP 01/03). *Eur. J. Cancer.* 2011; 47 (15): 2331-40.

[25] Johnson BE, Kabbinavar F, Fehrenbacher L, et al. ATLAS: Randomized, Double-Blind, Placebo-Controlled, Phase IIIB Trial Comparing Bevacizumab Therapy With or Without Erlotinib, After Completion of Chemotherapy, With Bevacizumab for First-Line Treatment of Advanced Non-Small-Cell Lung Cancer. *J. Clin. Oncol.* 2013; 31 (31): 3926-34.

[26] Zhu CQ, da Cunha Santos G, Ding K, et al. Role of KRAS and EGFR as biomarkers of response to erlotinib in National Cancer Institute of Canada Clinical Trials Group Study BR.21. *J. Clin. Oncol.* 2008; 26 (26): 4268-75.

[27] Thatcher N, Chang A, Parikh P, et al. Gefitinib plus best supportive care in previously treated patients with refractory advanced non-small-cell lung cancer: results from a randomised, placebo-controlled, multicentre study (Iressa Survival Evaluation in Lung Cancer). *Lancet.* 2005; 366 (9496): 1527-37.

[28] Hirsch FR, Varella-Garcia M, Bunn PA, Jr., et al. Molecular predictors of outcome with gefitinib in a phase III placebo-controlled study in advanced non-small-cell lung cancer. *J. Clin. Oncol.* 2006; 24 (31): 5034-42.

[29] Kim ES, Hirsh V, Mok T, et al. Gefitinib versus docetaxel in previously treated non-small-cell lung cancer (INTEREST): a randomised phase III trial. *Lancet.* 2008; 372 (9652): 1809-18.

[30] Douillard JY, Shepherd FA, Hirsh V, et al. Molecular predictors of outcome with gefitinib and docetaxel in previously treated non-small-cell lung cancer: data from the randomized phase III INTEREST trial. *J. Clin. Oncol.* 2010; 28 (5): 744-52.

[31] Ciuleanu T, Stelmakh L, Cicenas S, et al. Efficacy and safety of erlotinib versus chemotherapy in second-line treatment of patients with advanced, non-small-cell lung cancer with poor prognosis (TITAN): a randomised multicentre, open-label, phase 3 study. *Lancet Oncol.* 2012; 13 (3): 300-8.

[32] Karampeazis A, Voutsina A, Souglakos J, et al. Pemetrexed versus erlotinib in pretreated patients with advanced non-small cell lung cancer: a Hellenic Oncology Research Group (HORG) randomized phase 3 study. *Cancer.* 2013; 119 (15): 2754-64.

[33] Garassino MC, Martelli O, Broggini M, et al. Erlotinib versus docetaxel as second-line treatment of patients with advanced non-small-cell lung cancer and wild-type EGFR tumours (TAILOR): a randomised controlled trial. *Lancet Oncol.* 2013; 14 (10): 981-8.

[34] Okano Y AM, Asami K, Fukuda M, et al. Randomized phase III trial of erlotinib (E) versus docetaxel (D) as second- or third-line therapy in patients with advanced non-

small cell lung cancer (NSCLC) who have wild-type or mutant epidermal growth factor receptor (EGFR): Docetaxel and Erlotinib Lung Cancer Trial (DELTA). ASCO: *J. Clin. Oncol.;* 2013; (suppl; abstr 8006).

[35] Zhou Q CY, Zhao M, Yang J, et al. Final results of CTONG 0806: a phase II trial comparing pemetrexed with gefitinib as second-line treatment of advanced non-squamous NSCLC patients with wild-type EGFR. *World Conference of Lung Cancer;* Sydney 2013.

[36] Hynes NE, Lane HA. ERBB receptors and cancer: the complexity of targeted inhibitors. *Nat. Rev. Cancer.* 2005; 5 (5): 341-54.

[37] Fujimoto N, Wislez M, Zhang J, Iet al. High expression of ErbB family members and their ligands in lung adenocarcinomas that are sensitive to inhibition of epidermal growth factor receptor. *Cancer Res.* 2005; 65 (24): 11478-85.

[38] Yonesaka K, Zejnullahu K, Lindeman N, et al. Autocrine production of amphiregulin predicts sensitivity to both gefitinib and cetuximab in EGFR wild-type cancers. *Clin. Cancer Res.* 2008; 14 (21): 6963-73.

[39] Busser B, Sancey L, Josserand V, et al. Amphiregulin promotes BAX inhibition and resistance to gefitinib in non-small-cell lung cancers. *Mol. Ther.* 2010; 18 (3): 528-35.

[40] Busser B, Sancey L, Josserand V, et al. Amphiregulin promotes resistance to gefitinib in nonsmall cell lung cancer cells by regulating Ku70 acetylation. *Mol. Ther.* 2010; 18 (3): 536-43.

[41] Liu X, Carlisle DL, Swick MC, Gaither-Davis A, Grandis JR, Siegfried JM. Gastrin-releasing peptide activates Akt through the epidermal growth factor receptor pathway and abrogates the effect of gefitinib. *Exp. Cell Res.* 2007; 313 (7): 1361-72.

[42] Chang MH, Ahn HK, Lee J, et al. Clinical impact of amphiregulin expression in patients with epidermal growth factor receptor (EGFR) wild-type nonsmall cell lung cancer treated with EGFR-tyrosine kinase inhibitors. *Cancer.* 2010; 117 (1): 143-51.

[43] Cappuzzo F, Hirsch FR, Rossi E, et al. Epidermal growth factor receptor gene and protein and gefitinib sensitivity in non-small-cell lung cancer. *J. Natl. Cancer Inst.* 2005; 97 (9): 643-55.

[44] Ishikawa N, Daigo Y, Takano A, et al. Increases of amphiregulin and transforming growth factor-alpha in serum as predictors of poor response to gefitinib among patients with advanced non-small cell lung cancers. *Cancer Res.* 2005; 65 (20): 9176-84.

[45] Masago K, Fujita S, Hatachi Y, et al. Clinical significance of pretreatment serum amphiregulin and transforming growth factor-alpha, and an epidermal growth factor receptor somatic mutation in patients with advanced non-squamous, non-small cell lung cancer. *Cancer Sci.* 2008; 99 (11): 2295-301.

[46] Vollebergh MA, Kappers I, Klomp HM, et al. Ligands of epidermal growth factor receptor and the insulin-like growth factor family as serum biomarkers for response to epidermal growth factor receptor inhibitors in patients with advanced non-small cell lung cancer. *J. Thorac. Oncol.* 2010; 5 (12): 1939-48.

[47] Addison CL, Ding K, Zhao H, et al. Plasma transforming growth factor alpha and amphiregulin protein levels in NCIC Clinical Trials Group BR.21. *J. Clin. Oncol.* 2010; 28 (36): 5247-56.

[48] Schlessinger J. Ligand-induced, receptor-mediated dimerization and activation of EGF receptor. *Cell.* 2002; 110 (6): 669-72.

[49] Nakamura H, Saji H, Ogata A, et al. Correlation between encoded protein overexpression and copy number of the HER2 gene with survival in non-small cell lung cancer. *Int. J. Cancer*. 2003; 103 (1): 61-6.
[50] Liu L, Shao X, Gao W, et al. The role of human epidermal growth factor receptor 2 as a prognostic factor in lung cancer: a meta-analysis of published data. *J. Thorac. Oncol.* 2010; 5 (12): 1922-32.
[51] Stephens P, Hunter C, Bignell G, et al. Lung cancer: intragenic ERBB2 kinase mutations in tumours. *Nature*. 2004; 431 (7008): 525-6.
[52] Mazieres J, Peters S, Lepage B, Cet al. Lung cancer that harbors an HER2 mutation: epidemiologic characteristics and therapeutic perspectives. *J. Clin. Oncol.* 2013; 31 (16): 1997-2003.
[53] Wang SE, Narasanna A, Perez-Torres M, et al. HER2 kinase domain mutation results in constitutive phosphorylation and activation of HER2 and EGFR and resistance to EGFR tyrosine kinase inhibitors. *Cancer Cell*. 2006; 10 (1): 25-38.
[54] Gandhi J, Zhang J, Xie Y, et al. Alterations in genes of the EGFR signaling pathway and their relationship to EGFR tyrosine kinase inhibitor sensitivity in lung cancer cell lines. *PLoS One*. 2009; 4 (2): e4576.
[55] Cappuzzo F, Varella-Garcia M, Shigematsu H, et al. Increased HER2 gene copy number is associated with response to gefitinib therapy in epidermal growth factor receptor-positive non-small-cell lung cancer patients. J Clin Oncol. 2005; 23 (22): 5007-18.
[56] Ise N, Omi K, Nambara D, Higashiyama S, Goishi K. Overexpressed HER2 in NSCLC is a possible therapeutic target of EGFR inhibitors. *Anticancer Res.* 2011; 31 (12): 4155-61.
[57] Hirata A, Hosoi F, Miyagawa M, et al. HER2 overexpression increases sensitivity to gefitinib, an epidermal growth factor receptor tyrosine kinase inhibitor, through inhibition of HER2/HER3 heterodimer formation in lung cancer cells. *Cancer Res.* 2005; 65 (10): 4253-60.
[58] Amann J, Kalyankrishna S, Massion PP, et al. Aberrant epidermal growth factor receptor signaling and enhanced sensitivity to EGFR inhibitors in lung cancer. *Cancer Res.* 2005; 65 (1): 226-35.
[59] Engelman JA, Janne PA, Mermel C, et al. ErbB-3 mediates phosphoinositide 3-kinase activity in gefitinib-sensitive non-small cell lung cancer cell lines. *Proc. Natl. Acad. Sci. USA*. 2005; 102 (10): 3788-93.
[60] Frolov A, Schuller K, Tzeng CW, et al. ErbB3 expression and dimerization with EGFR influence pancreatic cancer cell sensitivity to erlotinib. *Cancer Biol. Ther.* 2007; 6 (4): 548-54.
[61] Buck E, Eyzaguirre A, Haley JD, Gibson NW, Cagnoni P, Iwata KK. Inactivation of Akt by the epidermal growth factor receptor inhibitor erlotinib is mediated by HER-3 in pancreatic and colorectal tumor cell lines and contributes to erlotinib sensitivity. *Mol. Cancer Ther.* 2006; 5 (8): 2051-9.
[62] Cappuzzo F, Toschi L, Domenichini I, et al. HER3 genomic gain and sensitivity to gefitinib in advanced non-small-cell lung cancer patients. *Br. J. Cancer*. 2005; 93 (12): 1334-40.
[63] Ding L, Getz G, Wheeler DA, et al. Somatic mutations affect key pathways in lung adenocarcinoma. *Nature*. 2008; 455 (7216): 1069-75.

[64] Bellezza G, Del Sordo R, Colella R, et al. Co-expression of receptors of the HER family correlates with clinical outcome in non-small cell lung cancer (NSCLC). *Virchows Arch.* 2013; 463 (5): 663-71.
[65] Thiery JP. Epithelial-mesenchymal transitions in tumour progression. *Nat. Rev. Cancer.* 2002; 2 (6): 442-54.
[66] De Craene B, Berx G. Regulatory networks defining EMT during cancer initiation and progression. *Nat. Rev. Cancer.* 2013; 13 (2): 97-110.
[67] Garcia de Herreros A, Baulida J. Cooperation, amplification, and feed-back in epithelial-mesenchymal transition. *Biochim. Biophys. Acta.* 2012; 1825 (2): 223-8.
[68] Zeisberg M, Neilson EG. Biomarkers for epithelial-mesenchymal transitions. *J. Clin. Invest.* 2009; 119 (6): 1429-37.
[69] Yauch RL, Januario T, Eberhard DA, et al. Epithelial versus mesenchymal phenotype determines in vitro sensitivity and predicts clinical activity of erlotinib in lung cancer patients. *Clin. Cancer Res.* 2005; 11 (24 Pt 1): 8686-98.
[70] Thomson S, Buck E, Petti F, et al. Epithelial to mesenchymal transition is a determinant of sensitivity of non-small-cell lung carcinoma cell lines and xenografts to epidermal growth factor receptor inhibition. *Cancer Res.* 2005; 65 (20): 9455-62.
[71] Witta SE, Gemmill RM, Hirsch FR, et al. Restoring E-cadherin expression increases sensitivity to epidermal growth factor receptor inhibitors in lung cancer cell lines. *Cancer Res.* 2006; 66 (2): 944-50.
[72] Frederick BA, Helfrich BA, Coldren CD, et al. Epithelial to mesenchymal transition predicts gefitinib resistance in cell lines of head and neck squamous cell carcinoma and non-small cell lung carcinoma. *Mol. Cancer Ther.* 2007; 6 (6): 1683-91.
[73] Fuchs BC, Fujii T, Dorfman JD, et al. Epithelial-to-mesenchymal transition and integrin-linked kinase mediate sensitivity to epidermal growth factor receptor inhibition in human hepatoma cells. *Cancer Res.* 2008; 68 (7): 2391-9.
[74] Thomson S, Petti F, Sujka-Kwok I, Epstein D, Haley JD. Kinase switching in mesenchymal-like non-small cell lung cancer lines contributes to EGFR inhibitor resistance through pathway redundancy. *Clin. Exp. Metastasis.* 2008; 25 (8): 843-54.
[75] Byers LA, Diao L, Wang J, Saintigny P, Girard L, Peyton M, et al. An epithelial-mesenchymal transition gene signature predicts resistance to EGFR and PI3K inhibitors and identifies Axl as a therapeutic target for overcoming EGFR inhibitor resistance. *Clin. Cancer Res.* 2013; 19 (1): 279-90.
[76] Oloumi A, McPhee T, Dedhar S. Regulation of E-cadherin expression and beta-catenin/Tcf transcriptional activity by the integrin-linked kinase. *Biochim. Biophys. Acta.* 2004; 1691 (1): 1-15.
[77] Hannigan G, Troussard AA, Dedhar S. Integrin-linked kinase: a cancer therapeutic target unique among its ILK. *Nat. Rev. Cancer.* 2005; 5 (1): 51-63.
[78] Takanami I. Increased expression of integrin-linked kinase is associated with shorter survival in non-small cell lung cancer. *BMC Cancer.* 2005; 5: 1.
[79] Marks PA, Richon VM, Rifkind RA. Histone deacetylase inhibitors: inducers of differentiation or apoptosis of transformed cells. *J. Natl. Cancer Inst.* 2000; 92 (15): 1210-6.
[80] Bolden JE, Peart MJ, Johnstone RW. Anticancer activities of histone deacetylase inhibitors. *Nature reviews Drug discovery.* 2006; 5 (9): 769-84.

[81] Peinado H, Ballestar E, Esteller M, Cano A. Snail mediates E-cadherin repression by the recruitment of the Sin3A/histone deacetylase 1 (HDAC1)/HDAC2 complex. *Mol. Cell Biol.* 2004; 24 (1): 306-19.
[82] Witta SE, Jotte RM, Konduri K, et al. Randomized phase II trial of erlotinib with and without entinostat in patients with advanced non-small-cell lung cancer who progressed on prior chemotherapy. *J. Clin. Oncol.* 2012; 30 (18): 2248-55.
[83] Kakiuchi S, Daigo Y, Ishikawa N, et al. Prediction of sensitivity of advanced non-small cell lung cancers to gefitinib (Iressa, ZD1839). *Hum. Mol. Genet.* 2004; 13 (24): 3029-43.
[84] Tan EH, Ramlau R, Pluzanska A, Kuo HP, Reck M, Milanowski J, et al. A multicentre phase II gene expression profiling study of putative relationships between tumour biomarkers and clinical response with erlotinib in non-small-cell lung cancer. *Ann. Oncol.* 2010; 21 (2): 217-22.
[85] Balko JM, Potti A, Saunders C, Stromberg A, Haura EB, Black EP. Gene expression patterns that predict sensitivity to epidermal growth factor receptor tyrosine kinase inhibitors in lung cancer cell lines and human lung tumors. *BMC Genomics.* 2006; 7: 289.
[86] Coldren CD, Helfrich BA, Witta SE, et al. Baseline gene expression predicts sensitivity to gefitinib in non-small cell lung cancer cell lines. *Mol. Cancer Res.* 2006; 4 (8): 521-8.
[87] Bryant JL, Britson J, Balko JM, et al. A microRNA gene expression signature predicts response to erlotinib in epithelial cancer cell lines and targets EMT. *Br. J. Cancer.* 2012; 106 (1): 148-56.
[88] Chen G, Umelo IA, Lv S, et al. miR-146a inhibits cell growth, cell migration and induces apoptosis in non-small cell lung cancer cells. *PLoS One.* 2013; 8 (3): e60317.
[89] Kalinowski FC, Giles KM, Candy PA, et al. Regulation of epidermal growth factor receptor signaling and erlotinib sensitivity in head and neck cancer cells by miR-7. *PLoS One.* 2012; 7 (10): e47067.
[90] Ceppi P, Mudduluru G, Kumarswamy R, et al. Loss of miR-200c expression induces an aggressive, invasive, and chemoresistant phenotype in non-small cell lung cancer. Mol Cancer Res. 2010; 8 (9): 1207-16.
[91] Li J LX, Ren S, Chen X, Zhou C. EGFR wild-type NSCLC patients with high miR-200c expression can benefit from EGFR-TKI. *World Conference on Lung Cancer;* Sydney 2013.
[92] Cufi S, Bonavia R, Vazquez-Martin A, et al. Silibinin suppresses EMT-driven erlotinib resistance by reversing the high miR-21/low miR-200c signature in vivo. *Sci. Rep.* 2013; 3: 2459.
[93] Taguchi F, Solomon B, Gregorc V, et al. Mass spectrometry to classify non-small-cell lung cancer patients for clinical outcome after treatment with epidermal growth factor receptor tyrosine kinase inhibitors: a multicohort cross-institutional study. *J. Natl. Cancer Inst.* 2007; 99 (11): 838-46.
[94] Carbone DP, Ding K, Roder H, et al. Prognostic and predictive role of the VeriStrat plasma test in patients with advanced non-small-cell lung cancer treated with erlotinib or placebo in the NCIC Clinical Trials Group BR.21 trial. *J. Thorac. Oncol.* 2012; 7 (11): 1653-60.

[95] Lazzari C NS, Bami S, Aieta M, et al. Randomized proteomic stratified phase III study of second-line erlotinib (E) versus chemotherapy (CT) in patients with inoperable non-small cell lung cancer (PROSE). *J. Clin. Oncol.* 2013; 31 (suppl; abstr LBA8005)).

In: Fighting Lung Cancer through the HER Family ...
Editor: Diego Márquez-Medina
ISBN: 978-1-63321-092-9

Chapter 10

Treatment II. Treatment of Selected Non-Small Cell Lung Cancer Patients

Ramon Palmero
Medical Oncology Department,
Catalan Institute of Oncology of L'Hospitalet, Spain

Abstract

Tyrosine kinase inhibitors directed against the epidermal growth factor receptor (EGFR-TKI) were the first molecular-targeted agents to be approved for the treatment of advanced non-small-cell lung cancer (NSCLC) after failure of chemotherapy. Sensitizing mutations of the *EGFR* increase the efficacy of EGFR-TKI. In *EGFR*-mutant patients, response rate to EGFR-TKIs in exceed 60%, and progression-free survival is prolonged. However, overall survival did not significantly increase probably due to crossed over as post-progression therapy. First, second, and third line therapy, as well as maintenance therapy with EGFR-TKI are reviewed.

1. Introduction

Tyrosine kinase inhibitors directed against the epidermal growth factor receptor (EGFR-TKI) were the first molecular-targeted agents to be approved for the treatment of advanced non-small-cell lung cancer (NSCLC) after failure of chemotherapy. However, tumor response rate (RR) in unselected patients were below 20%, which was similar to standard second-line chemotherapy [1]. Some patient characteristics, such as female gender, East Asian origin, never-smoking, adenocarcinoma histology, and bronchioloalveolar subtype, were early associated with higher RR from treatment with EGFR-TKIs. But the groundbreaking finding was the identification, in such patients, of somatic mutations affecting hot-spots at the kinase domain of the *EGFR* gene [1-3], opening a brand new field of personalized medicine in lung cancer. In this chapter, we briefly review what we have learnt in the last ten years of therapeutic research in this setting.

2. Overall Response Rate

During the first year after the identification of the *EGFR* sensitizing mutations, several case series of patients of both Asian and Caucasian origin confirmed that the majority of *EGFR* mutated patients cluster among gefitinib or erlotinib responding patients (Table 1). This initially led to a first generation of single-arm clinical studies, from which we learnt that the tumor RR to EGFR-TKIs in patients with *EGFR*-mutant tumors consistently exceed 60%, higher than previously reported for chemotherapy in unselected NSCLC patients (Table 2). Recent data from randomized clinical trials have confirmed this striking antitumor activity, with overall RR ranging from 56% to 85% (Table 3).

Table 1. EGFR gene mutation rate among responders and non-responders to gefitinib and erlotinib treatment in NSCLC patients

Study characteristics				EGFR gene mutation rate	
Study	**TKI**	**N**	**Ethnic origin**	**Responders**	**Non-responders**
Lynch et al. (2004) [1]	Gefitinib	16^{s}	Caucasian	8/9	0/7
Paez et al. (2004) [2]	Gefitinib	9^{s}	Caucasian	5/5	0/4
Pao et al. (2004) [3]	Gefitinib	24^{s}	Caucasian	9/12	0/12
Pao et al. (2004) [3]	Erlotinib	36^{s}	Caucasian	8/10	0/26
Huang et al. (2004) [4]	Gefitinib	16^{c}	Chinese	7/9	1/7
Amann et al. (2005) [5]	Gefitinib	3^{s}	Caucasian	3/3	0
Han et al. (2005) [6]	Gefitinib	90^{c}	Korean	11/21	6/69
Mitsudomi et al. (2005) [7]	Gefitinib	59^{c}	Japanese	24/26	5/24
Kim et al. (2005) [8]	Gefitinib	27^{c}	Korean	6/8	0/19
Tokumo et al. (2005) [9]	Gefitinib	21^{c}	Japanese	8/10	1/11
Chou et al. (2005) [10]	Gefitinib	54^{c}	Chinese	17/21	6/16
Mu et al. (2005) [11]	Gefitinib	22^{c}	Chinese	7/7	3/15
Cortes-Funes et al. (2005) [12]	Gefitinib	83^{c}	Caucasian	6/10	4/66
Cappuzzo et al. (2005) [13]	Gefitinib	89^{c}	Caucasian	8/15	7/74
Takano et al. (2005) [14]	Gefitinib	66^{c}	Japanese	32/35	7/31
Tsao et al. (2005) [15]	Erlotinib	100^{c}	Caucasian	3/9	16/91

Table 2. Tumor RR to EGFR-TKIs in prospective single-arm trials with patients harboring EGFR mutations

Study	*n*	EGFR mut (*n*)	TKI	RR (%)	TTP (months)
Inoue et al. (2009) [16]	99	16	Gefitinib	75	9.7
Rosell et al. (2009) [17]	2,105	350	Erlotinib	71	14
Tamura et al. (2008) [18]	118	32	Gefitinib	75	NA
Sutani et al. (2006) [19]	100	38	Gefitinib	78	9.4
Sequist et al. (2007) [20]	98	31	Gefitinib	55	11.4

3. Progression-Free Survival

Following the initial observation of these unprecedented RR for lung cancer, the second breakthrough was the possibility of achieve long-term progression-free survival (PFS). A literature-based pooled analysis compiling data from retrospective and prospective trials published before June 2009 compared PFS between EGFR-TKI and chemotherapy in NSCLC with *EGFR* mutations [21]. A total of 54 studies were included: 12 evaluated erlotinib (365 patients), 39 evaluated gefitinib (1069 patients) and 9 evaluated chemotherapy (375 patients). In this hypothesis-generating analysis, patients with *EGFR*-mutated NSCLC appear to have a significantly longer PFS both treated with erlotinib (13.2 months) and gefitinib (9.8 months) than with cytotoxic chemotherapy (5.9 months).

All this compelling body of data showing high and durable antitumor activity of EGFR-TKIs in NSCLC patients harbouring *EGFR* sensitizing mutations led to the comparison of EGFR-TKIs with standard platinum-based chemotherapy in the first-line setting. Eight randomized controlled trials have been conducted, with two different strategies in their design (Table 3).

The first two trials, IPASS and FIRST-SIGNAL, included patients selected by *clinical* criteria previously associated with higher probability of carrying *EGFR* mutation: Asian ethnicity, adenocarcinoma histology, and light or never-smoking. Patients were randomly assigned to receive first-line gefinitib or platinum-based standard chemotherapy. And both studies showed similar results. In the subset of patients (261/42 out of 437/96 tested) with *EGFR* sensitizing mutations, PFS was significantly higher in the gefitinib arm. By contrast, in patients with *EGFR* wild type tumors, PFS was higher in the chemotherapy arm. Therefore, patient selection for EGFR-TKI should be based on *EGFR* mutation status rather than on clinical parameters. The importance of biomarker selection has been further confirmed by six other randomized studies with a *molecularly* selected population of 1450 patients, all of them with *EGFR* sensitizing mutations. Three different EGFR-TKIs (gefitinib, erlotinib and afatinib) were compared to 4 to 6 cycles of five different platinum-doublets (cis- or carbo- with paclitaxel, gemcitabine or pemetrexed). All but one trial (EURTAC) were conducted in East Asian populations. And all six trials consistently showed for EGFR-TKIs significantly higher RR and longer PFS than chemotherapy. Median PFS ranged from 9.2 to 13.1 months, which largely exceed what had been previously achieved with first-line platinum-based chemotherapy. Currently, EGFR-TKIs are the standard first-line therapy for patients with known activating mutations in the *EGFR* gene.

4. Overall Survival: Updated Trials

Overall survival (OS) has been the key endpoint for regulatory approval of standard cytotoxic chemotherapy in advanced-stage NSCLC, given the limited benefit in survival in any line of treatment. But arrival of personalized medicine poses a new challenge for clinicians and regulators. Benefit of targeted therapies can be independent of the line of therapy. For instance, the Spanish Lung Adenocarcinoma DataBase Study (SLADB) enrolled 217 *EGFR* mutated patients to receive erlotinib, regardless of the previous treatment received.

There were no differences in overall RR, PFS and OS between patients treated at first-line, second- line or third-line therapy.

Mature survival data are available in five of the eight randomized clinical trials of first-line EGFR-TKI versus chemotherapy listed in Table 3 [30-33]. And despite the clear benefit on RR and PFS, and after encouraging median OS over 2 years, none of these trials has found any significant difference in OS. The most argued explanation has been the large numbers of patients in the chemotherapy arms that crossed over to EGFR-TKI as post-progression therapy. Given the potential benefit of molecularly-targeted therapies, it would be unethical not to allow patients to cross over from the control arm to the experimental molecular-targeted drug group upon disease progression. In these trials, more than a half of the patients randomized to first-line chemotherapy received an EGFR-TKI as the second-line therapy. With such a portion of patients crossed over to the study group, overall survival will likely be similar between arms. Therefore, PFS would be the only rational endpoint for an effective targeted therapy. This question has been recently addressed by Lee and colleagues [34] with a meta-analytical approach and reached to similar conclusions. They calculated pooled estimates of treatment efficacy of EGFR-TKIs for the *EGFR* mutation positive subgroup in several randomized clinical trials of EGFR-TKI versus chemotherapy, among others, and found that EGFR-TKIs therapy statistically significantly delays disease progression in *EGFR* mutant patients but has no demonstrable impact on OS.

Table 3. Randomized controlled trials of front-line treatment with EGFR-TKI versus platinum-based chemoterapy in advanced-stage NSCLC patients

Study	**n (EGFRmut)**	**TKI**	**CT**	**ORR (%)**	**Median PFS *months (HR, 95%CI)***	**Median OS *months (HR, 95%CI)***	**Crossover CT-TKI**
IPASS [22]	1217 (261)	Gef	Cb + P	71 vs 47*	9.5 vs 6.3 (0.48, 0.36-0.64*)	21.6 vs 21.9 (1.00, 0.76 - 1.33)	64,3%
First-SIGNAL [23]	309 (42)	Gef	C + G	85 vs 38	8 vs 6.3 (0.54, 0.27-1.10, *p* = 0.086)	27.2 vs 25.6 (1.04, 0.50 - 2.18)	75,0%
WJTOG-3405 [24]	172	Gef	C + D	62 vs 32*	9.2 vs 6.3 (0.49, 0.34-0.71*)	35.5 vs 38.8 (1.18, 0.77 - 1.83)	90,7%
NEJ-002 [25]	230	Gef	Cb + P	74 vs 31*	10.8 vs 5.4 (0.3, 0.22-0.41*)	27.7 vs 26.6 (0.89, 0.63 - 1.24)	95,6%
OPTIMA L [26]	165	Erl	Cb + G	83 vs 36*	13.1 vs 4.6 (0.16, 0.1-0.26*)	30.4 vs 31.5 (1.08, 0.61 - 1.91)	71,0%
EURTAC [27]	174	Erl	C/Cb+ D/G	58 vs 15	9.7 vs 5.2 (0.37, 0.25-0.54*)	NMD	
LUX-Lung 3 [28]	345	Afa	C + Pe	56 vs 23*	11.1 vs 6.9 (0.58, 0.43-0.78*)	NMD	65,0%
LUX-ung 6 [29]	364	Afa	C + G	67 vs 23*	11 vs 5.6 (0.28*)	NMD	48,4%

Gef: gefitinib; Erl: erlotinib; Afa: afatinib. CT: chemotherapy, C: cisplatin; Cb: carboplatin, P: paclitaxel, G: gemcitabine, D: docetaxel, Pe: pemetrexed. * p values <0,001.

5. Quality of Life: Patient-Reported Outcomes in Randomized Clinical Trials

Health-related quality of life (QoL) is an important endpoint in clinical cancer research. Given the lack of survival difference between EGFR-TKIs and chemotherapy, improvement in quality of life and disease-related symptoms emerge as key issues through the decision making process in the first-line setting. To date, six of the eight randomized studies have reported assessment of QoL as a secondary endpoint [35-37].

Two studies (IPASS, OPTIMAL) evaluate global QoL using three different scales: Functional Assessment of Cancer Therapy-Lung (FACT-L), the Lung Cancer Symptoms Scale (LCSS) and the Trial Outcome Index (TOI). Both trials and all three scales found differences in the percentage of patients with a clinically relevant improvement in QoL: more than 70% of patients treated with an EGFR-TKI compared with 24-54% of patients with a first-line platinum-based chemotherapy.

Three studies (First-SIGNAL and the LUX-Lung 3 and 6 trials) analyzed QoL data from the European Organization for Research and Treatment of Cancer (EORTC) QoL questionnaires QLQ-C30 and LC-13. Analysis of the functional scales reported significantly better mean scores over time in global health status/QoL, physical, role, social and cognitive functioning in the EGFR-TKI arm in at least one or two of the three studies. There were no significant differences between emotional functions. In the analysis of the symptoms scales, differences in mean scores over time or in time to deterioration significantly favored EGFR-TKI over chemotherapy for cough, dyspnea, fatigue and pain in two of the three trials and for insomnia in one trial. Conversely, diarrhea, sore mouth and dysphagia were reported more frequently in the gefitinib arm.

Only one study (NEJ002) assessed QoL using the Care Notebook, and the primary endpoint of the QoL analysis was time to deterioration from baseline on each of the physical, mental, and life well-being QoL scales. Time to defined deterioration in physical (pain and dyspnea) and life well-being (daily functioning) significantly favored gefitinib over chemotherapy.

Overall, six different randomized trials using three different EGFR-TKI and different QoL assessment tools have confirmed first-line EGFR-TKI to be superior to chemotherapy for QoL.

6. Maintenance, Second and Third Line

Evidence about EGFR-TKI efficacy in unselected NSCLC patients have been previously explained. However, seven trials on second-line or subsequent treatment and three trials on maintenance treatment have reported PFS and/or OS data on molecularly-tested subgroup of patients. It must be pointed out that these results are based on a minority of patients for which *EGFR* status was known, that ranged from 12% up to 50%, of which only 10% or less were *EGFR* mutated. Nevertheless, both maintenance and second line trials found that EGFR treatment is associated with a reduction in the risk of disease progression in EGFR mutated patients. The magnitude of this effect seemed to be similar to that observed in the first-line setting.

Table 4. Clinical trials including EGFR-TKI beyond the first line of treatment

Study	% EGFRmut (pos/neg/unk)	TKI	CT	PFS HR (95%CI)
IFCT-GFPC 0502 (2010) [38, 39]	3/34/63	Erl/Gef	Placebo	0.32 (0.05-1.95)
SATURN (2010) [40]	6/44/50	Erl	Placebo	0.10 (0.04-0.25)
INFORM (2011) [41]	10/17/73	Gef	Placebo	0.17 (0.07-0.42)
ISEL (2005) [42]	2/11/87	Gef	Placebo	-
BR21 (2005) [43]	5/23/72	Erl	Placebo	-
INTEREST (2008) [44]	3/17/80	Gef	Doc	0.16 (0.05-0.50)
V-15–32 (2008) [45]	6/6/88	Gef	Doc	0.74 (0.22-2.47)
TITAN (2012) [46]	3/35/62	Erl	Pem/Doc	0.71 (0.13-3.92)
TAILOR (2012) [47]	0/100/0	Erl	Doc	-
KCSG-LU08-01 (2012) [48]	24/28/48	Gef	Pem	0.30 (0.13-0.71)

Conclusion

EGFR mutation is a predictive biomarker of RR and PFS benefit and improvement in quality of life with EGFR-TKIs treatment of advanced-stage NSCLC in all settings of the disease. These findings support the need for *EGFR* mutation assessment before initiation of treatment. EGFR-TKIs should be considered as front-line therapy in *EGFR* mutated advanced-stage NSCLC patients, in spite of the lack of survival advantage. Additional arguments, including assurance on drug exposure, better tolerance by patients with poor performance status, and deferral of whole-brain radiation therapy for patients with brain metastasis, support the general application of first-line EGFR-TKI, but are beyond the scope of this chapter.

References

[1] Lynch, TJ; Bell, DW; Sordella, R; et al. Activating mutations in the epidermal growth factor receptor underlying responsiveness of non–small-cell lung cancer to gefitinib. *N Engl J Med.*, 2004, 350 (21), 2129-39.

[2] Paez, JG; Jänne, PA; Lee, JC; et al. EGFR mutations in lung can- cer: correlation with clinical response to gefitinib therapy. *Science.*, 2004, 304 (5676), 1497-500.

[3] Pao, W; Miller, V; Zakowski, M; et al. EGF receptor gene mutations are common in lung cancers from "never smokers" and are associated with sensitivity of tumors to gefitinib and erlotinib. *Proc Natl Acad Sci U S A.*, 2004, 101 (36), 13306-11.

[4] Huang, SF; Liu, HP; Li, LH; et al. High frequency of epidermal growth factor receptor mutations with complex patterns in non-small cell lung cancers related to gefitinib responsiveness in Taiwan. *Clin Cancer Res.*, 2004, 10 (24), 8195-203.

[5] Amann, J; Kalyankrishna, S; Massion, PP; et al. Aberrant epidermal growth factor receptor signaling and enhanced sensitivity to EGFR inhibitors in lung cancer. *Cancer Res.*, 2005, 65 (1), 226-35.

[6] Han, SW; Kim, TY; Hwang, PG; et al. Predictive and prognostic impact of epidermal growth factor receptor mutation in non- small-cell lung cancer patients treated with gefitinib. *J Clin Oncol.*, 2005, 23 (11), 2493-501.
[7] Mitsudomi, T; Kosaka, T; Endoh, H; et al. (2005) Mutations of the epidermal growth factor receptor gene predict prolonged survival after gefitinib treatment in patients with non-small-cell lung cancer with postoperative recurrence. *J Clin Oncol.*, 2005, 23 (11), 2513-520.
[8] Kim, KS; Kosaka, T; Endoh, H; et al. Predictors of the response to gefitinib in refractory non-small cell lung cancer. *Clin Cancer Res.*, 2005, 23 (11), 2244-51.
[9] Tokumo, M; Toyooka, S; Kiura, K; et al. The relationship between epidermal growth factor receptor mutations and clinicopathologic features in non-small cell lung cancers. *Clin Cancer Res.*, 2005, 11 (3), 1167-73.
[10] Chou, TY; Chiu, CH; Li, LH; et al. (2005) Mutation in the tyrosine kinase domain of epidermal growth factor receptor is acpredictive and prognostic factor for gefitinib treatment 36 in patients with non-small cell lung cancer. *Clin Cancer Res.*, 2005, 11 (10), 3750-7.
[11] Mu, XL; Li, LY; Zhang, XT; et al. (2005) Gefitinib-sensitive mutations of the epidermal growth factor receptor tyrosine kinase domain in chinese patients with non-small cell lung cancer. *Clin Cancer Res.*, 2005, 11 (12), 4289-94.
[12] Cortes-Funes, H; Gomez, C; Rosell, R; et al. Epidermal growth factor receptor activating mutations in Spanish gefitinib- treated non-small-cell lung cancer patients. *Ann Oncol.*, 2005, 16 (7), 1081-6.
[13] Cappuzzo, F; Hirsch, FR; Rossi, E; et al. Epidermal growth factor receptor gene and protein and gefitinib sensitivityin non-small-cell lung cancer. *J Natl Cancer Inst.*, 2005, 97 (9), 643-55.
[14] Takano, T; Ohe, Y; Sakamoto, H; et al. Epidermal growth factor receptor gene mutations and increased copy numbers predict gefitinib sensitivity in patients with recurrent non-small-cell lung cancer. *J Clin Oncol.*, 2005, 23(28), 6829-37.
[15] Tsao, MS; Sakurada, A; Cutz, JC; et al. Erlotinib in lung cancer— molecular and clinical predictors of outcome. *N Engl J Med.*, 2005, 353 (2), 133-44.
[16] Inoue, A; Kobayashi, K; Usui, K; et al. First-line gefitinib for patients with advanced non-small-cell lung cancer harboring epidermal growth factor receptor mutations without indication for chemotherapy. *J Clin Oncol.*, 2009, 27 (9), 1394-400.
[17] Rosell, R; Moran, T; Queralt, C; et al. Screening for epidermal growth factor receptor mutations in lung cancer. *N. Engl J Med.*, 2009, 361 (10), 958-67.
[18] Tamura; K; Okamoto, I; Kashii, T; et al. Multicentre prospective phase II trial of gefitinib for advanced non-small cell lung cancer with epidermal growth factor receptor mutations: results of the West Japan Thoracic Oncology Group trial (WJTOG0403). *Br J Cancer.*, 2008, 98 (5), 907-14.
[19] Sutani, A; Nagai, Y; Udagawa, K; et al. Gefitinib for non-small-cell lung cancer patients with epidermal growth factor receptor gene mutations screened by peptide nucleic acid-locked nucleic acid PCR clamp. *Br J Cancer.*, 2006, 95 (11), 1483-9.
[20] Sequist, LV; Bell, DW; Lynch, TJ; Haber, DA. Molecular predictors of response to epidermal growth factor receptor antagonists in non-small-cell lung cancer. *J Clin Oncol.*, 2007, 25 (5), 587-95.

[21] Paz-Ares, L; Soulières, D; Melezínek, I; Moecks, J; Keil, L; Mok, T; Rosell, R; Klughammer, B. Clinical outcomes in non-small-cell lung cancer patients with EGFR mutations: pooled analysis. *J Cell Mol Med.*, 2010, 14(1-2), 51-69.
[22] Mok, TS; Wu, YL; Thongprasert, S; et al. Gefitinib or carboplatin-paclitaxel in pulmonary adeno- carcinoma. *N Engl J Med.*, 2009, 361 (10), 947-57.
[23] Han, JY; Par, K; Kim, SW; et al. First-SIGNAL: First-line single-agent iressa versus gemcitabine and cisplatin trial in never-smokers with adenocarcinoma of the lung. *J Clin Oncol.*, 2012, 30 (10), 1122-8.
[24] Mitsudomi, T; Morita, S; Yatabe, Y; et al. Gefitinib versus cisplatin plus docetaxel in patients with non-small-cell lung cancer harbouring muta- tions of the epidermal growth factor receptor (WJTOG3405): An open label, randomised phase 3 trial. *Lancet Oncol.*, 2010, 11 (2), 121-8.
[25] Maemondo, M; Inoue, A; Kobayashi, K; et al. Gefitinib or chemotherapy for non-small-cell lung cancer with mutated EGFR. *N Engl J Med.*, 2010, 362 (25), 2380-8.
[26] Zhou, C; Wu, YL; Chen, G; et al. Erlotinib versus chemotherapy as first-line treatment for patients with advanced EGFR mutation-positive non-small-cell lung cancer (OPTIMAL, CTONG-0802): A multicentre, open-label, randomised, phase 3 study. *Lancet Oncol.*, 2011, 12 (8), 735-42.
[27] Rosell, R; Carcereny, E; Gervais, R; et al. Erlotinib versus standard chemotherapy as first-line treatment for European patients with advanced EGFR mutation-positive non-small-cell lung cancer (EURTAC): A multicentre, open-label, randomised phase 3 trial. *Lancet Oncol.*, 2012, 13 (3), 239-46.
[28] Yang, JC-H; Schuler, MH; Yamamoto, N; et al. LUX-Lung 3: A randomized, open-label, phase III study of afatinib versus pemetrexed and cisplatin as first-line treatment for patients with advanced adenocarcinoma of the lung harboring EGFR-activating mutations. *J Clin Oncol.*, 2012, 30 (suppl), 480s abstr LBA7500.
[29] Wu, YL; Zhou, C; Hu, CP; et al. Afatinib versus cisplatin plus gemcitabine for first-line treatment of Asian patients with advanced non-small-cell lung cancer harbouring EGFR mutations (LUX-Lung 6), an open-label, randomised phase 3 trial. *Lancet Oncol.*, 2014, 15 (2), 213-22.
[30] Fukuoka, M; Wu, YL; Thongprasert, S; et al. Biomarker analyses and final overall survival results from a phase III, randomized, open-label, first-line study of gefitinib versus carboplatin/paclitaxel in clinically selected patients with advanced non-small-cell lung cancer in Asia (IPASS). *J Clin Oncol.*, 2011, 29 (21), 2866-74.
[31] Inoue, A; Kobayashi, K; Maemondo, M; et al. Updated overall survival results from a randomized phase III trial comparing gefitinib with carboplatin-paclitaxel for chemo-naïve non-small cell lung cancer with sensitive EGFR gene mutations (NEJ002). *Ann Oncol.*, 2013, 24 (1), 54-9.
[32] Mitsudomi, T; Morita, S; Yatabe, Y; et al. Updated overall survival results of WJTOG 3405, a randomized phase III trial comparing gefitinib (G) with cisplatin plus docetaxel (CD) as the first-line treatment for patients with non-small cell lung can-cer harboring mutations of the epidermal growth factor receptor (EGFR). *J Clin Oncol.*, 2012, 30, 485s (abstr 7521).
[33] Zhou, C; Wu, YL; Chen, G; et al. Updated efficacy and quality-of-life (QoL) analyses in OPTIMAL, a phase III, randomized, open-label study of first-line erlotinib versus gemcitabine/carboplatin in patients with EGFR-activating mutation-positive (EGFR Act

Mut+) advanced non-small cell lung cancer (NSCLC) *J Clin Oncol.*, 2011, 29 (suppl 20), 480s abstr 7520.

[34] Lee, CK; Brown, C; Gralla, RJ; et al. Impact of EGFR inhibitor in non-small cell lung cancer on progression-free and overall survival: a meta-analysis. *J Natl Cancer Inst.*, 2013, 105 (9), 595-605.

[35] Thongprasert, S; Duffield, E; Saijo, N; et al. Health-related quality-of-life in a randomized phase III first-line study of gefitinib versus carboplatin/paclitaxel in clinically selected patients from Asia with advanced NSCLC (IPASS). *J Thorac Oncol*, 2011, 6 (11), 1872-80.

[36] Zhou, C; Wu, YL; Chen, G; et al. Updated efficacy and quality-of-life (QoL) analyses in OPTIMAL, a phase III, randomized, open-label study of first-line erlotinib versus gemcitabine/carboplatin in patients with EGFR-activating mutation-positive (EGFR Act Mut+) advanced non-small cell lung cancer (NSCLC) *J Clin Oncol.*, 2011, 29 (suppl 20), 480s abstr 7520.

[37] Oizumi, S; Kobayashi, K; Inoue, A; et al. Quality of life with gefitinib in patients with EGFR-mutated non-small cell lung cancer: Quality of life analysis of North East Japan Study Group 002 Trial (NEJ02). *Oncologist.*, 2012, 17: 863-70.

[38] Bylicki, O; Ferlay, C; Chouaid, C; et al. Efficacy of pemetrexed as second-line therapy in advanced NSCLC after either treatment-free interval or maintenance therapy with gemcitabine or erlotinib in IFCT-GFPC 05-02 phase III study. *J Thorac Oncol.*, 2013, 8 (7), 906-14.

[39] Petrelli, F; Borgonovo, K; Cabiddu, M; Barni, S. Erlotinib as maintenance therapy in patients with advanced non-small cell lung cancer: a pooled analysis of three randomized trials. *Anticancer Drugs.*, 2011, 22 (10), 1010-9.

[40] Cappuzzo, F; Ciuleanu, T; Stelmakh, L; et al. Erlotinib as maintenance treatment in advanced non-small-cell lung cancer: a multicentre, randomised, placebo-controlled phase 3 study. *Lancet Oncol.*, 2010, 11 (6), 521-9.

[41] Zhang, L; Ma, S; Song, X; et al. Gefitinib versus placebo as maintenance therapy in patients with locally advanced or metastatic non-small-cell lung cancer (INFORM, C-TONG 0804), a multicentre, double-blind randomised phase 3 trial. *Lancet Oncol.*, 2012, 13 (5), 466-75.

[42] Hirsch, FR; Varella-Garcia, M; Bunn, PA, Jr. et al. Molecular predictors of outcome with gefitinib in a phase III placebo-controlled study in advanced non-small-cell lung cancer. *J Clin Oncol.*, 2006, 24 (31), 5034-42.

[43] Florescu, M; Hasan, B; Seymour, L; Ding, K; Shepherd, FA. A clinical prognostic index for patients treated with erlotinib in National Cancer Institute of Canada Clinical Trials Group study BR.21. *J Thorac Oncol.*, 2008, 3 (6), 590-8.

[44] Kim, ES; Hirsh, V; Mok, T; et al. Gefitinib versus docetaxel in previously treated non-small-cell lung cancer (INTEREST), a randomised phase III trial. *Lancet.*, 2008, 372 (9652), 1809-18.

[45] Maruyama, R; Nishiwaki, Y; Tamura, T; et al. Phase III study, V-15-32, of gefitinib versus docetaxel in previously treated Japanese patients with non-small-cell lung cancer. *J Clin Oncol.*, 2008, 26 (26), 4244-52.

[46] Ciuleanu, T; Stelmakh, L; Cicenas, S; et al. Efficacy and safety of erlotinib versus chemotherapy in second-line treatment of patients with advanced, non-small-cell lung

cancer with poor prognosis (TITAN), a randomised multicentre, open-label, phase 3 study. *Lancet Oncol.*, 2012, 13 (3), 300-8.

[47] Garassino, MC; Martelli, O; Broggini, M; et al. Erlotinib versus docetaxel as second-line treatment of patients with advanced non-small-cell lung cancer and wild-type EGFR tumours (TAILOR), a randomised controlled trial. *Lancet Oncol.*, 2013, 14 (10), 981-8.

[48] Sun, JM; Lee, KH; Kim, SW; et al. Gefitinib versus pemetrexed as second-line treatment in patients with nonsmall cell lung cancer previously treated with platinum-based chemotherapy (KCSG-LU08-01), an open-label, phase 3 trial. *Cancer.*, 2012, 118 (24), 6234-42.

In: Fighting Lung Cancer through the HER Family ... ISBN: 978-1-63321-092-9
Editor: Diego Márquez-Medina

Chapter 11

Future I. Still Unapproved Drugs

Rosario García Campelo, M.D., Joaquín Mosquera, M.D. and Aurea Molina, M.D.
Medical Oncology Unit, A Coruña University Hospital, Spain

Abstract

Lung cancer is the leading cause of cancer deaths and probably one of the most challenging cancers to treat. Platinum-based chemotherapy remains as the standard of treatment for most of advanced non-small cell lung cancer (NSCLC) patients, and although therapeutic improvements have been achieved in the last years, the benefits are quite modest.

One of the most important advances in NSCLC care has been the identification of oncogenic mutations that contribute to the pathogenesis of lung cancer, suggesting that some tumors can rely on a specific gene for their survival and proliferation, and the subsequent development of drugs targeted to these specific alterations. Activating mutations of the epidermal growth factor receptor (EGFR) have been the first molecular event that can be targeted with specific drugs in NSCLC.

The discovery of the first reversible EGFR small-molecule inhibitors (EGFR-TKI) in the past decade has changed the history of lung cancer treatment. EGFR inhibition has emerged to be an important strategy in the treatment of NSCLC. Novel EGFR-TKIs and mono-clonal antibodies targeting the EGFR pathway are being investigated in NSCLC, with promising results. In the future, a better understanding of the tumor heterogeneity as well as tumor resistance mechanisms will evolve more rational therapies and potential combinations of different targeted therapies.

1. Introduction

Lung cancer is a major cause of cancer death worldwide, largely because most patients have advanced stage disease at the time of diagnosis [1]. During the last five years due to the rapid and exciting discovery of many "driver mutations" in non-small cell lung cancer (NSCLC), novel paradigms of treatment have emerged in our daily clinical practice.

This oncogene addiction model, where key genetic alterations control cell survival and proliferation has led to an explosion of knowledge in the field of lung cancer biology, targeted therapies, and resistance mechanisms. The epidermal growth factor receptor (EGFR) has surfaced as one of those important targets for therapy in different solid tumors, including NSCLC. The EGFR is a member of a family of closely related receptors, including EGFR (ErbB1), human epidermal growth factor receptor-2 HER2/neu (ErbB2), HER3 (ErbB3), and HER4 (ErbB4). EGFR is overexpressed in the majority of NSCLC and its expression is inversely related to survival outcome [2]. The activation of this tyrosine kinase receptor leads to autophosphorylation of the intracellular domain of EGFR. Improper activation of EGFR tyrosine kinase results in increased malignant cell survival, proliferation, invasion, and metastasis [3]. Mutations of the *EGFR* gene have been identified in specimens from NSCLC patients who have dramatic responses to treatment with the reversible EGFR tyrosine kinase inhibitors (EGFR-TKI) gefitinib and erlotinib [4-6]. Randomized phase III clinical trials have demonstrated that personalizing first-line therapy by *EGFR* mutation status with these reversible EGFR-TKIs leads to improvement in progression-free survival (PFS) compared to conventional chemotherapy [7-10].

But despite the impressive initial response to treatment, disease progression generally occurs after 9 to 14 months of erlotinib or gefitinib therapy, driven in approximately 60% of cases by a second site *EGFR* point mutation that results in the substitution of threonine with methionine at amino acid position 790 (T790M) [11-13], so novel approaches, including new EGFR-TKIs (Table 1) and new combinations are needed and are being evaluated in the field of NSCLC.

2. Second Generation of Irreversible EGFR-TKI

Several theoretical advantages of the second-generation irreversible EGFR-TKIs over the first-generation reversible EGFR-TKIs are that some have a higher affinity for the EGFR kinase domain that may result in longer suppression of ERBB signaling than that resulting from reversible inhibitors. Second, the second-generation EGFR-TKIs also inhibit HER2, a common dimerization partner of EGFR, and some inhibit HER4 as well, to effect signaling transduction, thus allowing a more complete blockade of the EGFR signaling pathway. Third, second-generation EGFR-TKIs have modest *in vitro* activity against the T790M gatekeeper mutation and other rare mutations that render the first-generation reversible EGFR-TKIs ineffective [14].

Table 1. EGFR-TKI in development for NSCLC

AGENT	TARGET	PHASE
DACOMITINIB	EGFR, HER2, HER3, HER4	PHASE III
BMS-690514	EGFR, HER2, HER4, VEGFR 1-3	PHASE II
XL647	EGFR, HER2, VEFR.2, EphB4	PHASE II
AP26113	EGFR, ALK	PHASE II
CO-1686	EGFR T790M	PHASE II
AZD9291	EGFR T790M	PHASE II

2.1. Dacomitinib

Dacomitinib (PF-00299804) is an irreversible EGFR-TKI of HER1, HER2, and HER4. In preclinical studies, dacomitinib demonstrated higher potency HER kinase inhibition and greater anticancer activity in gefitinib and erlotinib sensitive and resistant cell line and in xenograft NSCLC models [15, 16]. Two phase I studies on dacomitinib in NSCLC were conducted in the US [17] and South Korea [18], respectively. The maximum tolerated dose (MTD) of dacomitinib was determined to be 45 mg once daily. The most common reported adverse event (AE) was diarrhea in both the US and Korean trials (78% and 61%, respectively) followed by rash (65% and 50%, respectively). The Korean trial included refractory to platinum-based chemotherapy and erlotinib or gefitinib, *EGFR* wild-type and *Kras* wild-type advanced NSCLC patients. A response rate (RR) of 15% and 6-month overall survival (OS) of 32% was reported in this trial. In the US trial, which included patients enriched for *HER* gene amplification, *EGFR/HER2* mutation, or *KRAS* wild-type, 2 out of 29 patients achieved durable PR.

Dacomitinib has also been investigated in the salvage treatment setting in advanced NSCLC patients after progression to chemotherapy and erlotinib treatment [19]. Sixty-six patients progressing on 1 or 2 regimens of chemotherapy and erlotinib, *KRAS* wild-type or known *EGFR*-sensitizing mutant tumor, were enrolled in this phase II trial. In the overall population, the overall RR was 5.2%; responders included 2 of 25 *EGFR* mutation-positive tumors, 1 of 3 *EGFR* wild-type with *HER2* amplification.

Median progression-free survival (PFS) was 12 weeks for the overall population and 18 weeks for patients with *EGFR* mutation-positive tumors. Common treatment-related AEs were of grade 1 or 2 severity, manageable with standard supportive care, and included diarrhea (G3, 12%), acneiform dermatitis (G3, 6%), exfoliative rash (G3, 3%), dry skin (G3, 0%), fatigue (G3, 3%), and stomatitis (G3, 2%). Six patients (9%) discontinued due to treatment-related AES. The National Cancer Institute of Canada is completing a randomized phase III trial (JBR-26) comparing dacomitinib to placebo in the third line setting or beyond where patients have failed chemotherapy and reversible EGFR-TKIs.

A phase II trial, compared dacomitinib versus erlotinib in 188 patients with advanced NSCLC after failing first line chemotherapy [20]. Median PFS was significantly prolonged with dacomitinib compared with erlotinib (2.86 months for patients treated with dacomitinib and 1.91 months for patients treated with erlotinib (hazard ratio [HR] 0.66, 95% CI 0.47-0.91; p= 0.012); in patients with KRAS wild-type tumors, median PFS was 3.71 months for patients treated with dacomitinib and 1.91 months for patients treated with erlotinib (HR 0.55, 95% CI 0.35-0.85; p= 0.006); and in patients with *KRAS* wild-type/*EGFR* wild-type tumors, median PFS was 2.21 months for patients treated with dacomitinib and 1.84 months for patients treated with erlotinib (HR 0.61, 95% CI 0.37-0.99; p= 0.043). Median overall survival (OS) was 9.53 months for patients treated with dacomitinib and 7.44 months for patients treated with erlotinib (HR 0.8, 95% CI 0.56-1.13; p= 0.205). Adverse events-related discontinuations were uncommon in both arms. Common treatment-related AEs were dermatologic and gastrointestinal, predominantly grade 1 to 2, and more frequent with dacomitinib. A randomized phase III registration trial comparing dacomitinib to erlotinib in unselected advanced NSCLC patients in the second-line treatment setting is being conducted to attempt to gain regulatory approval for dacomitinib (ARCHER 1009).

Regarding molecular defined populations, Dacomitinib has been investigated in the first-line treatment of patients who were never-smokers/former light-smokers, or patients who harbored *EGFR* mutations but with *KRAS* wild-type. Those 46 NSCLC patients harboring *EGFR* mutations achieved a RR of 74% and a median PFS was 17 months [21]. The phase III trial ARCHER 1050, comparing dacomitinib versus gefitinib in the first line setting of *EGFR* mutated advanced NSCLC is being conducted.

2.2. Afatinib

Afatinib (BIBW 2992; Boehringer Ingelheim; Ingelheim, Germany), an anilinoquinazoline derivative, is a highly selective, and irreversible ErbB family inhibitor of both EGFR and HER2 kinases [22]. Afatinib is being systemically investigated in several major trials in NSCLC (LUX-Lung trials) employing various treatment strategies similar to dacomitinib.

Afatinib was tested in Japanese patients in advanced NSCLC in a phase I/II trial (LUX-Lung 4) to ensure the MTD of 50 mg once daily achieved in non-Asian patients was similar for Asian patients [23]. This single-arm phase II trial was conducted in patients with stage IIIB to IV pulmonary adenocarcinoma who progressed after $\geq$ 12 weeks of prior erlotinib and/or gefitinib. Patients received afatinib 50 mg per day. Of 62 treated patients, 45 (72.6%) were *EGFR* mutation positive. Fifty-one patients (82.3%) fulfilled the criteria of acquired resistance to erlotinib and/or gefitinib. Of 61 evaluable patients, five (8.2%) had a confirmed objective RR. Median PFS was 4.4 months (95% CI 2.8-4.6 months), and median OS was 19 months (95% CI 14.9 months to not achieved). Two patients had acquired T790M mutations: L858R + T790M, and deletion in exon 19 + T790M; they had stable disease for 9 months and 1 month, respectively. The most common afatinib-related AEs were diarrhea (100%) and rash/acne (91.9%). Treatment-related AEs leading to afatinib discontinuation were experienced by 18 patients (29%). The LUX-Lung 1 phase IIB/III trial investigated afatinib versus placebo in 585 NSCLC patients who were progressing after prior treatment with at least 1 line of platinum-based chemotherapy and erlotinib or gefitinib [24]. Patients were clinically enriched by enrolling only those who derived a minimum of 12 weeks of disease control under a first-generation EGFR-TKI. However, afatinib did not meet the primary endpoint of extending OS compared to placebo (10.8 months versus 12 months; HR 1.08, 95% CI 0.86-1.35), presumably due to subsequent therapies; PFS was in favor of afatinib (3.3 months versus 1.1 months; HR 0.38; $p < 0.0001$), with some improvement in cancer-related symptoms. Diarrhea (87%) and rash/acne (78%) were reported as the two most common AEs in those patients receiving afatinib therapy. The LUX-Lung 2 trial, a phase II study, was conducted in those advanced NSCLC patients harboring activating *EGFR* gene mutations who had 0 or 1 line of prior chemotherapy but were naive for EGFR-TKIs [25]. The overall RR was similar with once daily dosing of 40 or 50 mg afatinib (60% for 40 mg versus 62% for 50 mg), but more side effects were observed in the group receiving 50 mg. Based on these findings, two large phase III trials were developed: the LUX-Lung 3, the so far largest registrational phase III trial in *EGFR* mutation-positive adenocarcinoma including 345 patients randomized to 40 mg once daily of afatinib versus a highly effective and tolerable chemotherapy doublet consisting of cisplatin and pemetrexed [26]. The trial was conducted throughout Asia, Europe, North/South America, and Australia, with 72% of enrolled patients having Asian ethnicity and 28% being non-Asians.

Treatment with afatinib led to a prolonged PFS (11.1 months versus 6.9 months; HR 0.58, 95% CI 0.43-0.78) compared to cisplatin/pemetrexed and a significantly higher overall RR (56% versus 23%; p< 0.0001), as assessed by independent review. The superiority of afatinib was consistent in all relevant subgroups. In those 308 patients with common *EGFR* mutations (exon 19 deletion or *EGFR* L858R) the median PFS was 13.6 months with afatinib versus 6.9 months with chemotherapy (HR 0.47, 95% CI 0.34-0.65). In those patients receiving the experimental arm, afatinib demonstrated a significant delay in time to deterioration of cancer-related symptoms such as cough (HR 0.6; p= 0.007) and dyspnea (HR 0.68; p= 0.015) and increased quality of life [27].

OS data have yet to be reported. Similarly to Lux-Lung 3, the Lux-Lung 6 [28] is a phase III that has been completed in Asian population including 364 patients randomly assigned to afatinib (N= 242), versus gemcitabine and cisplatin (N= 122). Median PFS was significantly longer in the afatinib group (11 months) than in the gemcitabine and cisplatin group (5.6 months; HR 0.28, 95% CI 0.2-0.39; p< 0.0001). The most common treatment-related grade 3 or 4 AEs in the afatinib group were rash or acne (14.6%), diarrhoea (5.4%), and stomatitis or mucositis (5.4%), Treatment-related serious AEs occurred in 15 (6.3%) patients in the afatinib group and nine (8%) patients in the gemcitabine and cisplatin group. Based on Lux-Lung 3 and Lux-Lung 6 phase III trials positive results, afatinib should be considered today as a new therapeutic option in the first-line setting for those advanced NSCLC harboring EGFR mutations.

3. Third Generation of EGFR-TKI

Despite these significant and positive results, clinical efficacy in *EGFR* mutant NSCLC patients is limited by acquired resistance, frequently driven by the *EGFR* T790M mutation. Relapsed NSCLCs with acquired T790M mutations seem to remain dependent on EGFR signaling for their growth, prompting substantial efforts to discover novel EGFR inhibitors that can overcome the effects of the T790M substitution.

3.1. CO-1686

CO-1686 is a novel, irreversible and orally delivered kinase inhibitor that specifically targets the mutant forms of *EGFR* including T790M while exhibiting minimal activity towards the wild-type receptor. Oral administration of CO-1686 as single agent induces tumor regression in *EGFR* mutated NSCLC tumor xenograft and transgenic models. Minimal activity of CO-1686 against the wild-type EGFR was observed [29]. CO-1686 is currently being evaluated in phase I/II clinical trials in *EGFR*-mutant NSCLC. Recently, preliminary results of an ongoing first-in-human dose finding study (3 + 3) of oral CO-1686 administered continuously in 21-day cycles was evaluated in *EGFR*-mutant NSCLC previously treated with an EGFR-TKI. For the 56 patients included, 70% were reported to be T790M+; treatment-related AEs (all grades) include nausea, diarrhea, fatigue, vomiting and decreased appetite. The majority of events were mild or moderate. At the highest evaluated dose, 900mg BID, a RR of 67% was achieved in evaluable T790M+ patients [30].

Additional evaluations of the optimal dose and formulation of CO-1686 are underway to further explore its potential for improved activity.

3.2. AZD9291

AZD9291 is a potent oral, irreversible inhibitor of the EGFR sensitizing and resistance mutations (T790M). In a phase I open label multicenter study, AZD9291 was shown to have mostly mild AEs, and no grade 3-4 serious AEs. Moreover, 89 patients received at least one dose, and no dose limiting toxicities were observed.

Promising efficacy has been observed at all doses studied thus far, including 9/18 patients with T790M who had confirmed or unconfirmed partial responses [31].

3.3. Other Non-Covalent Wild-Type Sparing Inhibitors of EGFR T790M

WZ4002 is a recently reported irreversible inhibitor that displays much improved selectivity against *EGFR* T790M over wild-type *EGFR* in preclinical studies [32]. Indeed, at concentrations as low as 10 nanomolar, WZ4002 inhibits ATP-dependent autophosphorylation of *EGFR* T790M without any observed effects on wild-type *EGFR*. However, at higher concentrations, this compound also inhibits wild-type *EGFR in vitro* and in cell line studies. Because of the irreversible nature of its inhibitory mechanism, prolonged administration of this agent could potentially affect wild-type *EGFR*, particularly in tissues where it accumulates.

The noncovalent indolocarbazole compounds, including Gö6976 and PKC412, seem to function as more selective inhibitors of *EGFR* T790M. Importantly, PKC412A structurally related reversible kinase inhibitor, that is currently undergoing phase III clinical testing as a FLT3 kinase inhibitor, was found to exhibit potent inhibition of *EGFR* T790M compound. PKC412A is at least 100-fold more potent against *EGFR* T790M than Gö6976 and is comparably potent with the irreversible EGFR-TKIs, but with 500-fold less activity against wild-type *EGFR* in drug-treated cells [33].

4. New Drugs Targeting EGFR Pathway

4.1. BMS-690514

BMS-690513 is a potent, reversible oral inhibitor of EGFR, HER-2 and -4, and vascular endothelial growth factor receptors 1 to 3 offering targeted inhibition of tumor growth and vascularization in a single agent. It has been tested in a phase I–IIa study designed to identify the MTD and assess safety, antitumor activity, pharmacokinetics and pharmacodynamics [34]. In phase IIa, erlotinib-naïve (cohort A) or erlotinib-resistant (cohort B) patients with advanced NSCLC received BMS-690514 once-daily at the MTD. In phase I (N= 28), the MTD was determined to be 200mg daily. In phase IIa (N= 62), the most frequent treatment-related AEs were diarrhoea and acneiform rash.

Disease control (over 4months) and objective RR, respectively, were 43.3% and 3.3% (cohort A) and 22.6% and 3.2% (cohort B).

Six of 21 (29%) NSCLC patients with wild-type *EGFR* achieved disease control versus 7 of 10 (70%) patients with *EGFR* mutations (including T790M).

4.2. XL647

XL647 is a kinase inhibitor that targets EGFR, HER2, vascular endothelial growth factor receptor-2 and EphB4. In a phase II study of XL-647 in the first-line setting, the RR in *EGFR*-mutant NSCLC was 88% [35].

In a subsequent phase II study in patients with acquired resistance to EGFR-TKIs, the RR was only 3% and none of the 12 patients with a known T790M mutation responded [36].

4.3. AP26113

The protein kinase inhibitor AP26113 targets both EGFR and ALK with preferential activity against mutant *EGFR* versus wild type. The first-in-human phase I study included 18 evaluable patients with an *EGFR* mutation but there was only one response [37]. Seven patients achieved stable disease, including four with T790M. The phase II portion of the study is ongoing and includes a cohort of patients with T790M.

5. EGFR Monoclonal Antibodies

Anti-EGFR monoclonal antibodies inhibit signal transduction binding to the surface of the EGFR and blocking the binding of EGF. Antibody receptor complexes are internalized, degraded, leading to EGFR downregulation on the surface of tumor cells. Monoclonal antibodies may also act via immunological mechanisms [38]. Several monoclonal antibodies directed against EGFR have been or are currently being evaluated in patients with NSCLC (Table 2).

5.1. Cetuximab

Cetuximab, a chimeric murine monoclonal antibody has been extensively studied in lung cancer patients. Although the addition of EGFR-TKIs to systemic chemotherapy in the first-line setting did not result in improved response or survival in any of the randomized clinical trials [39], the addition of the monoclonal antibody cetuximab to chemotherapy in advanced NSCLC has demonstrated improvements in overall RR and, in some studies significant, although modest, improvements in PFS and OS.

Lynch et al. [40] reported a significant improvement in overall RR with the addition of cetuximab to a carboplatin/ taxane regimen (BMS099 trial), although without significant prolongation of PFS or OS.

Table 2. Monoclonal anti-EGFR antibodies

	NATURE	PHASE
CETUXIMAB	Chimeric IgG1	Approved in CRC Phase III in NSCLC
PANITUMUMAB	Fully human IgG2	Approved in CRC Phase II in NSCLC
MATUZUMAB	Humanized IgG1	Phase II in NSCLC
NECITUMUMAB	Fully human IgG1	Phase III in NSCLC

Pirker et al. [41] reported results of similar magnitude in the First-Line Erbitux in Lung Cancer (FLEX) trial comparing chemotherapy (vinorelbine/cisplatin) with or without cetuximab as first- line treatment in patients with advanced NSCLC, who had tumors expressing even a minimum amount of EGFR (>1% cells). The study showed better survival for the treatment with chemotherapy plus cetuximab (median survival 11.3 months versus 10.1 months; HR 0.87, 95% CI 0.76–1; p= 0.04). Confirming the positive effect of adding cetuximab to conventional chemotherapy, a meta-analysis based on 2,018 patients from four randomized trials confirmed the efficacy of cetuximab when added to first-line platinum-based chemotherapy [42]. The benefit was seen for OS (median 10.3 months versus 9.4 months; HR 0.88; p< 0.009), PFS (median 4.7 months versus 4.5 months; HR 0.9; p= 0.045) and overall RR (32.2% versus 24.4%; p< 0.001).

To define patients benefiting most from cetuximab, the FLEX investigators analyzed the association of tumor EGFR expression level with clinical outcome [43]. High EGFR expression was scored for 345 (31%) evaluable patients and low for 776 (69%) patients. For patients in the high EGFR expression group, OS was longer in the chemotherapy plus cetuximab group than in the chemotherapy alone group (median 12 months versus 9.6 months; HR 0.73, 95% CI 0.58-0.93; p= 0.011), with no meaningful increase in side effects. No corresponding survival benefit for patients in the low EGFR expression group (median 9.8 months versus 10.3 months; HR 0.99, 95% CI 0.84-1.16; p= 0.88) was observed. The use of EGFR immunohistochemistry in the FLEX study seems to be an encouraging step towards personalized medicine for patient subgroups with advanced NSCLC who could potentially benefit from cetuximab, but further prospective validation of the FLEX findings is necessary. Indeed a large ongoing prospective phase 3 study comparing chemotherapy with and without cetuximab (SWOG 0819 study) is ongoing. Other potential biomarkers such as *Kras* mutation status or *EGFR* gene copy number detected by FISH have not been established as predictors of cetuximab benefits for advanced NSCLC patients.

5.2. Matuzumab

Matuzumab is a humanized IgG1 EGFR monoclonal antibody. A randomized phase II study compared pemetrexed plus matuzumab with pemetrexed alone as second-line therapy for patients with advanced NSCLC [44]. Pemetrexed was given at 500 mg/m^2 every 3 weeks, and matuzumab was given at either 800 mg weekly or 1,600 mg every 3 weeks. The RR was 11 % for patients treated with pemetrexed plus matuzumab and 5 % for those treated with pemetrexed alone.

Patients receiving weekly matuzumab had higher response rate (16% versus 2 %) and a trend towards longer survival (12.4 months versus 5.9 months) than those treated with matuzumab every 3 weeks. The combination of pemetrexed and matuzumab had an acceptable safety profile, with the most common grade 3/4 adverse event being neutropenia.

5.3. Panitumumab

Panitumumab is a fully human anti-EGFR IgG2 monoclonal. A randomized phase II trial in 175 patients with *EGFR*-positive advanced NSCLC could not demonstrate a benefit for panitumumab added to paclitaxel plus carboplatin compared to the same chemotherapy alone [45]. Rash, dry skin, pruritus, diarrhea, vomiting, stomatitis, and dizziness were more frequent in the panitumumab arm.

5.4. Necitumumab

Necitumunab is a fully human IgG1 monoclonal antibody targeting EGFR, having the potential benefit of lower hypersensitivity reaction risk as compared with cetuximab and also equivalent antibody-dependent cell-mediated cytotoxicity [46]. Recently, a phase III clinical trial (INSPIRE trial) evaluating the addition of necitumumab to pemetrexed and cisplatin in non-squamous NSCLC was prematurely closed due to concerns about the increased risk of thromboembolic events in the experimental arm [47].

Accrual in the phase III trial evaluating necitumumab in combination with cisplatin plus gemcitabine in patients with squamous cell NSCLC is still ongoing (SQUIRE trial, Clinical Trials.gov Identifier: NCT00981058).

6. Combination of EGFR-TKI and EGFR Monoclonal Antibodies

One of the most promising therapeutic approaches under evaluation for *EGFR* mutant advanced NSCLC patients includes the combination of afatinib plus cetuximab. Because the points of receptor inhibition for TKIs (intracellular tyrosine kinase domain) and monoclonal antibodies (extracellular domain) are different, improved inhibition may result from a combination approach. Indeed a phase Ib study, testing afatinib plus cetuximab combination therapy has shown promising activity: of 26 treated patients, 22 received the predefined MTD (afatinib 40 mg + cetuximab 500 mg/m^2).

Common AEs were grade 1/2 rash (35/46%) and diarrhea (50/19%), respectively, and three patients (11.5%) had grade 3 rash. Disease control was observed in all patients enrolled at the predefined MTD (tumor size reduction up to 76%). Confirmed partial responses were seen in 36% of the patients, including 29% confirmed partial responses in T790M+ NSCLC. An expansion cohort in an 80-patient population is ongoing [48].

7. HER2 Inhibition

HER2 is a member of the erbB receptor tyrosine kinase family, that forms homodimers and heterodimers with other members of the HER family, without a specific ligand for its receptor described. Involvement of HER2 in lung carcinogenesis has been known for many years, with different mechanisms such as HER2 protein overexpression or gene amplification [49, 50] although clinical research showed disappointing results when combining trastuzumab with conventional chemotherapy in those patients with HER2 immunohistochemistry positive lung cancer [51]. *HER2* mutations have been recently reported in 1.7% of NSCLC patients, 65 of 3,800 patients tested, and it was almost an exclusive driver mutation, more frequently found in never smokers, women and those patients with adenocarcinoma subtype. Twenty-two heavily pretreated individual patients included in this retrospective analysis receiving different HER2 targeted drugs were evaluated: Overall RR was 50%, and a median PFS of 5.1 months was obtained. Specifically, authors observed a disease control rate of 96% for trastuzumab-based therapies (N= 15), and 100% for afatinib (N= 4), but not response to lapatinib (N= 2) or to masatinib (N= 1) [52]. Despite these results, available data from the literature concerning HER2 targeted therapies in NSCLC are scarce.

The most promising compounds are irreversible TKIs targeting HER2 and EGFR, such as the already mentioned dacomitinib (PF-00299804), and afatinib (BIBW-2992). Of the three patients with an *HER2* mutation included in the previously mentioned publication from Maziéres et al. [52], those who later received afatinib, one patient achieved a response and the other two had stable disease. A separate report described three patients with *HER2*-mutant NSCLC treated with afatinib, all of whom responded [53]. An ongoing phase II study of afatinib monotherapy reported seven patients with *HER2* mutations and though no responses were seen, five patients maintained stable disease [54].

Dacomitinib is actively being explored in *HER2*-mutant NSCLC. A prospective, phase II study of dacomitinib (NCT00818441) includes a cohort of patients with an *HER2* mutation or amplification; Kris et al. recently reported an overall RR of 12% in patients with *HER2*-mutant lung cancers heavily pretreated, without no responses in *HER2*- amplified lung cancers included in this trial.Interestingly in a patient with an *HER2* amplified and mutated NSCLC tumor, dacomitinib plus trastuzumab provided a significant response [56]. Another pan-HER kinase inhibitor is neratinib (HKI-272) [57], which is now being studied in patients with *HER2*-mutant NSCLC in combination with weekly temsirolimus (NCT01 827267).

Conclusion

The focus of several recently completed and ongoing clinical trials has been targeting the EGFR pathway as a key oncogenic pathway in NSCLC. Novel small molecule inhibitors alone or in combination with other biologics targeted agents could be effective in overcoming resistance mechanisms in *EGFR* mutant NSCLC patients.

Also monoclonal antibodies directed against EGFR are being evaluated and may open new opportunities in the treatment of patients with NSCLC.

References

[1] Parkin, D. M., Bray, F., Ferlay, J., Pisani, P. Global cancer statistics, 2002. *CA Cancer J. Clin.* 2005; 55 (2): 74-108.

[2] Brabender, J., Danenberg, K. D., Metzger, R., et al. Epidermal growth factor receptor and HER2-neu mRNA expression in non-small cell lung cancer is correlated with survival. *Clin. Cancer Res.* 2001; 7: 1850–5.

[3] Kumar, A., Petri, E. T., Halmos, B., Boggon, T. A. Structure and clinical relevance of the epidermal growth factor receptor in human cancer. *J. Clin. Oncol.* 2008; 26 (10): 1742-51.

[4] Lynch, T. J., Bell, D. W., Sordella, R., et al. Activating mutations in the epidermal growth factor receptor underlying responsiveness of non-small cell lung cancer to gefitinib. *N. Engl. J. Med.* 2004; 350 (21): 2129-39.

[5] Paez, J. G., Jãnne, P. A., Lee, J. C., et al. EGFR mutations in lung cancer: correlation with clinical response to gefitinib therapy. *Science.* 2004; 304 (5676): 1497-500.

[6] Pao, W., Miller, V., Zakowski, M., et al. EGF receptor mutations are common in lung cancers from "never smokers" and are associated with sensitivity of tumors to gefitinib and erlotinib. *Proc. Natl. Acad. Sci. US* 2004; 101 (36):13306-11.

[7] Mitsudomi, T., Morita, S., Yatabe, Y., et al. Gefitinib versus cisplatin plus docetaxel in patients with non-small-cell lung cancer harboring mutations of the epidermal growth factor receptor (WJTOG3405): an open label, randomised phase 3 trial. *Lancet Oncol.* 2010; 11: 121–28.

[8] Maemondo, M., Inoue, A., Kobayashi, K., et al. Gefitinib or chemotherapy for non-small-cell lung cancer with mutated EGFR. *N. Engl. J. Med.* 2010; 362: 2380–88.

[9] Zhou, C., Wu, Y. L., Chen, G., et al. Erlotinib versus chemotherapy as first-line treatment for patients with advanced EGFR mutation-positive non-small-cell lung cancer (OPTIMAL, CTONG-0802): a multicentre, open-label, randomised, phase 3 study. *Lancet Oncol.* 2011; 12: 735–42.

[10] Rosell, R., Carcereny, E., Gervais, R., et al. Erlotinib versus standard chemotherapy as first-line treatment for European patients with advanced EGFR mutation-positive non-small-cell lung cancer (EURTAC): a multicentre, open-label, randomised phase 3 trial. *Lancet Oncol.* 2012; 13: 239–46.

[11] Sequist, L. V., Waltman, B. A., Dias-Santagata, D., et al. Genotypic and histological evolution of lung cancers acquiring resistance to EGFR inhibitors. *Sci. Transl. Med.* 2011; 3 (75): 75ra26.

[12] Pao, W., Miller, V. A., Politi, K. A., et al. Acquired resistance of lung adenocarcinomas to gefitinib or erlotinib is associated with a second mutation in the EGFR kinase domain. *PLoS Med.* 2005; 2: e73.

[13] Sharma, S. V., Bell, D. W., Settleman, J., Haber, D. A. Epidermal growth factor receptor mutations in lung cancer. *Nat. Rev. Cancer.* 2007; 7: 169-81.

[14] Ou, S. H. Second-generation irreversible epidermal growth factor receptor (EGFR) tyrosine kinase inhibitors (TKIs): A better mousetrap? A review of the clinical evidence. *Crit. Rev. Oncol. Hematol.* 2012; 83 (3): 407-21.

[15] Engelman, J. A., Zejnullahu, K., Gale, C. M., et al. PF00299804, an irreversible pan-ERBB inhibitor, is effective in lung cancer models with EGFR and ERBB2 mutations that are resistant to gefitinib. *Cancer Res*. 2007; 67: 11924-32.

[16] Gonzales, A. J., Hook, K. E., Althaus, I. W., et al. Antitumor activity and pharmacokinetic properties of PF-00299804, a second-generation irreversible pan-erbB receptor tyrosine kinase inhibitor. *Mol. Cancer Ther*. 2008; 7:1880-9.

[17] Janne, P. A., Schellens, J. H., Engelman, J. A., et al. Preliminary activity and safety results from a phase I clinical trial of PF-00299804, an irreversible pan-HER inhibitor, in patients (pts) with NSCLC. *J. Clin. Oncol*. 2008; 26: abstr 8027.

[18] Park, K., Heo, D. S., Cho, B., et al. PF-00299804 (PF299) in Asian patients (pts) with non-small cell lung cancer (NSCLC) refractory to chemotherapy (CT) and erlotinib (E) or gefitinib (G): a phase (P) I/II study. *J. Clin. Oncol*. 2010; 28: abstr. 7599.

[19] Reckamp, K. L., Giaccone, G., Camidge, D. R., et al. A phase 2 trial *Cancer* 2014 Feb. 5. doi: 10.1002/cncr.28561. [Epub. ahead of print].

[20] Ramalingam, S. S., Blackhall, F., Krzakowski, M., et al. Randomized phase II study of dacomitinib (PF-00299804), an irreversible pan-human epidermal growth factor receptor inhibitor, versus erlotinib in patients with advanced non-small-cell lung cancer. *J. Clin. Oncol*. 2012; 30 (27): 3337-44.

[21] Kris, M. G., Mok, T., Ou, S. H., et al. First-line dacomitinib (PF-00299804), an irreversible pan-HER tyrosine kinase inhibitor, for patients with EGFR-mutant lung cancers. *J. Clin. Oncol*. 2012; 30: abstr. 7530.

[22] Li, D., Ambrogio, L., Shimamura, T., et al. BIBW2992, an irreversible EGFR/HER2 inhibitor highly effective in preclinical lung cancer models. *Oncogene*. 2008; 27: 4702-11.

[23] Katakami, N., Atagi, S., Goto, K., et al. LUX-Lung 4: a phase II trial of afatinib in patients with advanced non-small-cell lung cancer who progressed during prior treatment with erlotinib, gefitinib, or both. *J. Clin. Oncol*. 2013; 31 (27): 3335-41.

[24] Miller, V. A., Hirsh, V., Cadranel, J., et al. Afatinib versus placebo for patients with advanced, metastatic non-small-cell lung cancer after failure of erlotinib, gefitinib, or both, and one or two lines of chemotherapy (LUX-Lung 1): a phase 2b/3 randomised trial. *Lancet Oncol*. 2012; 13 (5): 528-38.

[25] Yang, J. C., Shih, J. Y., Su, W., et al. Afatinib for patients with lung adenocarcinoma and epidermal gorwth factor receptor mutations (LUX-Lung 2): a phase II trial. *Lancet Oncol*. 2012; 13 (5): 539-48.

[26] Sequist, L. V., Yahn, J. C., Yamamoto, N., et al. Phase III study of afatinib or cisplatin plus Pemetrexed in patients with metastatic lung adenocarcinoma with EGFR mutations. *J. Clin. Oncol*. 2013; 31 (27): 3327-34.

[27] Yang, J. C., Hirsh, V., Schuler, M., et al. Symptom control and quality of life in LUX-Lung 3: a phase III study of afatinib or cisplatin/pemetrexed in patients with advanced lung adenocarcinoma with EGFR mutations. *J. Clin. Oncol*. 2013; 31 (27): 3342-50.

[28] Wu, Y. L., Zhou, C., Hu, C. P., et al. Afatinib versus cisplatin plus gemcitabine for first-line treatment of Asian patients with advanced non-small-cell lung cancer harbouring EGFR mutations (LUX-Lung 6): an open-label, randomised phase 3 trial. *Lancet Oncol*. 2014; 15 (2): 213-22.

[29] Walter, A. O., Sjin, R. T., Haringsma, H. J., et al. Discovery of a mutant-selective covalent inhibitor of EGFR that overcomes T790M-mediated resistance in NSCLC. *Cancer Discov*. 2013; 3 (12): 1404-15.

[30] Soria, J. C., Sequist, L., Gadgeel, S., et al. First-In-Human evaluation of CO-1686, an irreversible, highly selective tyrosine kinase inhibitor of mutations of EGFR (activating and T790M). *J. Thorac. Oncol*. 2013; 8 (Suppl. 2): abstr. O03.06.

[31] Ranson, M., Pao, W., Kim, D. W., et al. AZD9291: an irreversible, potent and selective tyrosine kinase inhibitor (TKI) of activating (EGFR+) and resistance (T790M) mutations in advanced NSCLC. The AURA study. *J. Thorac. Oncol*. 2013; 11-034 (suppl. 2); abstr. P1.11-034.

[32] Zhou, W., Ercan, D., Chen, L., et al. Novel mutant-selective EGFR kinase inhibitors against EGFR T790M. *Nature*. 2009; 462: 1070-4.

[33] Lee, H. J., Schaefer, G., Heffron, T. P., et al. Noncovalent Wild-type–Sparing Inhibitors of EGFR T790M. *Cancer Discov*. 2013; 3: 168-81.

[34] Soria, J. C., Baselga, J., Hanna, N., et al. Phase I-IIa study of BMS-690514, an EGFR, HER-2 and -4 and VEGFR-1 to -3 oral tyrosine kinase inhibitor, in patients with advanced or metastatic solid tumours. *Eur. J. Cancer*. 2013; 49 (8): 1815-24.

[35] Rizvi, N. A., Kris, M. G., Miller, V. A., et al. Activity of XL647 in clinically selected NSCLC patients (pts) enriched for the presence of EGFR. *J. Clin. Oncol*. 2008; 26: abstr. 8053.

[36] Pietanza, M. C., Lynch, T. J. Jr, Lara, P. N. Jr, et al. XL647-a multitargeted tyrosine kinase inhibitor: results of a phase II study in subjects with non-small cell lung cancer who have progressed after responding to treatment with either gefitinib or erlotinib. *J. Thorac. Oncol*. 2012; 7: 219-26.

[37] Camidge, D. R., Bazhenova, L., Salgia, R., et al. First-in-human dose-finding study of the ALK/EGFR inhibitor AP26113 in patients with advanced malignancies: updated results. *J. Clin. Oncol*. 2013; 31: abstr 8031.

[38] Kurai, J., Chikumi, H., Hashimoto, K., et al. Antibody-dependent cellular cytotoxicity mediated by cetuximab against lung cancer cell lines. *Clin. Cancer Res*. 2007; 13: 1552-61.

[39] Wheatley-Price, P., Shepherd, F. A. Epidermal growth factor receptor inhibitors in the treatment lung cancer: Reality and hopes. *Curr. Opin. Oncol*. 2008; 20: 162-75.

[40] Lynch, T. J., Patel, T., Dreisbach, L., et al. Cetuximab and 1st-line taxane/ carboplatin chemotherapy in advanced non–small-cell lung cancer: Results of the randomized phase multicenter III trial BMS099. *J. Clin. Oncol*. 2010; 28 (6): 911-7.

[41] Pirker, R., Pereira, J. R., Szczesensa, A., et al. Cetuximab plus chemotherapy in patients with advanced non–small-cell lung cancer (FLEX): An open-label randomized phase III trial. *Lancet*. 2009; 373: 1525-31.

[42] Pujol, J. L., Pirker, R., Lynch, T. J., et al. Meta-analysis of individual patient data from randomized trials of chemotherapy plus cetuximab as first-line treatment for advanced non-small cell lung cancer. *Lung Cancer*. 2014; 83 (2): 211-8.

[43] Pirker, R., Pereira, J. R., von Pawel, J., et al. EGFR expression as a predictor of survival for first-line chemotherapy plus cetuximab in patients with advanced non-small-cell lung cancer: analysis of data from the phase 3 FLEX study. *Lancet Oncol*. 2012; 13 (1): 33-42.

[44] Schiller, J. H., von Pawel, J., Schütt, P., et al. Pemetrexed with or without matuzumab as second-line treatment for patients with stage IIIB/IV non-small cell lung cancer. *J. Thorac. Oncol.* 2010; 5: 1977-85.

[45] Crawford, J., Swanson, P., Prager, D., et al. Panitumumab, a fully human antibody, combined with paclitaxel and carboplatin versus paclitaxel and carboplatin alone for first line advanced non-small cell lung cancer (NSCLC): a primary analysis. *Eur. J. Cancer* Suppl. 2005; 3: 324: abstr. 1123.

[46] Dienstmann, R., Felip, E. Necitumumab in the treatment of advanced non-small cell lung cancer: translation from preclinical to clinical development. *Expert Opin. Biol. Ther.* 2011; 11 (9): 1223-31.

[47] Paz-Ares, L., Miziara, J. E., Losonczy, G., et al. Randomized Phase-3 trial (INSPIRE) of Necitumumab plus Cisplatin-Pemetrexed versus Cisplatin-Pemebrexed alone as First-Line Therapy in Stage IV Non-Squamous NSCLC. *J. Thorac. Oncol.* 2013; 8 (Suppl. 2): O03.02.

[48] Janjigian, Y. Y., Groen, H. J., Horn, L., et al. Activity and tolerability of afatinib (BIBW 2992) and cetuximab in NSCLC patients with acquired resistance to erlotinib or gefitinib. *J. Clin. Oncol.* 2011; 29: abstr. 7525.

[49] Hirsch, F. R., Varella-Garcia, M., Franklin, W. A., et al. Evaluation of HER-2/neu gene amplification and protein expression in non-small cell lung carcinomas. *Br. J. Cancer.* 2002; 86: 1449-56.

[50] Heinmöller, P., Gross, C., Beyser, K., et al. HER2 status in non-small cell lung cancer. *Clin. Cancer Res.* 2003; 9: 5238-43.

[51] Zinner, R. G., Glisson, B. S., Fossella, F. V., et al. Trastuzumab in combination with cisplatin and gemcitabine in patients with Her2-overexpressing, untreated, advanced non-small cell lung cancer: Report of a phase II trial and findings regarding optimal identification of patients with Her2-overexpressing disease. *Lung Cancer.* 2004; 44: 99-110.

[52] Maziéres, J., Peters, S., Lepage, B., et al. Lung Cancer that harbors and HER2 Mutation: Epidemiologic characteristics and Therapeutic Perspectives. *J. Clin. Oncol.* 2013; 31 (16): 1997-2004.

[53] De Grève, J., Teugels, E., Geers, C., et al. Clinical activity of afatinib (BIBW 2992) in patients with lung adenocarcinoma with mutations in the kinase domain of HER2/neu. *Lung Cancer.* 2012; 76: 123-7.

[54] De Greve, J., Moran, T., Graas, M. P., et al. Phase II study of afatinib, an irreversible ErbB family blocker, in demographically and genotypically defined non-small cell lung cancer (NSCLC) patients. *J. Clin. Oncol.* 2013; 31: abstr. 8063.

[55] Kris, M., Camidge, R., Giaccone, G., et al. Results with Dacomitinib (PF-00299804), an irreversible pan-her tyrosine kinase inhibitor, in a Phase II cohort of patients with HER2 mutant of amplified lung cancers. *J. Thorac. Oncol.* 2013; 8 (Suppl. 2): abstract P1.11-032.

[56] Kelly, R. J., Carter, C., Giaccone, G., et al. Personalizing therapy in an epidermal growth factor receptor–tyrosine kinase inhibitor–resistant non–small-cell lung cancer using PF-00299804 and trastuzumab. *J. Clin. Oncol.* 2010; 28: e507–e510.

[57] Shimamura, T., Ji, H., Minami, Y., et al. Non-small-cell lung cancer and Ba/ F3 transformed cells harboring the ERBB2 G776insV_G/C mutation are sensitive to the dual-specific epidermal growth factor receptor and ERBB2 inhibitor HKI-272. *Cancer Res*. 2006; 66: 6487-91.

In: Fighting Lung Cancer through the HER Family … ISBN: 978-1-63321-092-9
Editor: Diego Márquez-Medina

Chapter 12

Future II. Targeted Therapies in Early-Stage Non-Small Cell Lung Cancer

Elsa Dalmau Pórtulas, M.D., Ph.D.
and Marta Ferrer Cardona, M.D.
Medical Oncology Department,
Parc Taulí University Hospital of Sabadell, Spain

Abstract

Although the benefit of adjuvant chemotherapy in early stage non-small cell lung cancer (NSCLC) has been amply demonstrated, there is a high risk of relapse after surgery and overall survival remains poor at 5 years. New targeted therapies such as epidermal grow factor receptor tyrosine kinase inhibitors (EGFR-TKI) have shown important activity in advanced disease and are now being studied for incorporation into postoperative treatments.

The first randomized trials designed to demonstrate a survival benefit with EGFR-TKI in the adjuvant setting are showing disappointing results probably due to a lack of stratification by mutation status.

New phase 2 and 3 studies are ongoing to answer if these targeted therapies improve outcomes over chemotherapy in selected *EGFR* mutation positive patients with surgically resected NSCLC. Induction chemotherapy has shown only a small but significant survival benefit in early stages of NSCLC but the use of systemic treatment in neoadjuvant setting has some potential benefits. Its use gives quicker answers to assess sensibility to drugs, can improve resecability and permits to attack micrometastatic disease prematurely. Some phase 2 trials and case reports with EGFR-TKIs as neoadjuvant therapy in stage I-IIIA NSCLC have showed encouraging results in selected population but there isn't still sufficient evidence to use them outside clinical trials.

1. Introduction

Lung cancer is the most common cancer worldwide, accounting for 13% (1.6 million) of the total cases and 18% (1.4 million) of the deaths in 2008 [1]. Overall mortality is 87% and 5-year survival is 12.2% in Europe and 10.7% in Spain [2].

Surgical resection remains the standard of care for patients with early stage non-small cell lung cancer (NSCLC) (stage I-IIIA). However, prognosis varies depending on the stage. The 5-year survival rate for lung cancer is 73% for cases detected when the disease is still very localized and decreases to 24% in IIIA stage [3]. Distant metastases occur in nearly 60% of patients in stages I to IIIA NSCLC after complete resection and most of them will ultimately die within 5 years [4]. Based on this data, it is important to progress in the development of new strategies to improve the prognosis of these patients.

2. Adjuvant Treatment

Numerous trials have been carried out to demonstrate the benefit of adjuvant chemotherapy or radiotherapy to reduce the risk of recurrence and improve NSCLC survival rates. The most recent studies have concluded that adjuvant chemotherapy conferred a survival advantage in patients with resected NSCLC [5-7].

Two meta-analyses were conducted to pool data from these trials. The update of the 1995 NSCLC collaborative group individual data meta-analysis was based on 34 trials that compared surgery with chemotherapy versus surgery alone in 8,447 patients.

The results showed a benefit of chemotherapy on survival (HR 0.86, 95% CI 0.81-0.92; $p < 0.0001$) with an absolute improvement of 4% at 5 years. No significant differences were observed in the relative effect of chemotherapy by stage [8]. The LACE meta-analysis collected individual patient data from five studies with a total of 4584 patients who had undergone complete resection. A 5-year absolute benefit of 5.4% on overall survival (OS) was observed with adjuvant cisplatin-based chemotherapy with a HR of 0.89 (95% CI 0.82-0.96; $p = 0.005$). The HR of death varied by disease stage (0.92 for stage IB, and 0.83 for stages II and III). Stage IA was associated with a potential harm of adjuvant chemotherapy with a HR of 1.41 [9, 10]. A subgroup analysis no pre-planned with all the patients randomized to cisplatin-vinorelvine or observation also showed a significant interaction between this regimen and stage with a great benefit in stage III. However, even with chemotherapy, survival rates remain poor at 5 years [10].

On the other hand, the lower percentage of compliance is an important limitation for the use of adjuvant chemotherapy with up to 67% of patients in adjuvant clinical trials being non-compliant [5, 7, 9, 11-14]. The most common reasons given for premature discontinuation, dose reduction or delay of adjuvant chemotherapy are patient choice or unacceptable toxicity. Evidence of 9% of G3-4 febrile neutropenia and 2% of toxic deaths in ANITA trial for example, urge us to assess the risk-benefit of treatment, especially in earliest stages [7].

Research has focused on developing new therapeutic strategies to improve survival in patients with early-stage of NSCLC after complete resection and to reduce chemotherapy related toxicity.

2.1. Epidermal Growth Factor Receptor Tyrosine Kinase Inhibitors in Adjuvant Setting

Currently, we know that certain subgroups of patients with particular clinical characteristics have a greater response to epidermal grow factor receptor tyrosine kinase inhibitors (EGFR-TKIs) gefitinib (IRESSA) and erlotinib (TARCEVA) and it has been widely proved that *EGFR* sensitive mutations are the most important factor associated with sensitivity to EGFR-TKIs. Several phase III trials, in the setting of first line metastatic NSCLC, have demonstrated the benefit on overall response (OR) and progression-free survival (PFS) of EGFR-TKIs over chemotherapy in selected populations [15-21]. Furthermore, all these studies have shown lower incidences of grade 3-4 toxicities than those seen with chemotherapy.

However, the role for EGFR-targeted therapy as postoperative treatment has not been established. Some subgroups of patients may be likely to benefit from anti-EGFR therapy in this setting, and some series suggest a benefit of these treatments after complete resection in *EGFR*-mutated patients, but no randomized trials directing this therapy in selected population have been performed to date.

The first trial that tried to demonstrate the benefit of EGFR-TKIs in maintenance therapy after a radical treatment included patients with inoperable stage IIIA or IIIB NSCLC. The SWOG-0023 study randomized patients to receive gefitinib or placebo orally after concurrent cisplatin-etoposide and thoracic radiation followed by three cycles of docetaxel. The planned accrual target was 840 patients and the authors hypothesized that gefitinib would produce a 33% increase in median survival time. But the trial was closed prematurely on the recommendation of an unplanned interim analysis that was prompted after the negative results of the ISEL study. With only 620 patients registered, those patients receiving gefitinib had a median survival time of 23 months compared with 35 months for patients receiving placebo (HR 0.633, 95% CI 0.44-0.91; p= 0.013). An imbalance of additional patient characteristics (such smoking history) or an imbalance of tumor-related characteristics such as *EGFR* mutations not captured in this study might explain the negative results of gefitinib maintenance added to the incomplete accrual caused by the premature closure [22].

Only one phase III trial has been published for patients with early stages of NSCLC after complete resection [23]. The NCIC CTG BR19 study was a multicentric, prospective, randomized, placebo-controlled trial of gefitinib in patients with completely resected stages IB-IIIA NSCLC. The study was activated in 2002 but was closed early in April 2005 with discontinuation of study medication after the negative results of the ISEL and SWOG-0023 studies. As a result, BR19 accrued 503 of the planned 1,242 patients with a median duration of active study therapy of less than 5 months. Toxicity in general was mild. Grade 3 to 4 diarrhea, skin effects, fatigue and nausea were more frequent in gefitinib-treated patients. The most common serious adverse event in both cohorts was dyspnea, occurring in 13% and 7% of patients on gefitinib and placebo, respectively. With a median disease-free survival (DFS) of 4.2 years on gefitinib and not reached on the placebo arm (HR 1.22, 95% CI 0.93-1.61; p= 0.15) and a median OS of 5.1 years on gefitinib and not reached for placebo patients (HR 1.24, 95% CI 0.94-1.64; p= 0.14) gefitinib remained not significant and potentially harmful in the adjuvant setting. It should be stressed that the study eligibility criteria were not based on clinical or molecular characteristics. The majority of patients enrolled in BR19 were former or current smokers, almost 30% had squamous cell histology and more than half were males. An exploratory molecular analysis was performed to demonstrate the clinical benefit of adjuvant gefitinib in the subgroup of patients with sensitive mutations but patient population was not enriched for the presence of *EGFR* mutations. In consequence only 15 patients (4%) had sensitive mutations of 359 that could be analyzed. DFS (HR 0.95, 95% CI 0.3-3.01; p= 0.93) and OS (HR 0.57, 95% CI 0.14-2.33; p= 0.43) did not differ between gefitinib treatment and placebo in the subgroup of patients with *EGFR*-mutated tumors, but analyses are limited by the low mutation rate. Taking into account that the study was underpowered, with a brief duration of exposure to gefitinib and no stratification by mutation status, it is not possible to draw conclusions about the benefit of the study drug in *EGFR*-mutated patients with resected NSCLC.

The Randomized, Double-Blind Trial in Adjuvant NSCLC with Tarceva (RADIANT) is another phase 3 trial that compares 2 years of adjuvant erlotinib or 2 years of placebo in 945 patients with resected stage IB-IIIA NSCLC who have overexpression of EGFR protein by immunohistochemistry or *EGFR* gene amplification by fluorescence in situ hybridization. Although *EGFR* mutations are not a prerequisite for study entry, *EGFR* mutation analysis is performed in all patients. At the 2009 ASCO meeting, the RADIANT investigators presented the results of the biomarker analyses from the first 655 patients enrolled which showed an *EGFR* mutation-positive rate of 12%, which suggests that in the final result there will be approximately 38 *EGFR* mutation-positive patients on the placebo arm and about 76 on the erlotinib arm [24]. The estimated study completion date is June 2016, but based on this number of mutated patients, it is unlikely to demonstrate a significant benefit of genotype-directed adjuvant therapy in patients with *EGFR* mutations and resected NSCLC.

Only retrospective cohort studies have been carried-out with exclusively selected *EGFR*-mutated tumors and adjuvant EGFR-TKI therapy with published results.

Investigators from the Memorial-Sloan Kettering Cancer Center analyzed retrospective series of 167 patients with resected stages I-III NSCLC between 2002 and 2008, which were *EGFR* exon 19 or 21 mutation-positive. Of these, 33% (56 patients) received postoperative EGFR-TKI therapy. Twenty-one of the adjuvant TKI-treated patients were enrolled in a phase II trial and received gefitinib for 21 days before surgery and again postoperatively for up 2 years. In a multivariate analysis after adjusting for sex, pathologic stage, surgery type and application of cisplatin-based chemotherapy, an improved 2-year DFS was observed in patients who received perioperative EGFR-TKI therapy compared to those who did not (89 versus 72%) (HR 0.53, 95% CI 0.28-1.03; p= 0.06). A trend toward more favorable OS in patients treated with erlotinib/gefitinib was also seen with a 2-year OS of 96% compared with 90% for patients who were not treated with EGFR-TKI therapy (HR 0.62, 95% CI 0.26-1.51; p= 0.296) [25].

The same investigators presented an update of the prior study including 286 patients with resected lung adenocarcinoma from 2002 to October 2010 and *EGFR* mutation positive identified at the time of surgery of which 84 were treated with adjuvant gefitinib or erlotinib. Patients with *EGFR*-mutant lung cancer who received EGFR-TKI therapy demonstrated a longer DFS than those who did not receive adjuvant erlotinib or gefitinib (HR 0.43, 95% CI 0.26-0.72; p= 0.001). A numerically superior OS was also observed with adjuvant EGFR-TKI, but the difference was not significant (HR 0.50, 95% CI 0.23-1.08; p= 0.076) [26]. It is important to note that patients with *EGFR* mutation who were treated with EGFR-TKIs tended to have a higher stage of the disease and were also more likely to have received up to four cycles of chemotherapy. This bias might underestimate the value of the targeted treatment in reducing the risk of death. In the same publication, the authors performed an update of their database made up of all the patients with complete resected stage I-III lung cancer and *EGFR* mutation analyzed who had undergone surgery between 2002 and 2009. In this case, all patients who received an EGFR-TKI at any time during their treatment course were included in the analysis. *EGFR*-mutant disease at exon 19 or 21 was identified in 222 of 1,118 patients of which 24% received adjuvant EGFR-TKI, 9% received EGFR-TKI only at recurrence and 5% received it both in the adjuvant setting and at recurrence. OS was improved in the mutation positive subgroup compared with patients who did not have *EGFR* mutation (HR 0.51, 95% CI 0.34-0.76; p= 0.002). Nevertheless, taking into account that 83 patients in the EGFR-mutated subgroup received adjuvant EGFR-TKI and/or EGFR-TKI at recurrence, it is difficult to establish whether *EGFR* mutation is a prognostic or a predictive factor for sensibility to EGFR-TKI treatment [26].

At present, phase II and phase III studies with surgically resected stage II-IIIA *EGFR* mutation-positive adenocarcinoma are ongoing in Japan and in China. Two of them, the ADJUVANT and IMPACT trials, are randomized phase III studies comparing gefitinib 250 mg daily for 2 years with adjuvant cisplatin and vinorelbine chemotherapy in patients with *EGFR* mutation whose primary endpoint is DFS.

The preliminary results of a phase 2 study with selected *EGFR* mutated patients were presented at ASCO 2012. The SELECT (Surgically resected EGFR-mutant Lung cancer with adjuvant Erlotinib Cancer Treatment) trial is a single-arm, prospective study of two years of adjuvant erlotinib in 100 patients with resected, stage IA to IIIA *EGFR* mutation positive NSCLC. The primary endpoint is to reach a 2-year DFS > 89% based on the results of the retrospective cohort series of the Memorial-Sloan Kettering Cancer Center. Only results for the first 36 patients showed a DFS of 94% compared to the historical control of 72% with a median follow-up of 2.7 months [27].

Thus, although EGFR-TKI is presently the most potent drug for *EGFR*-positive patients with superiority over platinum-doublet in terms of efficacy, safety and tolerability in first-line metastatic NSCLC, it remains unclear whether these targeted therapies improve outcomes over chemotherapy in the adjuvant setting. Their apoptotic effect may have a role in eradicating minimal residual disease, but patients who have no evidence of disease might develop resistance to the most effective treatment for this way. On the other hand, it is important to define the optimal duration of adjuvant EGFR-TKI therapy because the quality of life of patients while on therapy also needs to be considered if treatment has to be given over a prolonged period of time. Furthermore, another unanswered question is whether EGFR TKI may be a substitute to standard adjuvant therapies or a complement. A subgroup analysis from the National Cancer Institute of Canada JBR.10 study identified *EGFR* mutations in 43 patients of 221 analyzed. The benefit of adjuvant chemotherapy on DFS was numerically higher in patients with sensitizing mutations (exon 19 deletions or L858R mutations) (HR 0.44, 95% CI 0.11-1.70; p= 0.22) than in the subgroup with *EGFR* wild-type tumors (HR 0.76, 95% CI 0.56-1.04; p= 0.08) [28]. The phase 3 randomized trials that are currently ongoing will be useful to answer all these questions.

3. Neoadjuvant Treatment

Some potential benefits of neoadjuvant or induction therapy have been used to design clinical trials in this setting. Treatment administration prior to surgery provides quicker answers to assess sensibility of drugs with the measurement of pathologic or radiologic treatment response that can be used to plan adjuvant therapy. Moreover, effective neoadjuvant treatment would facilitate surgery and resecability by shrinking the primary tumor and reducing possibly involved lymph nodes [29, 30]. On the other hand, considering that the presence of micrometastatic disease after surgery has a poorer prognosis [31], the use of systemic treatments in earliest times may be useful to attack these micrometastases prematurely.

A 2005 meta-analysis of 7 randomized controlled trials featuring 988 patients reported that neoadjuvant chemotherapy is associated with an absolute survival benefit of 6% at 5 years compared with surgery alone [32]. An update was published in 2010 adding 6 more randomized clinical trials. The combined HR in terms of OS of these 13 trials was 0.84 (95% CI 0.77-0.92), which was a statistically significant result (p= 0.0001) and, as a whole, was in favor of neoadjuvant chemotherapy. When only patients with stage III were considered, the combined HR of neoadjuvant chemotherapy was the same (HR 0.84) [33]. As patients with stage I-II disease were hardly represented in the trials included in these meta-analyses, it was not possible to draw any conclusion for this subgroup. More recently, the NATCH trial found no statistical difference in 5-year DFS (p= 0.71) between preoperative chemotherapy (38.3%), adjuvant chemotherapy (36.6%) or surgery alone (34.1%) in patients with predominantly stage I disease [34]. Thus, treatment with neoadjuvant chemotherapy in earliest stages does not seem to provide any benefit on survival. In addition, toxicity and decreased compliance persist, with up to 32% in neoadjuvant clinical trials being noncompliant and, in daily practice, only half of patients accepting adjuvant therapy [35-38]. Therefore, it is important to find more acceptable and less toxic treatments with improved efficacy for the early NSCLC population. Another important goal in the neoadjuvant treatment is to achieve a pathologic complete response. In breast cancer, pathologic complete response is the current drug development paradigm because it has been used as a surrogate for OS. In lung cancer, some investigators have studied the association between pathologic responses and overall survival in patients with resected NSCLC after neoadjuvant chemotherapy. A series from the MD Anderson was used to assess the ability of histopathologic criteria to predict survival and chemotherapy response in 192 patients with NSCLC treated with neoadjuvant chemotherapy. The presence of ≤10% viable tumor cells after neoadjuvant chemotherapy in the resected specimens predicted better DFS and OS, even when controlled for stage [39]. In the last World Conference on Lung Cancer, Chaft presented the results of a series of at least 46 patients with pathologically confirmed IIIAN2 disease who underwent surgery and ultimately underwent R0 resection. Major pathologic response defined as ≤10% viable tumor tissue was clearly related with overall survival identifying patients with good clinical outcomes after neoadjuvant chemotherapy (HR 0.26, 95% CI 0.07-0.95) [40]. Taking into account that histopathologic response may serve as a surrogate end point for survival and may potentially have a role to define more accurate subsequent therapeutic management, it is important to evaluate novel chemotherapeutic and biologic therapies in selected populations to achieve major pathologic responses.

3.1. EGFR-TKI in Neoadjuvant Setting

Given the activity of EGFR-TKIs in advanced disease, there is potentially a subset of patients with early NSCLC who may benefit from neoadjuvant EGFR-TKIs. Their low toxicity profile and the possibility of rapid tumor response suggest that this form of therapy may be used for induction therapy. Although no data published so far has supported the use of EGFR-TKIs as neoadjuvant therapy in stage I-IIIA NSCLC, some phase 2 trials with gefitinib or erlotinib have showed encouraging results.

Investigators from The Princess Margaret Hospital explored the impact of gefitinib on clinical response in a phase II trial that included at least 36 patients with clinical stage I disease with tumor size ≥10 mm who received gefitinib once daily for up to 28 days prior to surgery. Patients who experienced a partial response were allowed to continue adjuvant gefitinib for up to 2 years. Four patients (11%) had partial response and 15 patients (43%) had some tumor reduction. *EGFR* mutations were detected in 6 patients (17%) and although all of them showed reduction in tumor size, only half achieved partial response [41]. The only significant predictor of partial response was the presence of an *EGFR* mutation. Only 3 patients developed grade 3 toxicities (rash, diarrhea and ALT elevation) but did not require either dose reduction or discontinuation. At the time of the publication 78% of patients remained disease free, including all four patients with PR. Rizvi et al. designed another phase II trial to prospectively correlate radiographic response rate to gefitinib (≥ 25% decrease in bidimensional measurements in 21 days) with the presence of sensitizing *EGFR* mutations in enriched population [42]. Eligible patients had pathologically confirmed clinical stage I or II NSCLC with clinical features that predict for EGFR-TKI response and received gefitinib orally daily for at least 21 days before surgery. For patients that demonstrated a radiographic response and/or patients with mutations in the protein tyrosine kinase domain of EGFR, gefitinib was recommended for 2 additional years. A bidimensional response of 25% or more was obtained in 21 of 50 treated patients (42%). Seventeen of 21 patients with a response had an *EGFR* mutation and three of the 4 with an *EGFR* mutation who did not meet the criteria for response had lesion size changes of more than 10%. During preoperative treatment, toxicities were mild. Only one patient had grade 3 diarrheas and one patient discontinued treatment due to grade 2 rash. With a median follow-up of 44.1 months, there were no statistically significant differences in PFS between patients who received adjuvant gefitinib and those who did not or by presence or absence of an *EGFR* mutation.

Another trial performed in the Netherlands analyzed the pathologic response in 60 patients with clinical $T_{1\text{-}3}N_{0\text{-}1}$ NSCLC (29 of whom fulfilled the criteria of enriched population) who received neoadjuvant erlotinib daily during 3 weeks before resection. Specimens of 11 patients (18%) showed pathologic partial response with morphologic signs of therapy-induced regression or necrosis of 50% to 90% of the tumor mass, including 8 of 29 in the enriched population.Pathologic response was scored as more than 95% necrosis in three patients (5%), all in the enriched population. *EGFR* mutations were found in seven of 56 patients with NSCLC, five of them in the enriched population. Three patients with an *EGFR* mutation had a pathologic partial response and 4 patients had a metabolic response. Toxicity in general was mild, although in seven patients, mostly skin rash was reason for patients to stop treatment [43]. Some case reports provide more experience about the use of neoadjuvant

EGFR-TKIs in NSCLC patients harboring *EGFR* mutations, some of them in patients with locally advanced disease [44-46] (Table 1).

Table 1. Summary of Studies with EGFR-TKI as Neoadjuvant Treatments

Author /Study	Phase trial	N	Stage	Scheme	OR(%)	Comments
Lara-Guerra H	II	36	I	Gefitinib x 4 w → surgery	11% (RECIST)	EGFR M+ 17% Correlation with response 50%
Rizvi NA	II	50	I-II	Gefitinib x 3 w →surgery	42% (≥25% decrease in bidimensional measurements)	EGFR M+ 42% Correlation with response 80%
Schaake EE	II	60	I-IIIA	Erlotinib x 3 w →surgery	23% (>50% necrosis)	EGFR M+ 13% Correlation with response 43%
Liu M	Case report	1	IIIB	Getininib x 1 mo → surgery	pCR	EGFR M+ E21
Kappers I	Case report	1	IIIA	Erlotinib x 3 w →surgery	CR (PET/CT) Microscopic 1.5 mm	EGFR M+ E19
Ong M	Case report	1	IIIAN2	Erlotinib x 3 mo →surgery	PR (CT)	EGFR M+ E21

EGFR M+ Epidermal Grow Factor Receptor Mutation positive; E21 exon 21; E19 exon 19; OR overall response; w weeks; mo months; pCR pathologic complete response; CR complete response; PR partial response.

Several ongoing phase II trials are presently being conducted to evaluate the role of EGFR TKIs in the neoadjuvant setting. The EMERGING trial, for example, is a phase II-III study that investigates the efficacy and safety of erlotinib versus gemcitabine plus cisplatin as neoadjuvant treatment in patients with stage IIIA-N2 NSCLC with *EGFR* activating mutations.

Currently, the role of neoadjuvant chemotherapy in early stages of NSCLC remains unclear and there is a need for further treatment improvements, especially for patients with stage I disease. Although some encouraging results have been obtained with preoperative EGFR-TKIs in *EGFR* mutation-positive patients, there isn't still sufficient evidence to use EGFR-TKIs outside clinical trials.

References

[1] Jemal A, Bray F, Center MM, Ferlay J, Ward E, Forman D. Global cancer statistics. *CA Cancer J. Clin.* 2011; 61 (2): 69-90.

[2] Sant M, Allemani C, Santaquilani M, Knijn A, Marchesi F, Capocaccia R. EUROCARE-4. Survival of cancer patients diagnosed in 1995-1999. Results and commentary. *Eur. J. Cancer.* 2009; 45 (6): 931-91.

[3] Goldstraw P, Crowley J, Chansky K, et al. The IASLC Lung Cancer Staging Project: proposals for the revision of the TNM stage groupings in the forthcoming (seventh) edition of the TNM Classification of malignant tumours. *J. Thorac. Oncol.* 2007; (8): 706-14.

[4] Ikeda N, Nagase S, Ohira T. Individualized adjuvant chemotherapy for surgically resected lung cancer and the roles of biomarkers. *Ann. Thorac. Cardiovasc. Surg.* 2009; 15 (3): 144-9.

[5] Arriagada R, Bergman B, Dunant A, Le Chevalier T, Pignon J-P, Vansteenkiste J. Cisplatin-based adjuvant chemotherapy in patients with completely resected non-small-cell lung cancer. *N. Engl. J. Med.* 2004; 350 (4): 351-60.

[6] Winton T, Livingston R, Johnson D, et al. Vinorelbine plus cisplatin vs. observation in resected non-small-cell lung cancer. *N. Engl. J. Med.* 2005; 352 (25): 2589-97.

[7] Douillard JY, Rosell R, De Lena M, et al. Adjuvant vinorelbine plus cisplatin versus observation in patients with completely resected stage IB-IIIA non-small-cell lung cancer (Adjuvant Navelbine International Trialist Association [ANITA]): a randomised controlled trial. *Lancet Oncol.* 2006; 7 (9): 719-27.

[8] NSCLC Meta-analyses Collaborative Group, Arriagada R, Auperin A, et al. Adjuvant chemotherapy, with or without postoperative radiotherapy, in operable non-small-cell lung cancer: two meta-analyses of individual patient data. *Lancet.* 2010; 375 (9722): 1267-77.

[9] Pignon JP, Tribodet H, Scagliotti GV, et al. Lung adjuvant cisplatin evaluation: a pooled analysis by the LACE Collaborative Group. *J. Clin. Oncol.* 2008; 26 (21): 3552-3559.

[10] Douillard JY, Tribodet H, Aubert D, et al. Adjuvant cisplatin and vinorelbine for completely resected non-small cell lung cancer: subgroup analysis of the Lung Adjuvant Cisplatin Evaluation. *J. Thorac. Oncol.* 2010; 5 (2): 220-8.

[11] Strauss GM, Herndon JE 2nd, Maddaus MA, et al. Adjuvant paclitaxel plus carboplatin compared with observation in stage IB non-small-cell lung cancer: CALGB 9633 with the Cancer and Leukemia Group B, Radiation Therapy Oncology Group, and North Central Cancer Treatment Group Study Groups. *J. Clin. Oncol.* 2008; 26 (31): 5043-51.

[12] Aljubran A, Leighl N, Pintilie M, Feld R, Burkes R, Shepherd F. Compliance of adjuvant chemotherapy in non-small cell lung cancer (NSCLC); no longer an issue. *J. Clin. Oncol.* 2006, ASCO Annual Meeting Proceedings (Post-Meeting Edition); 24: 7154.

[13] Scagliotti GV, Fossati R, Torri V, et al. Randomized study of adjuvant chemotherapy for completely resected stage I, II, or IIIA non-small-cell lung cancer. *J. Natl. Cancer Inst.* 2003; 95 (19): 1453-6.

[14] Kassam F, Shepherd FA, Johnston M, et al. Referral patterns for adjuvant chemotherapy in patients with completely resected non-small cell lung cancer. *J. Thorac. Oncol.* 2007; 2 (1): 39-43.

[15] Mok TS, Wu YL, Thongprasert S, et al. Gefitinib or carboplatin-paclitaxel in pulmonary adenocarcinoma. *N. Engl. J. Med.* 2009; 361 (10): 947-57.

[16] Han JY, Park K, Kim SW, et al. First-SIGNAL: first-line single-agent iressa versus gemcitabine and cisplatin trial in never-smokers with adenocarcinoma of the lung. *J. Clin. Oncol.* 2012; 30 (10): 1122-8.

[17] Mitsudomi T, Morita S, Yatabe Y, et al. Gefitinib versus cisplatin plus docetaxel in patients with non-small-cell lung cancer harbouring mutations of the epidermal growth factor receptor (WJTOG3405): an open label, randomised phase 3 trial. *Lancet Oncol.* 2010; 11 (2): 121-28.

[18] Maemondo M, Inoue A, Kobayashi K, Sugawara S, et al. Gefitinib or chemotherapy for non-small-cell lung cancer with mutated EGFR. *N. Engl. J. Med.* 2010; 362 (25): 2380-8.

[19] Zhou C, Wu YL, Chen G, et al. Erlotinib versus chemotherapy as first-line treatment for patients with advanced EGFR mutation-positive non-small-cell lung cancer (OPTIMAL, CTONG-0802): a multicentre, open-label, randomised, phase 3 study. *Lancet Oncol.* 2011; 12 (8): 735-42.

[20] Rosell R, Carcereny E, Gervais R, et al. Erlotinib versus standard chemotherapy as first-line treatment for European patients with advanced EGFR mutation-positive non-small-cell lung cancer (EURTAC): a multicentre, open-label, randomised phase 3 trial. *Lancet Oncol.* 2012; 13 (3): 239-246.

[21] Sequist LV, Yang JC, Yamamoto N, et al. Phase III study of afatinib or cisplatin plus pemetrexed in patients with metastatic lung adenocarcinoma with EGFR mutations. *J. Clin. Oncol.* 2013; 31 (27): 3327-34.

[22] Kelly K, Chansky K, Gaspar LE, et al. Phase III trial of maintenance gefitinib or placebo after concurrent chemoradiotherapy and docetaxel consolidation in inoperable stage III non-small-cell lung cancer: SWOG S0023. *J. Clin.Oncol.* 2008; 26 (15): 2450-6.

[23] Goss GD, O'Callaghan C, Lorimer I, et al. Gefitinib versus placebo in completely resected non-small-cell lung cancer: results of the NCIC CTG BR19 study. *J. Clin. Oncol.* 2013; 31 (27): 3320-6.

[24] Richardson F, Richardson K, Sennello G, et al. Biomarker analysis from completely resected NSCLC patients enrolled in an adjuvant erlotinib clinical trial (RADIANT). *J. Clin. Oncol.* 2009 ASCO Annual Meeting Proceedings (Post-Meeting Edition); 27: 7520.

[25] Janjigian YY, Park BJ, Zakowski MF, et al. Impact on disease-free survival of adjuvant erlotinib or gefitinib in patients with resected lung adenocarcinomas that harbor EGFR mutations. *J. Thorac. Oncol.* 2011; 6 (3): 569-75.

[26] D'Angelo SP, Janjigian YY, Ahye N, et al. Distinct clinical course of EGFR-mutant resected lung cancers: results of testing of 1118 surgical specimens and effects of adjuvant gefitinib and erlotinib. *J. Thorac. Oncol.* 2012; 7 (12): 1815-22.

[27] Neal J, Pennell N, Govindan R. The SELECT study: a multicenter phase II trial of adjuvant erlotinib in resected epidermal growth factor receptor (EGFR) mutation-

positive non-small cell lung cancer. *J. Clin. Oncol.* 2012 ASCO Annual Meeting Proceedings (Post-Meeting Edition); 30: 7010.
[28] Tsao M-S, Sakurada A, Ding K, et al. Prognostic and predictive value of epidermal growth factor receptor tyrosine kinase domain mutation status and gene copy number for adjuvant chemotherapy in non-small cell lung cancer. *J. Thorac. Oncol.* 2011; 6 (1): 139-47.
[29] De Marinis F, Gebbia V, De Petris L. Neoadjuvant chemotherapy for stage IIIA-N2 non-small cell lung cancer. *Ann. Oncol.* 2005; 16 (Suppl 4): iv116-22.
[30] Pujol JL, Le Chevalier T, Ray P, et al. Neoadjuvant chemotherapy of locally advanced non-small cell lung cancer. *Lung. Cancer.* 1995; 12 (Suppl 1): S107-18.
[31] Gu CD, Osaki T, Oyama T, et al. Detection of micrometastatic tumor cells in pN0 lymph nodes of patients with completely resected nonsmall cell lung cancer: impact on recurrence and Survival. *Ann. Surg.* 2002; 235 (1): 133-9.
[32] Burdett S, Stewart LA, Rydzewska L. A systematic review and meta-analysis of the literature: chemotherapy and surgery versus surgery alone in non-small cell lung cancer. *J. Thorac. Oncol.* 2006; 1 (7): 611-21.
[33] Song WA, Zhou NK, Wang W, et al. Survival benefit of neoadjuvant chemotherapy in non-small cell lung cancer: an updated meta-analysis of 13 randomized control trials. *J. Thorac. Oncol.* 2010; 5 (4): 510-6.
[34] Felip E, Rosell R, Maestre JA, et al. Preoperative chemotherapy plus surgery versus surgery plus adjuvant chemotherapy versus surgery alone in early-stage non-small-cell lung cancer. *J. Clin. Oncol.* 2010; 28 (19): 3138-45.
[35] Ramnath N, Sommers E, Robinson L, Nwogu C, Sharma A, Cantor A, Bepler G. Phase II study of neoadjuvant chemotherapy with gemcitabine and vinorelbine in resectable non-small cell lung cancer. *Chest.* 2005; 128 (5): 3467-74.
[36] Depierre A, Milleron B, Moro-Sibilot D, et al. Preoperative chemotherapy followed by surgery compared with primary surgery in resectable stage I (except T1N0), II, and IIIa non-small-cell lung cancer. *J. Clin. Oncol.* 2002; 20 (1): 247-53.
[37] Bepler G, Sommers KE, Cantor A, et al. Clinical efficacy and predictive molecular markers of neoadjuvant gemcitabine and pemetrexed in resectable non-small cell lung cancer. *J. Thorac. Oncol.* 2008; 3 (10): 1112-8.
[38] Gilligan D, Nicolson M, Smith I, et al. Preoperative chemotherapy in patients with resectable non-small cell lung cancer: results of the MRC LU22/NVALT 2/EORTC 08012 multicentre randomised trial and update of systematic review. *Lancet.* 2007; 369 (9577): 1929-37.
[39] Pataer A, Kalhor N, Correa AM, et al. Histopathologic response criteria predict survival of patients with resected lung cancer after neoadjuvant chemotherapy. *J. Thorac. Oncol.* 2012; 7 (5): 825-32.
[40] Chaft JE, Hellmann MD, Rusch VW, Travis WD, Kris MG. Major pathologic response (≤10% viable tumor) following neoadjuvant chemotherapy as a surrogate for overall survival in patients with pathologically documented stage IIIA (N2) lung adenocarcinomas. 14th World Conference on Lung Cancer 2013.
[41] Lara-Guerra H, Waddell TK, Salvarrey MA, et al. Phase II Study of Preoperative Gefitinib in Clinical Stage I Non-Small-Cell Lung Cancer. *J. Clin. Oncol.* 2009; 27 (36): 6229-36.

[42] Rizvi NA, Rusch V, Pao W, et al. Molecular characteristics predict clinical outcomes: prospective trial correlating response to the EGFR tyrosine kinase inhibitor gefitinib with the presence of sensitizing mutations in the tyrosine binding domain of the EGFR gene. *Clin. Cancer Res. 2011*; 17 (10): 3500-6.

[43] Schaake EE, Kappers I, Codrington HE, et al. Tumor Response and Toxicity of Neoadjuvant Erlotinib in Patients With Early-Stage Non-Small-Cell Lung Cancer. *J. Clin. Oncol.* 2012; 30 (22): 2731-8.

[44] Liu M, Jiang G, He W, Zhang P, Song N. Surgical Resection of Locally Advanced Pulmonary Adenocarcinoma After Gefitinib Therapy. *Ann. Thorac. Surg.* 2011; 92 (1): e11-12.

[45] Kappers I, Klomp HM, Burgers JA, Van Zandwijk N, Haas RL, van Pel R. Neoadjuvant (Induction) Erlotinib Response in Stage IIIA Non-Small-Cell Lung Cancer. *J. Clin. Oncol.* 2008; 26 (25): 4205-7.

[46] Ong M, Kwan K, Kamel-Reid S, Vincent M. Neoadjuvant erlotinib and surgical resection of a stage iiia papillary adenocarcinoma of the lung with an L861Q activating EGFR mutation. *Curr. Oncol.* 2012; 19 (3): e222-6.

In: Fighting Lung Cancer through the HER Family …
Editor: Diego Márquez-Medina
ISBN: 978-1-63321-092-9

Chapter 13

Resistance I. Acquired Resistance to Epidermal Growth Factor Receptor Tyrosine Kinase Inhibitors in *EGFR*-mutant Non-Small Cell Lung Cancer

Jordi Remón, M.D. and Pilar Lianes, M.D., Ph.D.
Medical Oncology Department, Hospital of Mataró, Spain

Abstract

The discovery of mutated oncogenes has changed the standard approach in advanced non-small cell lung cancer (NSCLC) patients and opened up a new era for the development of personalized treatment for those patients with sensitizing mutation of the Epidermal Growth Factor Receptor (*EGFR*). Nevertheless, the occurrence of clinical resistance limits the long-term results of these novel agents. The identification of these mechanisms of acquired resistance (AR) to EGFR tyrosine kinase inhibitors (TKI) is crucial to develop potential therapeutic strategies to overcome resistance. However, in up to 30% of cases, the underlying mechanisms of AR are still unexplained. In this chapter we will focus on the AR mechanisms to EGFR-TKI and some therapeutic strategies currently under study to overcome resistance, and briefly in the mechanisms of primary resistance to EGFR-TKI.

1. Introduction

Somatic mutations in the Epidermal Growth Factor Receptor (*EGFR*) are present in approximately 10-16% of Caucasian European patients diagnosed with metastatic lung adenocarcinoma [1, 2]. These mutations result in enhanced EGFR signaling and confer hypersensitivity to first- and second-generation of tyrosine kinase inhibitors (TKI) in advanced non-small cell lung cancer (NSCLC).

EGFR is a tyrosine kinase receptor and a crucial component of cell signaling pathway activation. These pathways include: the Ras-Raf-Mek pathways, that transduce signals related with proliferative activity, and the phosphoinositide 3-kinase (PI3K)-AKT-mammalian target of rapamycin (mTOR) pathway, that transduces survival signals, largely linked to an anti-apoptotic effect. Unlikely to wild-type EGFR cells, the *EGFR*-mutant cells, selectively transduce through survival signals on which they are dependent. Inhibition of these signals by TKIs contributes to the efficacy of the drug [3].

Six randomized phase III trials have demonstrated that first-generation EGFR-TKI such as erlotinib or gefitinib, improve the response rate (RR) and the progression free survival (PFS), compared with upfront platinum combination chemotherapy [4-10] (Table 1) in *EGFR* mutant advanced lung cancer patients. Recently in two randomized phase III trials (LUX-Lung 3 [11] and LUX-Lung 6 [12] trials), second-generation EGFR-TKI such as afatinib, which is an irreversible inhibitor against all EGFR family members and in preclinical data against T790M mutation [13], has also demonstrated better outcome in RR and PFS compared with two different regimens of chemotherapy, one of them including pemetrexed, as first line treatment in *EGFR* mutant patients. However, any of these trials have improved overall survival (OS) with EGFR-TKI compared with upfront chemotherapy. FASTACT2 trial is the first randomized phase III trial in Asiatic population that has demonstrated a significant improvement in OS with first-generation EGFR-TKI in unselected and selected population when it is intercalated with chemotherapy followed by maintenance treatment with EGFR-TKI compared with first line chemotherapy [14].

Despite the initial dramatic outcome to EGFR-TKI monotherapy, resistance inevitable develops. Resistance to targeted therapies can be categorized as primary (ie, intrinsic) resistance or secondary (ie, acquired) resistance. Patients with primary resistance are initially refractory to treatment, whereas acquired resistance (AR) denotes disease progression after an initial response. Criteria for AR were recently proposed for *EGFR* mutant NSCLC [15]. Indeed, most of NSCLC patients with *EGFR*-activating mutation develop AR after less than 1-year treatment initiation (Table 1). Therefore is critical to identify the underlying mechanisms of EGFR-TKI resistance to develop more effective treatment strategies.

2. Primary Resistance to EGFR-TKI

A subset of lung adenocarcinomas shows primary resistance to EGFR-TKI therapy, even in presence of an activating mutation in *EGFR*. Primary resistance may be due in part to: first, differential TKI sensitivities across various *EGFR* mutations, such as exon 20 insertions that accounted for at least 9% of all *EGFR* mutated tumors [16, 17] and unlikely to "classic" *EGFR* mutations in exon 19 deletions and L858R, confers poorer prognosis by resistance to first- [18] and second-generation EGFR-TKI [19]; second, secondary genetic alterations that co-occur with sensitizing *EGFR* mutations, such as T790M mutation [20], and its presence has been significantly associated with poorer outcome on TKI therapy, or *MET* amplification [21]; third, the presence of other genetic alterations which affect signaling downstream from EGFR, such as mutations of *KRAS* [22], *PIK3CA* [23], and loss of PTEN expression [24, 25]; fourth, heterogeneity of EGFR-TKI response as a consequence of differences within cellular apoptotic machinery such us BIM, a pro-apoptotic protein which is upregulated in response to

EGFR-TKI [26] and whose levels correlate with the degree of apoptotic response. High pretreatment BIM RNA levels in *EGFR* mutant patients were associated a longer PFS after EGFR-TKI treatment [27].

Table 1. Randomized phase III trials of first- or second-generation EGFR TKI compared with chemotherapy as first-line treatment in EGFR-mutant advanced NSCLC

Author		Study	N	RR (%)	PFS (mo)	OS (mo)
Mok [4]	GEFITINIB	IPASS	261	71.2 vs. 47.3	9.5 vs. 6.3	21.6 vs. 21.9
Han [5]	GEFITINIB	First-SIGNAL	42	84.6 vs. 37.5	8.4 vs. 6.7	27.2 vs. 25.6
Mitsudomi [6, 7]	GEFITINIB	WJTOG 3405	177	62.1 vs. 32.2	9.2 vs. 6.3	35.5 vs. 38.8
Maemondo [8]	GEFITINIB	NEJGSG 002	228	73.7 vs. 30.7	10.8 vs. 5.4	27.7 vs. 26.6
Zhou [9]	ERLO	OPTIMAL	154	83 vs. 36	13.7 vs. 4.6	22.6 vs. 28.8
Rosell [10]	ERLO	EURTAC*	173	58 vs. 15	9.7 vs. 5.2	19.3 vs. 19.5
Sequist [11]	AFAT	LUX-Lung 3**	345	56 vs. 23	11.1 vs. 6.9	HR 1.12
Wu [12]	AFAT	LUX-Lung 6	364	67 vs. 23	11 vs. 5.6	HR 0.95

* First phase III study including Western patients. ** 26% of white patients included.
ERLO.: Erlotinib; Afat. Afatinib; RR: Response Rate; PFS: Progression Free Survival; OS: Overall Survival; mo: months.

3. Acquired Resistance to EGFR-TKI

Several mechanisms of AR have been yet reported, which could be grouped in four main categories: first, the presence of secondary mutations in *EGFR*; second, the presence of parallel activation of downstream signaling pathways (by-pass tracks activation); third, a phenomenon of a phenotypic transformation; and fourth, the occurrence of genetic alterations in addition to the *EGFR* mutation (Figure 1). The mechanisms and frequencies of AR to EGFR-TKI in Asian population are comparable tot-those observed in Western populations [28].

However, approximately up to 30% of cases, the AR mechanisms are still unexplained. Currently, tumor rebiopsy at recurrence is becoming increasingly important due to the potential therapeutic consequence in the clinical setting, a direct change in therapy or better prediction of prognosis [29, 30]. However, not all patients are suitable for performing a rebiopsy at AR time or there is no optimal tissue sample. Recent studies have shown that genomic alterations in solid cancers can be characterized by massively parallel sequencing of circulating cell-free tumor DNA released from cancer cells into plasma, representing a non-invasive liquid biopsy [31]. These liquid biopsies could enable the investigation of AR mechanisms and allows the investigators to monitor the evolution of resistance over the time [32].

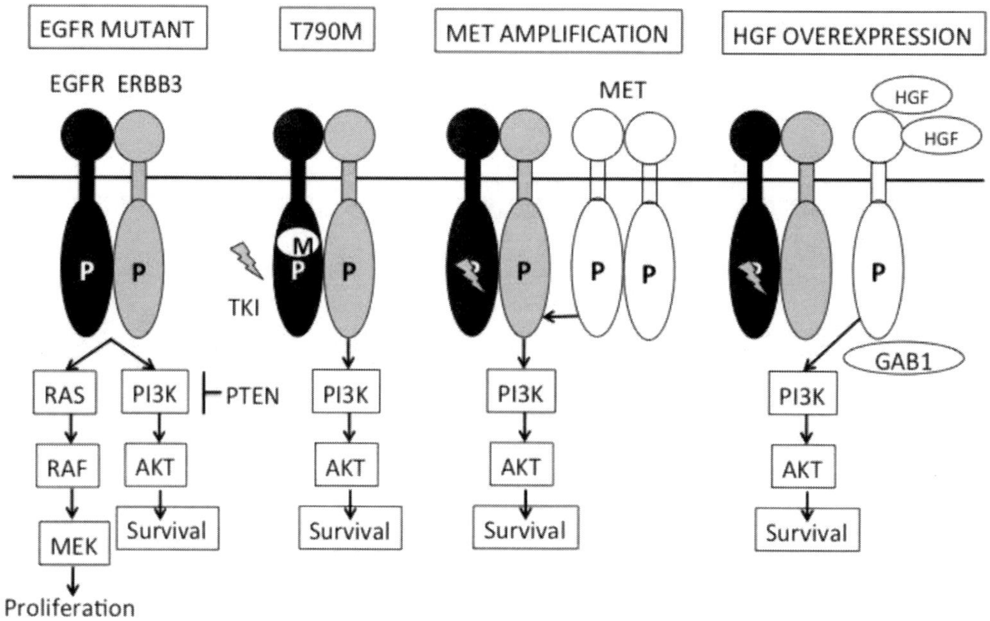

Figure 1. Main mechanisms of AR to EGFR-TKI in EGFR-mutant NSCLC cells.

Given that the growth and survival signals are so dependent upon EGFR activation, it is understandable that cells would overcome this inhibition by developing resistance mechanisms that reactivate EGFR despite the presence of the EGFR-TKI. *EGFR* mutant lung cancers maintain a certain degree of sensitivity to TKI despite the development of AR. In a pilot study, which included 13 patients (8 *EGFR*-mutant patients) with AR to EGFR-TKI, a CT-scan and positron emission tomography imaging were performed at baseline, after a period of 3 weeks free of TKI, and after 3 weeks of resuming the TKI. Tumor volume and metabolic activity increased significantly when the TKI was stopped and decreased when TKI was restarted, suggesting the dependence of these tumors even when resistance appears [33].

4. Mechanisms of AR to EGFR-TKI in EGFR-Mutant Patients

4.1. Presence of Second-Site Mutations in EGFR

In *EGFR* mutant NSCLC, the earliest reports of TKI resistance identified an analogous secondary mutation in exon 20 of *EGFR*, leading to a threonine-to-methionine substitution within the gatekeeper residue at position 790 (T790M) [34, 35]. Approximately 50-60% of cases with AR to EGFR-TKI therapy carry a secondary T790M mutation in the kinase domain of the EGFR that coexists with the *EGFR* activating mutation [36, 37]. It has suggested that the incidence of T790M mutation in resistant cell lines is undetected based on most commonly used detection methods because it can be present in a very low proportion of EGFR alleles, and this allelic dilution can obscure detection of the T790M mutation [38]. Higher sensitivity assays, such as high-performance liquid chromatography, mass spectrometry, and locked nucleic acid PCR techniques, have been proposed as alternative methods. Based on 64 patients tested by the combination of standard DNA sequencing and the highly sensitive locked nucleic acid PCR/sequencing assay developed to detect low levels (0.1% of the total DNA) of mutant EGFR T790M, the authors were able to estimate a T790M mutation prevalence of 70% [39].

The T790M mutation causes resistance because alters the proper binding of the drug to the ATP pocket of EGFR and restores the affinity for ATP at the level of wild-type EGFR, re-establishing ATP as the favored substrate rather than EGFR-TKI [40]. In vitro studies, cells carrying *EGFR* activating mutation proliferate faster (1.22 times) than resistant clones harboring T790M, conferring a more indolent tumor growth [41], which translates in a more indolent tumor phenotype. Clinical data on patients carrying acquired T790M mutation had longer post-progression survival than those without T790M, 19 months and 12 months, respectively. Also, T790M mutation positive patients were more likely to progress in an existing site of disease and had higher performance status than T790M mutation negative patients [42].

Preclinical data with irreversible TKI was encouraging showing activity against lung cancer cells harboring *EGFR* activating mutations concomitantly with the T790M resistance mutation [43, 44]. However, the results from clinical data with irreversible EGFR-TKI have been very disappointing respect to RR and PFS even in selected patients, with no responses in patients whose tumors harbored the T790M mutation, due to dosage limitation related to the toxicity when wild-type EGFR was also inhibited [45]. In fact, in two in vitro assays, T790M was the main factor that significantly abrogated the efficacy of two different irreversible pan-ERBB inhibitors, afatinib [46] and dacomitinib [47]. In the clinic, afatinib showed lower outcome for those *EGFR* mutated patients with primary T790M mutations (PFS 2.9 months, OS 14.9 months) in a retrospective analysis from LUX-Lung 2, LUX-Lung 3 and LUX-Lung 6 trials [48]. In the LUX-Lung 1 phase III, afatinib versus placebo in 697 unselected patients previously treated with an EGFR-TKI, demonstrated a 2-months improvement in PFS (3.3 months versus 1.1 months; HR 0.38, 95% CI 0.31-0.48; $p< 0.0001$) although no significant benefit in OS was observed (10.8 months versus 12 months; HR 1.08, 95% CI 0.86-1.35; $p= 0.74$) [49]. Similar activity was reported in the LUX-Lung 4 trial, where afatinib showed a modest activity in patients with advanced NSCLC who progressed while receiving treatment with reversible EGFR-TKI [50]. These findings suggest that afatinib administered at conventional doses may not be efficient to suppress NSCLC clones harboring *EGFR* T790M mutation.

Based on the new phase III trials, LUX-Lung 3 [11] and LUX-Lung 6 [12] results; AR also is a major clinical issue in those *EGFR* mutant patients treated with upfront irreversible EGFR-TKI. However, currently, there is no extensive clinical data available which points at the mechanistic basis of afatinib resistance.

The T790M mutation enables cancer cells to maintain oncogenic EGFR signalling in the presence of current EGFR-TKI, suggesting that tumor growth and proliferation remains dependent on EGFR (Figure 1). Previous studies have shown that intensification of the EGFR inhibition with the addition of monoclonal antibodies (mAB) targeting EGFR pathway such as cetuximab to the irreversible EGFFR TKI have shown promising synergistic activity in EGFR mutant xenografts [51]. This hypothesis has been confirmed in a phase I/II clinical trial testing afatinib plus cetuximab in 100 *EGFR* mutated heavily pre-treated patients with or without T790M mutation, with an encouraging RR of 32% and a median PFS of 4.6 months irrespective of the T790M mutational status, suggesting that afatinib plus cetuximab combination should be further explored [52]. It is worth mentioning that although the combination of reversible TKI with mAB shown *in vitro* activity in T790M positive cells [53], the combination of erlotinib and cetuximab has no clinical efficacy [54].

In vitro, afatinib significantly induced downregulation of thymidylate synthase expression in gefitinib-resistant NSCLC cell lines. The combination of afatinib with 5-fluorouracil or pemetrexed synergistically inhibited the proliferation of NSCLC xenograft with T790M mutation greater than either agent alone, suggesting that the addition of thymidylate synthase-targeting drugs to afatinib may be a promising strategy to overcome EGFR-TKI resistance in NSCLC with the T790M mutation [55].

The new T790M specific inhibitor WZ-4002 is also under investigation, and unlikely irreversible TKI, has demonstrated to induce greater growth inhibition *in vitro* and *in vivo* against T790M than against wild-type EGFR [56], suggesting a better toxicity profile. However, the activity of this drug in the clinical setting remains to be clarified and resistance to WZ4002 has been yet described in multiple complementary models, through aberrant activation of extracellular signal-regulated kinase (ERK) through MAPK amplification [57]. The FLT3 receptor inhibitor, an indolocarbazole compound, is also under investigation as potent and reversible inhibitor of EGFR T790M that do not inhibit wild-type EGFR in the context of T790M-mediated drug resistance in NSCLC [58]. New drugs in clinical trials with a preclinical higher activity against T790M mutation and lower toxicity compared to first and second TKI generation are ongoing, such as CO1686 [59] and AZD9291 [60] with a promising activity regardless of T790M mutational status.

In addition to EGFR T790M mutation, other mutations have been associated with AR: the T854A in exon 21 [61], L747S [62], and D761Y [63], both in exon 19. However, the frequency of these mutations appears to be very low in comparison with the T790M mutation.

4.2. Parallel Activation of Downstream Signaling Pathways

Other mechanisms of AR to EGFR-TKI consist of the activation of parallel pathways in which the key downstream targets of EGFR are activated independently of EGFR-TKI (Figure 1). These mechanisms include: *MET* amplification and Hepatocyte Growth Factor (HGF) overexpression. Others additional bypass tract have been recently reported such as: *HER2* amplification, *BRAF* mutation and IGFR pathway.

4.3. *MET* Amplification

The second most common EGFR-TKI resistance mechanism is related to *MET* amplification that occurs in about 20% [64] of patients with AR (half of whom with concomitant T790M mutation). Interestingly, *MET* amplified subclones were identified at low frequencies in untreated specimens and the dominant mechanism of resistance at the time of disease progression was *MET* amplification, suggesting that EGFR-TKI might select for dominant pre-existing cells with *MET* amplification during the acquisition of EGFR-TKI resistance [65]. However, in more recent studies of AR to EGFR-TKI, *MET* amplification has been identified in only 5%-11% of specimens [36, 37], perhaps reflecting differences in testing methodology and thresholds compared with those of earlier reports [66]. *MET* proto-oncogene encodes a transmembrane tyrosine kinase receptor that binds to the HGF. The binding induces receptor dimerization ERBB3 phosphorylation and PI3K/AKT activation, thus causing a persistent activation of the downstream pathway, overcoming the inhibition by EGFR-TKI (Figure 1) [67]. Thus, concomitant inhibition of both EGFR and MET would be required to overcome resistance to EGFR inhibitors by *MET* amplification [64]. Moreover, in preclinical models, MET inhibitors can overcome MET-mediated resistance, even in cells that harbour the T790M mutation [65].

In order to overcome the resistance mechanisms related to *MET* amplification, several c-MET inhibitors such as tivantinib, foretinib, cabozantanib (XL184), crizotinib and MET mAB have been explored [68], however, no one of these trials were specifically designed in *EGFR* mutant patients with AR to EGFR-TKI [69, 70].

XL184 is a potent MET/VEGFR2/RET inhibitor, with preclinical activity only in combination with erlotinib or gefitinib in xenograft models harbouring *MET* amplification [71]. A phase Ib/II trial of XL184 with or without erlotinib in EGFR-TKI resistant NSCLC patients (NCT 00596648) has reached the final data collection date for primary outcome and results are pending. *In vitro*, MET kinase inhibitor crizotinib in combination with new generation EGFR inhibitors (afatinib or WZ4002) had a synergistic effect in resistant EGFR-TKI lung cancer cell lines [72]. A phase I study (NCT01121575) to evaluate the combination of the MET inhibitor crizotinib with the pan-ERBB inhibitor, dacomitinib, in patients with NSCLC is ongoing. A planned expansion cohort of this trial will include patients with known AR to EGFR-TKI.

4.4. HGF Overexpression

The HGF, the ligand of the MET receptor, is produced by tumor cells or by the fibroblasts infiltrating tumor microenvironment [73]. Unlikely to *MET* amplification, overexpression of HGF induces drug resistance to EGFR-TKI in a dose-dependent manner, because it stimulates the PI3K/AKT signalling pathway through MET phosphorylation through Gab1 signalling, independent of ERBB3 phosphorylation (Figure 1), making cancer cells independent from the EGFR pathway. As a consequence, EGFR-TKIs are not effective in tumor control [19]. In some patients with paired tumor specimens without evidence of EGFR T790M or *MET* amplification, HGF expression was significantly greater in resistant specimen compared to pretreatment specimen (p= 0.025), supporting a role for HGF alone in promoting drug resistance [74].

In a Japanese study, the HGF overexpression, the T790M mutation and *MET* amplification were detected in 61, 52 and 9% of tumors with AR to EGFR-TKI, respectively. Moreover, HGF overexpression was significantly higher in tumors with AR than in sensitive tumors, and 50% of tumors with AR simultaneously overexpressed HGF with T790M and *MET* amplification [75], and provide the rationale for targeting HGF and the MET pathway in *EGFR* mutant patients with AR to EGFR-TKI. In other Asiatic study with tumor specimens obtained from 19 matched specimens before and after gefitinib treatment, HGF measured by immunohistochemistry had a prognostic value, and those patients with weak HGF expression tended to have lower 5-year OS compared with those patients with HGF overexpression (22.2% versus 75%; p= 0.259) [76].

Among strategies to overcome HGF-induced EGFR-TKI resistance in *EGFR* mutant tumors include the E7050, a dual MET/VEGF receptor-2 kinase inhibitor, which overcome HGF-induced resistance in *EGFR* mutant lung cancer cell lines through the inhibition of the MET/Gab1/PI3K-AKT pathway [77]. Crizotinib (PF02341066), a MET kinase inhibitor, plus gefitinib successfully prevented the emergence of EGFR-TKI resistance in cell lines after transient exposure to HGF, suggesting that crizotinib overcomes HGF-induced resistance [78]. Also, the BEZ235, a novel PI3K-mTOR inhibitor, which *in vitro* inhibits tumor growth circumventing resistance triggered by HGF, even as a single agent treatment [79]. Other strategies target the Heat shock protein90 (HSP 90) a molecular chaperone for several proteins including EGFR and MET. HSP90 inhibitors may overcome HGF-triggered resistance to EGFR-TKIs *in vitro* and *in vivo* [80]. Recently a new HSP90 inhibitor, AUY922, has been tested as a single agent in a phase II trial that included 19 *EGFR*-mutant patients with a progressive disease after EGFR-TKI treatment. The RR was 26% and PFS at 18 weeks was 46.6 [81]. A combination of AUY922 plus erlotinib is currently being tested in patients with AR to EGFR-TKI (NCT01259089) and the preliminary RR is 13% [82].

4.5. Others Bypass Pathways

Several additional bypass tracts have been implicated in EGFR-TKI resistance.

a) *HER2 amplification* by FISH was identified in 12% of tumors with AR to EGFR-TKI versus only 1% of untreated tumors. Notably, this new mechanism of AR is mutually exclusive with T790M mutation [83]. The presence of *HER2* amplification defines a clinical subset population with a more adverse prognosis and rapid progression [84]. When amplified, *HER2* is believed to function in parallel to the inhibited EGFR to reactivate common downstream signalling pathways. Interestingly, in preclinical models the combination of afatinib and cetuximab significantly inhibited HER2 phosphorylation. These results suggest that HER2 could be involved in the sensitivity or resistance of *EGFR*-mutant NSCLC providing a rationale to assess its status and target HER2 in such tumors.
b) *BRAF mutation*: The RAS/RAF/MEK/MAPK signaling pathway downstream of EGFR plays a role in lung cancer tumorigenesis. Two *BRAF* mutations were identified in 195 tumor samples (1%) with AR to EGFR-TKI. In one case of *BRAF* mutation (V600E) coexisted with T790M mutation and EGFR exon 19 deletion, while in the other *BRAF* mutation (G469A) concurred only with the sensitive *EGFR* mutation [85].
c) *IGFR*: In vitro data have shown that the insulin-like growth factor-1 receptor (IGF-1R) may also mediated resistance to EGFR-TKI by activating downstream targets that bypass dependency in EGFR [86]. Recently, *in vitro* has been described a resistance to irreversible EGFR-TKI by involving the IGF-1R pathway [87].

4.6. Phenotypic Transformation

Little is known about this mechanism of AR that includes changes in tumor histology on development of resistance to EGFR-TKIs from NSCLC to small-cell lung cancer (SCLC); and the transition from epithelial to mesenchymal phenotype (EMT). In one study of 37 *EGFR* mutant patients with AR, repeat biopsies identified SCLC in five patients (14%), all of whom had adenocarcinoma at baseline [36]. This histologic shift maintained the original *EGFR*-sensitizing mutation and responded to standard SCLC chemotherapy but samples were negative for T790M mutation and *MET* amplification, although one patient developed a new *PIK3CA* mutation concomitantly with SCLC-switch. Other recent analysis of 155 tumor specimens at the time of AR to EGFR-TKI reported that small cell histologic transformation occurred in only 3% of cases [37]. Although pulmonary alveolar cells have been found to transform occasionally to small cell morphology when loss of p53 and Rb1 is induced [88], the biological mechanism of the SCLC transformation is unknown. This finding indicated that resistance to EGFR-TKI in *EGFR* mutant positive patients is dynamic, and repeat biopsy on progression may help guide subsequent treatment.

Another histologic change observed in EGFR-TKI-resistant specimens is an EMT [89]. Three out of seven patients from the same Sequist's study who did not develop any identifiable mutations showed EMT at the time of EGFR-TKI resistance [36]. EMT is a phenomenon characterized by loss of epithelial phenotype and development of a more spindle-like mesenchymal morphology, with a loss of epithelial markers such as E-cadherin and gain of mesenchymal markers such as vimentin or fibronectin [90]. Actually, increased expression of E-cadherin has been associated with clinical activity of EGFR-TKI in NSCLC patients [91, 92] whereas EMT is associated with enhanced motility, invasiveness and EGFR-TKI resistance *in vitro* [93] and *in vivo* [36]. Unlikely to E-cadherin expression, N-cadherin expression was upregulated in erlotinib-resistant lung cancer cell lines and it was associated with acquisition of EMT phenotypes and enhanced invasion [94].

The biology underlying for the acquisition of EMT phenotype transformation and its impact on resistance remains unclear. Some studies have found that an upregulation of Notch-1 expression in gefitinib-resistant PC9/AB2 lung cancer cells promotes an EMT phenotype. Moreover, silencing Notch-1 by using siRNA reversed the EMT phenotype and restored sensitivity to gefitinib [95]. The aberrant expression of transforming growth factor (TGF)-β is also a potent inducer of EMT. In erlotinib-resistant cell lines, the blockade of the TGF-β signalling pathway combined with continuous EGFR inhibition had synergic effect [96]. TGF- β-1 induces histone deacetylase-6 (HDAC-6), which deacetylates alpha-tubulin that correlates with the expression of EMT markers in lung human epithelial cells [97]. In gefitinib-resistant cell lines, combination of gefitinib with an HDAC inhibitor (MS-275) enhances TKI sensitivity as a result of E-cadherin expression [98]. Thus, combining EGFR-TKI with drugs that induce E-cadherin expression could delay the emergence of EGFR-TKI resistance. In a phase II trial in non-molecular selected population, entinostat, an HDAC inhibitor, combined with erlotinib after progression to chemotherapy, showed increased OS and PFS compared to erlotinib monotherapy in NSCLC tumors with high E-cadherin expression levels at time of diagnosis [99]. In preclinical models was reported that ERK 1/2 mitogen-activated protein kinase 3/1 (MAPK3/1), signaling played a key role in directing the mesenchymal character of NSCLC cells and that blocking ERK signaling was sufficient to heighten therapeutic responses to EGFR inhibitors. MEK1/2 (MAPKK1/2) inhibition promoted an epithelial phenotype in NSCLC cells, preventing induction of EMT by exogenous TGF-β. Moreover, in cells exhibiting de novo or acquired resistance to the EGFR inhibitor gefitinib, MEK inhibition enhanced the sensitivity to gefitinib and slowed cell migration. These effects only occurred, however, if MEK was inhibited for a period sufficient to trigger changes in EMT marker expression [100]. Furthermore, treatment with selective MEK inhibitors, such as selumetinib or MSC19363669B, had a markedly antitumor activity in resistant cell lines, indicating a key role of the MEK/MAPK pathway in the EMT [101]. Finally, silibinin meglumine, a water-soluble form of milk thistle silymarin, efficiently prevented the loss of markers associated with a polarized epithelial phenotype as well as the *de novo* synthesis of proteins associated with the mesenchymal morphology of transitioning cells [102]. Future trials combining silibinin plus EGFR-TKI in patients with *EGFR* mutant tumors would be of interest.

It is unknown whether mesenchymal-like cells exist prior TKI therapy or are induced upon drug treatment. Recently, the activation of AXL receptor tyrosine kinase by overexpression or upregulation of its ligand GAS6, confers AR to EGFR-TKI in preclinical models. AXL pathway has been found associated with increased levels of tumor vimentin, thus suggesting that AXL may mediate the acquisition of an EMT phenotype in EGFR-TKI resistant patients. Approximately 20% of the EGFR-TKI resistant tumors show increased AXL expression, in co-occurrence with T790M, but not MET overexpression [103]. These preliminary data identify AXL as a promising therapeutic target whose inhibition could prevent or overcome AR to EGFR-TKI. AXL inhibitors, such as SGI-7079, combined with erlotinib reversed erlotinib resistance in mesenchymal lines expressing AXL [104].

4.7. Additional Genetic Alterations

As mentioned before, the analysis of clinical specimens is crucial to underline the mechanism of resistance of the 30% of tumors in which is not yet defined.

a) *PIK3CA and PTEN mutation*: The phosphatidyl insositol 3-kinase (PIK3)-AKT pathway is a key downstream signaling pathway from EGFR. Phosphatase and tensine homolog (PTEN) is a molecule that negatively regulates this pathway. Mutation in *PIK3CA* was identified in 5% of *EGFR*-mutant lung cancers that developed AR to EGFR-TKI [36] and in 2% of untreated lung adenocarcinoma in coexistence with other oncogenic mutations in 70% of cases [105]. Moreover, *EGFR*-mutant patients with high PIK3CA expression are more suitable for gefitinib treatment [106]. The combination of EGFR-TKI and PI3KCA inhibitor may be challenging because of overlapping toxicities, but these combinations are currently being tested in different clinical trials [107]. Recently, the combination of gefitinib plus BKM120, a pan-class I PI3K inhibitor, has reported antitumor activity in patients with AR to EGFR-TKI but 40% of patients had late grade 3 toxicities such as rash and diarrhea. Molecular analyses not revealed *PI3KCA* mutation among patients included [108]. *PTEN* is a tumor suppressor gene that negatively regulates PIK3CA. In preclinical models, loss of PTEN expression contributes to TKI resistance in NSCLC [109]. Cells with knockdown of PTEN, with constitutive PIK3CA activation, have a deficient homologous recombinant DNA repair and increased sensitivity to cisplatin and PARP inhibitors [110]. These results might suggest a possible therapeutic effect of PARP inhibitors in tumors with AR to EGFR-TKI by *PTEN* mutant mechanism.

b) *MAPK1 amplification*: MAPK1 amplification was described in approximately 5% of clinical specimens from patients with AR to EGFR-TKI. T790M mutation and *MET* amplification were mutually exclusive with MAPK1 amplification [111]. MEK inhibitors reverse resistance in tumors with AR to EGFR-TKI [112].

c) *JAK2*: The Signal Transducer and Activator of Transcription (STAT) family, composed of seven proteins, is involved in signal transduction. STAT3 is reported to be a critical mediator of oncogenic effects of EGFR mutations [113]. STATs exist within the cytoplasm in inactivate state and is activated upstream by JAK proteins which phosphorylate the receptor and STAT proteins. The phosphorylated STAT protein binds to another phosphorylated STAT protein (dimerizes) and translocates into the cell nucleus, where it binds to DNA and promotes transcription of genes [114]. In a preclinical cell line model, activation of JAK2 caused acquired EGFR-TKI resistance. Combined treatments of erlotinib plus a JAK2 inhibitor (JSI-124) restored sensitivity to erlotinib in PC-9/ERB3 cells and reduced tumors in a murine xenograft model [115].

d) *Loss of activating EGFR mutant gene*: Loss of activating *EGFR*-mutant gene contributes to AR to EGFR-TKI in lung cancer cells by gaining addiction to both HER2/HER3 and PI3K/AKT signalling pathway [116].

e) *Stem-cell properties acquisition*: aldehyde dehydrogenase isoform 1 (ALDH1A1) overexpression and self-renewal capability has been described as mechanism of AR to EGFR-TKI in *EGFR*-mutant cell lines [117].

f) *Integrin β1/Src/AKT-driven by pass:* In erlotinib resistant lung cancer cells harboring *EGFR* mutation an overexpression of Src and Integrin β1 was observed. Silencing Integrin β1 restored erlotinib sensitivity and reduced activation of Src/AKT after erlotinib treatment [118].

g) *Loss of an EGFR-amplified chromosome 7*: caused AR in *EGFR* mutated lung cancer cell lines exposed to relatively low concentration of erlotinib [119].

h) *CRKL amplification*: was identified as contributing to EGFR-TKI resistance; this cell line model can be utilized to study this resistance mechanism [120].

In some patients, tumor progression may be caused by several mechanisms and the re-biopsy of a single lesion may be insufficient to get an accurate molecular diagnosis. Occasionally, multiple different resistance mechanisms are found within the same biopsy specimen [36, 39]. Moreover, overlap among mechanisms of AR was seen in 4% of patients [37], underscoring the potential for clonal divergence across metastatic sites. In these patients combined treatment, targeting simultaneously different mechanisms of resistance, might be most appropriate strategy whether there is no increase in toxicity. The identification of a drug resistance mechanism in pretreatment tumor specimens may provide a window the opportunity to specifically target that resistance mechanism before its emergence. However, it would be critical to learn whether upfront treatment with combination therapy would be well tolerated and whether it would produce more clinical benefit than either agent alone or treatment at the time of relapse [75].

Conclusion

Several mechanisms of AR to EGFR-TKI in *EGFR*-mutant NSCLC patients have been reported. However, there is no standard treatment at the progressive disease on EGFR-TKI therapy based on molecular diagnosis. Rebiopsies at progression may help to select molecular treatment or evaluate the emergence of a phenotypic transformation. Clinical patterns of EGFR-TKI failure can help the clinician to select the best therapeutic strategy.

References

[1] Rosell R, Moran T, Queralt C, et al. Screening for epidermal growth factor receptor mutations in lung cancer. *N Engl J Med.* 2009; 361: 958-67.

[2] Gahr S, Stoehr R, Geissinger E, et al. *EGFR* mutational status in a large series of Caucasian European NSCLC patients: data from daily practice. *Br J Cancer.* 2013; 109:1821-8.

[3] Sordella R, Bell DW, Haber DA, Settleman J. Gefitinib-sensitizing *EGFR* mutations in lung cancer activate anti-apoptotic pathways. *Science.* 2004; 305 (5687): 1163-7.

[4] Fukoka M, Wu YL, Thongprasert S, et al. Biomarker analyses and final overall survival results from a phase III, randomized, open-label, first-line study of gefitinib versus carboplatin/paclitaxel in clinically selected patients with advanced non-small-cell lung cancer in Asia (IPASS). *J Clin Oncol.* 2011; 29: 2866-74.

[5] Han JY, Par K, Sim SW, et al. First-SIGNAL: First-line single-agent iressa versus gemcitabine and cisplatin trial in never-smokers with adenocarcinoma of the lung. *J Clin Oncol.* 2012; 30: 1122-8.

[6] Mitsudomi T, Morita S, Yatabe Y, et al. Gefitinib versus cisplatin plus docetaxel in patients with non-small-cell lung cancer harbouring mutations of epidermal growth factor receptor (WJTOG 3405): An open label, randomized phase 3 trial. *Lancet Oncol.* 2010; 11: 121-8.

[7] Mitsudomi T, Morita S, Yatabe Y, et al. Up-dated overall survival results of WJTOG 3405, a randomized phase III trial comparing gefitinib with cisplatin plus docetaxel as the first-line treatment for patients with advanced non-small-cell lung cancer harboring mutations of the epidermal growth factor receptor. *J Clin Oncol,* 2012; 30 (suppl; abstract 7521).

[8] Inoue A, Kobayashi K, Maemondo M, et al. Updated overall survival results from a randomized phase III trial comparing gefitinib with carboplatin-paclitaxel for chemo-naïve lung cancer with sensitive *EGFR* gene mutation (NEJ002). *Ann Oncol.* 2013; 24: 54-9.

[9] Zhou C, Wu YL, Chen G, et al. Erlotinib versus chemotherapy as first-line treatment for patients with advanced *EGFR* mutation-positive non-small-cell lung cancer (OPTIMAL, CTONG-0802): A multicenter, open-label, randomized, phase 3 study. *Lancet Oncol.* 2011; 12: 735-42.

[10] Rosell R, Carcereny E, Gervais R, et al. Erlotinib versus standard chemotherapy as first-line treatment for European patients with advanced *EGFR* mutation-positive non-

small-cell lung cancer (EURTAC): A multicenter, open-label, randomized phase 3 trial. *Lancet Oncol.* 2012; 13: 239-46.

[11] Sequist LV, Yang JC, Yamamoto N, et al. Phase III study of afatinib or cisplatin plus pemetrexed in patients with metastatic lung adenocarcinoma with *EGFR* mutation. *J Clin Oncol.* 2013; 31: 3327-34.

[12] Wu YL, Zhou C, Hu Ch-P, et al. LUX-Lung 6: A randomized, open-label, phase III study of afatinib versus gemcitabine/cisplatin as first-line treatment for Asian patients with *EGFR* mutation-positive advanced adenocarcinoma of the lung. *J clin Oncol* 2013; 31 (suppl; abstract 8016)

[13] Solca F, Dahl G, Zoephel A, et al. Target binding properties and cellular activity of afatinib (BIBW2992), an irreversible ErbB family blocker. *J Pharmacol Exp Ther.* 2012; 343: 342-50.

[14] Wu YL, Lee JS, Thongprasert S, et al. Intercalated combination of chemotherapy and erlotinib for patients with advanced stage non-small-cell lung cancer (FASTACT-2): a randomised, double-blind trial. *Lancet Oncol.* 2013; 14: 777-86.

[15] Jackman D, Pao W, Riely GJ, et al. Clinical definition of acquired resistance to epidermal growth factor receptor tyrosine kinase inhibitors in non-small cell lung cancer. *J Clin Oncol.* 2010; 28: 357-60.

[16] Arcila ME, Nafa K, Chaft JE, et al. EGFR exon 20 insertion mutations in lung adenocarcinoma: prevalence, molecular heterogeneity, and clinicopathologic characterisitics. *Mol Cancer Ther.* 2013; 12: 220-9.

[17] Oxnard GR, Lo PC, Nishino M, et al. Natural history and molecular characteristics of lung cancers harboring EGFR exon 20 insertion. *J Thorac Oncol.* 2013; 8: 179-84.

[18] Wu JY, Wu SG, Yang CH, et al. Lung cancer with epidermal growth factor receptor exon 20 mutations is associated with poor gefitinib treatment response. *Clin Cancer Res.* 2008; 14: 4877-82.

[19] Yang JC, Schuler M, Massey D, et al. Activity of afatinib in uncommon epidermal growth factor receptor mutations: findings from three trials of afatinib in EGFR mutation-positive lung cancer. *IASLC.* 2013 (O03.05).

[20] Rosell R, Molina MA, Costa C, et al. Pretreatment EGFR T790M mutation and BRCA1 mRNA expression in erlotinib-treated advanced non-small cell lung cancer patients with *EGFR* mutation. *Clin Cancer Res.* 2011; 17: 1160-8.

[21] Turke AB, Zejnullahu K, Wu YL, et al. Pre-existence and clonal selection of *MET* amplification in *EGFR* mutant NSCLC. *Cancer Cell.* 2010; 17: 77-88.

[22] Pao W, Wang TY, Riely GJ, et al. *KRAS* mutations and primary resistance of lung adenocarcinomas to gefitinib or erlotinib. *PLoS Med.* 2005; 2: e17.

[23] Kawano O, Sasaki H, Endo K, et al. PIK3CA mutation status in Japanese lung cancer patients. *Lung Cancer.* 2006; 54: 209–15.

[24] Sos ML, Koker M, Weir BA, et al. PTEN loss contributes to erlotinib resistance in EGFR-mutant lung cancer by activation of Akt and EGFR. *Cancer Res.* 2009;69: 3256–61.

[25] Vivanco I, Rohle D, Versele M, et al. The phosphatase and tensin homolog regulates epidermal growth factor receptor (EGFR) inhibitor response by targeting EGFR for degradation. *Proc Natl Acad Sci USA.* 2010; 107: 6459–64.

[26] Gong Y, Somwar R, Politi K, Balak M, Chmielecki J, Jiang X, Pao W. induction of BIM is essential for apoptosis triggered by EGFR kinase inhibitors in mutant *EGFR*-dependent lung adenocarcinomas. *PLoS med.* 2007; 4: e294.

[27] Rosell R, Massuti B, Costa C, et al. Concomitant actionable mutations and overall survival in *EGFR* mutant non-small-cell lung cancer patients included in the EURTAC trial. *Ann Oncol.* 2012; 23 (suppl 9, abstract 929).

[28] Ji W, Choi CH-M, Rho JK, et al. Mechanisms of acquired resistance to EGFR-tyrosine kinase inhibitor in Korean patients with lung cancer. *BMC Cancer.* 2013; 13: 606.

[29] Kuiper JL, Heideman D, Thurnnisen E, et al. Rebiopsy in TKI-resistance: a retrospective analysis. *J Clin Oncol.* 2013; 31 (Abstract 8065).

[30] Vergnenegre A, Beratrd H, Do P, et al. Feasibility and clinical impact of re-biopsy in advanced non-small cell lung cancer: a prospective multicentric study in real world setting (GFPC study 12-01). *IASLC.* 2013 (MO07.09).

[31] Murtaza M, Dawson SJ, Tsui DW, et al. Non-invasive analysis of acquired resistance to cancer therapy by sequencing of plasma DNA. *Nature.* 2013; 497: 108-12.

[32] Nakamura T, Sueoka-Aragane N, Iwanaga K, et al. A noninvasive system for monitoring resistance to epidermal growth factor receptor tyrosine kinase inhibitors with plasma DNA. *J Thorac Oncol.* 2011; 6: 1639-48.

[33] Riely GJ, Kris MG, Zhao B, et al. Prospective assessment of discontinuation and re-initiation of erlotinib or gefitinib in patients with acquired resistance to erlotinib or gefitinib followed by the addition of everolimus. *Clin Cancer Res.* 2007; 13: 5150-5.

[34] Kobayashi S, Boggon TJ, Dayaram T, et al. *EGFR* mutation and resistance of non-small-cell lung cancer to gefitinib. *N Engl J Med.* 2005; 352: 786-92.

[35] Pao W, Miller VA, Politi KA, et al. Acquired resistance of lung adenocarcinomas to gefitinib or erlotinib is associated with a second mutationin the EGFR-kinase domain. *PLoS Med.* 2005; 2: e73.

[36] Sequist LV, Waltman BA, Dias-Santagata D, et al. Genotyping and histological evolution of lung cancers acquiring resistance to EGFR inhibitors. *Sci Transl Med.* 2011; 3 (75): 75ra26.

[37] Yu HA, Arcila ME, Rekhtman N, et al. Analysis of tumor specimens at the time of acquired resistance to EGFR-TKI therapy in 155 patients with *EGFR*-mutant lung cancers. *Clin Cancer Res.* 2013; 19: 2240-7.

[38] Engelman JA, Mukohara T, Zenjullahu K, et al. Allelic dilution obscures detection of a biologically significant resistance mutation in *EGFR*-amplified lung cancer. *J Clin Invest.* 2006; 116: 2695-706.

[39] Arcila ME, Oxnard GR, Nafa K, et al. Rebiopsy of lung cancer patients with acquired resistance to EGFR inhibitors and enhanced detection of the T790M mutation using a locked nucleic acid-based assay. *Clin Cancer Res.* 2011; 17: 1169-80.

[40] Yun CH, Mengwasser KE, Toms AV, et al. The T790M mutation in *EGFR* kinase causes drug resistance by increasing the affinity for ATP. *Proc Natl Acad Sci USA.* 2008; 105: 2070-5.

[41] Chmielecki J, Foo J, Oxnard GR, et al. Optimizing of dosing for *EGFR*-mutant non-small cell lung cancer with evolutionary cancer modelling. *Sci Transl Med.* 2011; 3: 90ra59.

[42] Oxnard GR, Arcila ME, Sima CS, et al. Acquired resistance to EGFR tyrosine kinase inhibitor in *EGFR*-mutant lung cancer: distinct natural history of patients with tumors harboring the T790M mutation. *Clin Cancer Res.* 2011; 17: 1616-22.
[43] Kwak EL, Sordella R, Bell DW, et al. Irreversible inhibitors of the EGF receptor may circumvent acquired resistance to gefitinib. *Proc Natl Acad Sci USA.* 2005; 102: 7665-70.
[44] Engelman JA, Zejnullahu K, Gale CM, et al. PF00299804, an irreversible pan-ERBB inhibitor, is effective in lung cancer models with EGFR and ERBB2 mutations that are resistant to gefitinib. *Cancer Res.* 2007; 67: 11924-32.
[45] Sequist LV, Besse B, Lynch TJ, et al. Neratinib, an irreversible pan-ErbB receptor tyrosine kinase inhibitor: results of a phase II trial in patients with advanced non-small-cell lung cancer. *J Clin Oncol.* 2010; 28: 3076-83.
[46] Kim Y, Ko J, Cui Z, et al. The EGFR T790M mutation in acquired resistance to an irreversible second genration EGFR inhibitor. *Mol Cancer Ther.* 2012; 11: 784-91.
[47] Ercan D, Zejnullahu K, Yonesaka K. Amplification of EGFR T790M causes resistance to an irreversible EGFR inhibitor. *Oncogene.* 2010; 29: 2346-56.
[48] Miller VA, Hirsh V, Cadranel J, et al. Afatinib versus placebo for patients with advanced, metastatic non-small-cell lung cancer after failure of erlotinib, gefitinib, or both, and one or two lines of chemotherapy (LUX-Lung 1): a phase 2b/3 randomised trial. *Lancet Oncol.* 2012; 13: 528-38.
[49] Katakami N, Atagi S, Goto K, et al. LUX-Lung 4: a phase II trial of afatinib in patients with advanced non-small-cell lung cancer who progressed during prior treatment with erlotinib, gefitinib, or both. *J Clin Oncol.* 2013; 31: 3335-41.
[50] Regales L, Gong Y Shen R, et al. Dual targeting of EGFR can overcome a major drug resistance in mouse model of *EGFR*-mutant lung cancer. *J Clin Invest.* 2009; 119: 3000-10.
[51] Janjigian YY, Smit EF, Horn L, et al. Activity of afatinib / cetuximab in patients with *EGFR*-mutant non-small cell lung cancer and acquired resistance to EGFR inhibitors. *ESMO.* 2012 (abstract 12270).
[52] Wang M, Zhao J, Zhang LM, et al. Combined erlotinib and cetuximab overcome the acquired resistance to epidermal growth factor receptor tyrosine kinase inhibitor in non-small-cell lung cancer. *J Cancer Res Clin Oncol.* 2012; 138: 2069-77.
[53] Janjigian YY, Azzoli CG, Krug LM, et al. Phase I/II of cetuximab and erlotinib in patients with lung adenocarcinoma and acquired resistance to erlotinib. *Clin Cancer* Res. 2011; 17: 2521-7.
[54] Takezawa K, Okamoto I, Tanizaki J, et al. Enhanced anticancer effect of the combination of BIBW2992 and thymidylate synthase-targeted agents in non-small cell lung cancer with the T790M mutation of epidermal growth factor receptor. *Mol Cancer Ther.* 2010; 9: 1647-56.
[55] Zhou W, Ercan D, Chen L, et al. Novel mutant-selective EGFR kinase inhibitors against EGFR T790M. *Nature.* 2009; 462: 1070-4.
[56] Blakely CM, Bivona TG. Resiliency of lung cancer to EGFR inhibitor treatment unveiled, offering opportunities to divide and conquer EGFR inhibitor resistance. *Cancer Discovery.* 2012; 2: 872-5.
[57] Lee HJ, Schaefer G, Heffron TP, et al. Non-covalent wild-type-sparing inhibitors of EGFR T790M. *Cancer Discover.* 2013; 3: 168-81.

[58] Soria JC, Sequist LV, Shirish M, et al. First in-human evaluation of CO-1686, an irreversible, highly selective tyrosine kinase inhibitor of mutations of EGFR (activating and T790M*). IASLC.* 2013 (Abstract O03.06).

[59] Ranson M, Pao W, Kim D, et al. *AZD9291:* An irreversible, potent and selective tyrosine kinase inhibitor of activting *EGFR* and resistance T790M mutations in advanced NSCLC. *IASLC.* 2013 (Abstract P1.11-034).

[60] Bean J, Riely GJ, Malak M, et al. Acquired resistance to epidermal growth factor receptor kinase inhibitors associated with a novel T854A mutation in patients with *EGFR*-mutant lung adenocarcinoma. *Clin Cancer Res.* 2008; 22: 7519-25.

[61] Costa DB, Schumer ST, Tenen DG, Kobayashi S. Differential response to Erlotinib in Epidermal Growth Factor Receptor (EGFR)-mutate lung cancers with acquired resistance to gefitinib carrying the L747S or T790M secondary mutation. *J Clin Oncol.* 2008; 26: 1182-4.

[62] Balak MN, Gong Y, Riely GJ, et al. Novel D761Y and common secondary T790M mutations in epidermal growth factor receptor mutant lung adenocarcinoma with acquired resistance to kinase inhibitors. *Clin Cancer Res.* 2006; 12: 6494-01.

[63] Engelman JA, Zejnullahu K, Mitsudomi T, et al. *MET* amplification leads to gefitinib resistance in lung cancer by activating ERBB3 signalling. *Science.* 2007; 316: 1039-43.

[64] Bean J, Brennan C, Shih JY, et al. *MET* amplification occurs with or without T790M mutation in *EGFR*-mutant lung cancer tumors with acquired resistance to gefitinib or erlotinib. *Proc Natl Acad Sci USA.* 2007; 104: 20932-7.

[65] Oxnard GR, Arcila ME, Chmielecki J, et al. New strategies in overcoming acquired resistance to epidermal growth factor receptor tyrosine kinase inhibitors in lung cancer. *Clin Cancer Res.* 2011; 17: 5530-7.

[66] Robinson KW, Sandler AB. The role of MET receptor tyrosine kinase in non-small cell lung cancer and clinical development of targeted anti-MET agents. *The Oncologist.* 2013; 18: 115-22.

[67] Sgambato A, Casaluce F, Maione P. The c-MET inhibitors: a new class f drugs in the battle against advanced non-small cell lung cancer. *Curr Pharm Des.* 2012; 37: 6155-68.

[68] Sequist LV, von Pawel J, Garmey EG, et al. Randomized phase II study of erlotinib plus tivantinib versus erlotinib plus placebo in previously treated non-small cell lung cancer. *J Clin Oncol.* 2011; 29: 3307-15.

[69] Spigel DR, Ervin TJ, Ramlau R, et al. Final efficacy results from OAM4558g, a randomized phase II study evaluating MetMab or placebo in combination with erlotinib in advanced NSCLC. *J Clin Oncol.* 2011 (Abstract 7505).

[70] Jänne PA, Wax M, Leach JW, et al. Targeting MET with XL184 to reverse EGFR tyrosine kinase inhibitor resistance in NSCLC: impact of preclinical studies on clinical trial design. *Eur J Cancer Suppl.* 2008; 6: 174.

[71] Nanjo S, Yamada T, Mishihara H, et al. Ability of the Met kinase inhibitor crizotinib and new generation EGFR inhibitors to overcome resistance to EGFR inhibitors. *PLoS One.* 2013; 8: e84700.

[72] Gusenbauer S, Vlaicu P, Ullrich A. HGF induces novel EGFR functions involved in resistance formation to tyrosine kinase inhibitors. *Oncogene.* 2013; 32: 3846-56.

[73] Yano S, Wang W, Li Q, et al. Hepatocyte growth factor induces gefitinib resistance of lung adenocarcinoma with epidermal growth factor receptor-activating mutation. *Cancer Res.* 2008; 68: 9479-87.

[74] Turke AB, Zejnullahu K, Wu YL, et al. Pre-existence and clonal selection of *MET* amplification in *EGFR* mutant NSCLC. *Cancer Cell.* 2010; 17: 77-88.

[75] Yano S, Yamada T, Takeuchi S, et al. Hepatocyte growth factor expression in *EGFR*-mutant lung cancer with intrinsic and acquired resistance to tyrosine kinase inhibitors in a Japanese cohort. *J Thorac oncol.* 2011; 6: 2011-7.

[76] Uramoto H, Yamada T, Yano S, Kondo N, Hasegawa S, Tanaka F. Prognostic value of acquired resistance-related molecules in Japanese patients with NSCLC treated with an EGFR TKI. *Anticancer Res.* 2012; 32: 3785-90.

[77] Takeuchi S, Wang W, Li Q, et al. Dual inhibition of MET kinase and angiogenesis to overcome HGF-induced EGFR TKI resistance in *EGFR* mutant lung cancer. *Am J Pathol.* 2012; 181: 1034-43.

[78] Chen X, Zhou JY, Zhao J, Chen JJ, Ma SN, Zhou JY. Crizotinib overcomes hepatocyte growth factor mediated resistance to gefitinib in *EGFR* mutant non-small cell lung cancer cells. *Anticancer Drugs.* 2013; 24: 1039-46.

[79] Sano T, Takeuchi S, Nakagawa T, et al. The novel phosphoinositide 3-Kinase-mammalina target of rapamycin inhibitor, BEZ235, circumvetes erlotinib resistance of epidermal growth factor receptor mutant lung cancer cells triggered by hepatocyte growth factor. *Int J Cancer.* 2013; 133: 505-13.

[80] Koizumi H, Yamada T, Takeuchi S, et al. HSP90 inhibition overcomes HGF-triggering resistnace to EGFR TKI in *EGFR*-mutant lung cancer by decreasing client protein expression and angiogenesis. *J Thorac Oncol.* 2012; 7: 1078-85.

[81] Felip E, Carcereny E, Barlesi F, et al. Phase II activity of the HSP90 inhibitor in patients with ALK-rearranged (ALK+) or *EGFR*-mutated advanced non-small cell lung cancer. *ESMO.* 2012 (Abstract 4380).

[82] Johnson ML, Hart ME, Rademaker A, et al. A phase II of HSP90 inhibitor AUY922 and erlotinib for patients with EGFR-mutant lung cancer and acquired resistance to EGFR tyrosine kinase inhibitors. *J Clin Oncol.* 2013; 31 (Abstract 8036).

[83] Takezawa K, Pirazzoli V, Arcila ME, et al. HER2 amplification: a potential mechanism of acquired resistance to EGFR inhibitor in *EGFR*-mutant lung cancers that lack the second-site EGFR T790M mutation. *Cancer Discover.* 2012; 2: 922-33.

[84] Altavilla G, Arrigo C, Tomasello Ch, et al. Ocurrence of HER2 amplification in EGFR-mutant lung adenocarcinoma with acquired resistance to EGFR-TKIS. *J Clin Oncol.* 2013; 31 (Abstract 8047).

[85] Ohashi K, Sequist LV, Arcila ME, et al. Lung cancers with acquired resistance to EGFR inhibitors occasionally harbour *BRAF* gene mutations but lack mutations in KRAS, NRAS, or MEK1. *PNAS* 2012; 109: E2127-33.

[86] Guix M, Faber AC, Wang SE, et al. Acquired resistance to EGFR tyrosine kinase inhibitors in cancer cells is mediated by loss of IGF-binding proteins. *J Clin Investigation.* 2008; 118: 2609-19.

[87] Cortot AB, Repellin CE, Shimamura T, et al. Resistance to irreversible EGF receptor tyrosine kinase inhibitors through multistep mechanism involving the IGF1R pathway. *Cancer Res.* 2013; 73: 834-43.

[88] Sutherland KD, Proost N, Brouns I, Adriaensen D, Song JY, Berns A. Cell of origin of small cell lung cancer: inactivation of Trp53 and Rb1 in distinct cell types of adult mouse lung. *Cancer Cell.* 2011; 19 (6): 754–64.

[89] Chung JH, Rho JK, Xu X, et al. Clinical and molecular evidences of epithelial to mesenchymal transition in acquired resistance to EGFR-TKIs. *Lung Cancer.* 2011; 73: 176-82.

[90] Uramoto H, Iwata T, Onitsuka T, Shimokawa H, Hanagiri T, Oyama T. Epithelial-mesenchymal transition in EGFR-TKI acquired resistant lung adenocarcinoma. *Anticancer Res.* 2010; 30: 2513-7.

[91] Coldren CD, Helfrich BA, Witta SE, et al. Baseline gene expression predicts sensitivity to gefitinib in non-small cell lung cancer cell lines. *Mol Cancer Res.* 2006; 4: 521-8.

[92] Yaunch RL, Januario T, Eberhard DA, et al. Epithelial versus mesenchymal phenotype determines in vitro sensitivity and predicts clinical activity of erlotinib in lung cancer patients. *Clin Cancer Res.* 2005; 11: 8686-98.

[93] Suda K, Tomizawa K, Fujii M, et al. Epithelial to mesenchymal transition in an epidermal growth factor receptor-mutant lung cancer cell line with acquired resistance to erlotinib. *J Thorac Oncol.* 2011; 6: 1152-61.

[94] Zhang X, Liu G, Kang Y, Dong Z, Qian Q, Ma X. N-cadherin expression is associated with acquisition of EMT phenotype and with enhanced invasion in erlotinib-resistant lung cancer cell lines. *PLoS One.* 2013; 8: e57692.

[95] Xie M, He CS, Wei SH, Zhang L. Notch-1 contributes to epidermal growth factor receptor tyrosine kinase inhibitor acquired resistance in non-small cell lung cancer in vitro and in vivo. *Eur J Cancer.* 2013; 49: 3559-72.

[96] Serizawa M, Takahasi T, Yamamoto N, Koh Y. Combined treatment with erlotinib and a transforming growth factor β Type I receptor inhibitor effectively supress the enhanced motility of erlotinib-resistant non-small-cell lung cancer cells. *J Thorac Oncol.* 2013; 8: 259-69.

[97] Shan B, Yao TP, Nguyen HT, et al. requirement of HDAC6 for transforming growth factor-beta-1-induced epithelial-mesenchymal transition. *J Biol Chem.* 2008; 283: 21065-73.

[98] Witta SE, Gemmill RM, Hirsch FR, et al. Restoring E-cadherin expression increases sensitivity to epidermal growth factor receptor inhibitors in lung cancer cell lines. *Cancer Res.* 2006; 66: 944-50.

[99] Witta SE, Jotte RM. Konduri L, et al. Randomized phase II trial of erlotinib with and without entinostat in patients with advanced non-small-cell lung cancer who progressed on prior chemotherapy. *J Clin Oncol.* 2012; 30: 2248-55.

[100] Buonato JM, Lazzara MJ. ERK1/2 Blockade Prevents Epithelial-Mesenchymal Transition in Lung Cancer Cells and Promotes Their Sensitivity to EGFR Inhibition. *Cancer Res.* 2014; 74: 309-19.

[101] Morgillo F, Cascone T, D'Aiuto E, et al. Antitumor efficacy of MEK inhibitors in human lung cancer cells and their derivates with acquired resistance to different tyrosine kinase inhibitors. *B J Cancer.* 2011; 105: 382-92.

[102] Cufi S, Bonavia R, Vazquez-Martin A, et al. Silibinin meglumine, a water-soluble form of milk thistle silymarin, is an orally active anti-cancer agent that impedes the epithelial-to-mesenchymal transition (EMT) in EGFR-mutant non-small-cell lung carcinoma cells. *Food Chem Toxicol.* 2013; 60: 360-8.

[103] Zhang Z, Lee JC, Lin L, et al. Activation of the AXL kinase causes resistance to EGFR-targeted therapy in lung cancer. *Nature Genetics*. 2012; 44: 852-60.
[104] Byers LA, Diao L, Wang J, et al. An epithelial-mesenchymal transition gene signature predicts resistance to EGFR and PI3K inhibitors and identifies AXL as a therapeutic target overcoming EGFR inhibitor resistance. *Clin Cancer Res*. 2013; 19: 279-90.
[105] Chaft JE, Arcila ME, Paik PK, et al. Coexistence of PIK3CA and other oncogene mutations in lung adenocarcinoma-rationale for comprehensive mutation profiling. *Mol Cancer Ther*. 2012; 11: 485-91.
[106] Endoh H, Yatabe Y, Kosaka T, Kuwano H, Mitsudomi T. PTEN and PIK3CA expression is associated with prolonged survival after gefitinib treatment in *EGFR*-mutated lung cancer patients. *J Thorac Oncol*. 2006; 1: 629-34.
[107] Gadgeel SM, Wozniak A. Preclinical rational for PI3K/AKT/mTOR pathway inhibitors as therapy for epidermal growth factor receptor inhibitor-resistant non-small-cell lung cancer. *Clin Lung Cancer*. 2013; 14: 322-32.
[108] Tan DSW, Lim KH, Tai WM, et al. A phase Ib safety and tolerability study of a pan class I PI3K inhibitor buparlisib (BKM120) and gefitinib in EGFR TKI-resistant NSCLC. *J Clin Oncol*. 2013; 31 (Abstract 8107).
[109] Yamamoto C, Basaki Y, Kawahara A, et al. Loss of PTEN expression by blocking nuclear translocation of EGFR1 in gefitinib-resistant lung cancer cell harbouring epidermal growth factor receptor-activating mutations. *Cancer Res*. 2010; 70: 8715-25.
[110] Mendes-Pereira AM, Martin SA, Brough R, et al. Synthetic lethal targeting of PTEN mutant cells with PARP inhibitors. *EMBO Mol Med*. 2009; 1: 315-22.
[111] Ercan D, Xu C, Yanagita M, et al. Reactivation of ERK signaling causes resistance to EGFR kinase inhibitors. *Cancer Discover*. 2012; 2: 934-47.
[112] Huang MH, Lee JH, Chang YJ, Tsai HH, Lin YL, Lin AM, Yang JC. MEK inhibitors reverse resistance in epidermal growth factor receptor mutation lung cancer cells with acquired resistance to gefitinib. *Mol Oncol* 2013; 7: 112-20.
[113] Alvarez JV, Greulich H, Sellers WR, Meyerson M, Frank DA. Signal transducer and activator of transcription 3 is required for the oncogenic effects of non-small-cell lung cancer-associated mutations of the epidermal growth factor receptor. *Cancer Res*. 2006; 66 (6): 3162-8.
[114] Song L, Rawal B, Nemeth JH, Haura EB. JAK1 activates STAT3 activity in non-small-cell lung cancer cells and IL-6 neutralizing antibodies can supress JAK1-STAT3 signalling. *Mol Cancer Ther*. 2011; 10: 481-94.
[115] Harada D, Takigawa N, Ochi N, et al. JAK2-related pathway induces acquired erlotinib resistance in lung cancer cells harboring an epidermal growth factor receptor-activating mutation. *Cancer Sci*. 2012; 103: 1795-802.
[116] Tabara K, Kanda R, Sonoda K, et al. Loss of activating *EGFR* mutant gene contributes to acquired resistance to EGFR tyrosine kinase inhibitors in lung cancer cells. *PLoS One*. 2012; 7: e41017.
[117] Shien K, Toyooka S, Yamamoto H, et al. Acquired resistance to EGFR inhibitors is associated with a manifestation of stem cell-like properties in cancer cells. *Cancer Res*. 2013; 15: 3051-61.
[118] Kanda R, Kawahara A, Watari K, et al. Erlotinib resistance in lung cancer cells mediated by Integrin β1/Src /AKT-driven bypass signalling. *Cancer Res*. 2013; 73: 6243-53.

[119] Furugaki K, Iwai T, Moriya Y, Harada N, Fujimoto-Ouchi K. Loss of an EGFR-amplified chromosome 7 as a novel mechanism of acquired resistance to EGFR-TKIs in *EGFR* mutated NSCLC cells. *Lung Cancer.* 2014; 83: 44-50.

[120] Serizava M, Takahashi T, Yamamoto N, Noh Y. Genomic aberrations associated with erlotinib resistance in non-small cell lung cancer cells. *Anticancer Res.* 2013; 33: 5223-33.

In: Fighting Lung Cancer through the HER Family …
Editor: Diego Márquez-Medina
ISBN: 978-1-63321-092-9

Chapter 14

Resistance II. Conventional Salvage Therapies for the Resistance to Anti-Human Epidermal Growth Factor Receptor Treatments

Diego Márquez-Medina, M.D., Ph.D.
Medical Oncology Department, Arnau de Vilanova
University Hospital of Lleida, Spain

Abstract

Selected patients with Non-small cell lung cancer (NSCLC) clearly benefit from modern tyrosine kinase inhibitors of the epidermal growth factor receptor (EGFR-TKI). Therefore, in order to prolong their profit, physicians have to control the acquired resistance to these drugs in prior responders. Regular practices to bypass or to overcome secondary resistance to EGFR-TKI are reviewed in patients with different failure modes: Initial or dramatic refractivity, generalized gradual progression, and limited oligo-progression. The advantages and disadvantages of EGFR-TKI maintenance, switching to chemotherapy or to a new TKI, addition of chemotherapy to EGFR-TKI, and local therapies as salvage treatments for acquired resistance to EGFR-TKI are exhaustively described and discussed in the present chapter.

1. Background

Non-small cell lung cancer (NSCLC) is the most common and lethal malignancy worldwide. NSCLC produces 18% and 28% of cancer deaths in the European Economic Community and the United States of America, respectively [1], almost more than colon and breast cancer taken together. The majority of NSCLC cells over-express the epidermal growth factor receptor (EGFR) in their surface, and 10-20% harbor sensitizing conformational mutations in this receptor that increase the efficacy of modern tyrosine kinase inhibitors against its inner portion [2, 3] (EGFR-TKI).

Strategies to select sensitive NSCLC patients to reversible EGFR-TKIs have been extensively explored during the last decade, and as a result the presence of sensitizing *EGFR* mutations is the most reliable predictor of efficacy. The response rate to reversible EGFR-TKIs ranges from 9% in unselected NSCLC patients to 30-40% in clinically selected patients, and to 40-70% in *EGFR*-mutant patients [3-9]. Reversible EGFR-TKIs have been universally introduced in the daily practice, on account of which clinicians face the new challenge of managing acquired resistance to these drugs in order to prolong the efficacy in prior responder patients. The absence of a great long-term benefit from any other systemic conventional treatment warrants the maximum exploitation from EGFR-TKIs in advanced NSCLC.

In the previous chapter, Dr. Remón reviewed both the molecular changes that lead to primary and acquired resistance to EGFR-TKIs, and various experimental treatments to reverse them. The following sections are aim to describe common daily practices usable to reverse these EGFR-TKI resistance.

2. Clinical Modes of EGFR-TKI Failure

Resistance to EGFR-TKIs is an emerging health problem. Diverse advanced NSCLCs are currently treated or are applying for being medicated with EGFR-TKIs. However, they will inevitably progress in a mean time of 12-14 months even in those patients with a prior benefit from the drug [2, 5, 6, 10-15]. Clinical strategies to overcome primary or acquired resistance to EGFR-TKIs have not been well defined yet, and physicians are compelled to use all their skills to prolong the benefit in the absence of clear data from the ongoing trials.

An accurate diagnosis of progression is basic to define salvage strategies. Modified RECIST and PERCIST criteria have to be exhaustively applied in CT- and PET-Scans to outline the mode of TKI-failure. The analysis of those eventual molecular changes leading to the resistance should be done if available. Factors that could compromise the efficacy of EGFR-TKI such as a bad compliance, current smoking, or proton-pump inhibitors intake should be excluded or discussed with the patients.

The election of a certain salvage strategy for the TKI-resistance warrants to address the case one to one, and to consider: 1) Patients' peculiarities such as age, comorbidity, performance status, wishes and expectations; 2) Characteristics of the disease like symptomatology, stage and location, or forecast of response to eventual salvage therapies; 3) Aspects of the center such as the availability of clinical trials, lab portfolio, access to advanced techniques of radiation or surgery, or physicians' experience; and 4) Particularities of the salvage therapy like degree of toxicity, responsiveness, and cost-benefit. Moreover, all those items could be combined to configure different clinical EGFR-TKI failure modes despite the hidden molecular mechanism of resistance.

2.1. The Jackman Criteria

In 2010, Jackman et al. [3] proposed diverse clinical criteria to distinguish acquired from primary resistance to reversible EGFR-TKIs. Correspondingly, patients with acquired resistance are those progressing in the course of treatment with erlotinib or gefitinib, harboring any sensitizing *EGFR*-mutation and/or presenting a prior benefit from the drug such as either RECIST or WHO objective response, or significant stabilization for more than six months.

However, caution must be applied to the Jackman criteria. Exclusive symptomatic improvements without objective radiologic response have to be assumed with deliberation as a benefit from EGFR-TKI. Many of them are due to a toxicity recovery from previous therapies, or to the presence of smooth symptomatic progressions. On the other hand, the development of highly symptomatic newly brain metastases while on EGFR-TKI therapy does not always preclude an acquired resistance to the drug. They could be either on account of poor penetration of the TKIs in the central nervous system, or associated to a maintained extra-cranial disease control.

The absence of sensitizing EGFR-mutations does not preclude primary resistance to EGFR-TKI therapy too. The Jackman criteria have a positive predictive value of 66% for sensitizing *EGFR*-mutations [3]. Notwithstanding, wild type patients and those with non-analyzed *EGFR* can respond to reversible EGFR-TKIs, and second-third line erlotinib is currently approved for the treatment of any advanced NSCLC, regardless of the presence of sensitizing *EGFR*-mutations, obtaining the same benefit as conventional chemotherapy.

Nevertheless, the effect of erlotinib is higher in some clinically enriched subsets of wild type and unknown *EGFR* patients. For instance, female gender, Asian race, no smoking habit, and non-squamous histology increase the sensibility to EGFR-TKI. In the French ERMETIC trial [19], clinical selection of non-smoking women with lung adenocarcinoma was as effective and cost-efficient as laboratory detection of sensitizing EGFR-mutations to predict benefit from EGFR-TKIs. The profit from EGFR-TKI in some wild type and non-analyzed patients were partially related to the presence of uncommon un-detected *EGFR*-mutations in the tumors [16]. Uncommon *EGFR*-mutations represent 14.5% and 12.4% of mutations in Caucasian [17] and Asian [18] patients, respectively. A Taiwanese series [18] of 78 NSCLC with uncommon *EGFR*-mutations reported 48.4% response rate, and 5 months median progression-free survival (PFS) when treated with erlotinib or gefitinib. Response rate and PFS increased to 57.1% and 6 months, respectively, when only G719 and L861-mutations were taken into account.

2.2. Three Main Failure Modes

In 2012, Yang et al. [20] reported three clinical patterns of EGFR-TKI failure: Dramatic, gradual, and local mode. Firstly, the dramatic failure represents a generalized, fast and aggressive progression that commonly leads to a symptomatic worsening. Secondly, the gradual failure reproduces a better outcome and describes those slow, generalized, and commonly asymptomatic progressions. Finally, the local failure depicts those progressions confined to a limited number of tumor sites, while the rest of them remains controlled by the EGFR-TKI therapy.

Moreover, other papers [21] have focused on the timing concept and distinguished: 1) Initial refractivity in patients that never respond to EGFR-TKI who usually exhibit generalized and dramatic progression. This initial refractivity occurs in over 80% of wild type and 30% of *EGFR*-mutant NSCLCs; 2) Generalized-progression after a prior response to EGFR-TKI. These patients tend to progress gradually, and not dramatically, and; 3) Solitary or oligo-progression confined to a limited number of tumor sites or to the apparition of newly metastatic sites whereas the rest of the tumor spread is controlled by the EGFR-TKI.

The definition of those clinical failure modes is basic to adapt the salvage strategies, and to prolong the benefit from EGFR-TKIs [2,3,6,13,21]. In this regard, modern diagnostic techniques could be helpful. For instance, the 18F-FDG PET/CT is effective at detecting active foci of NSCLC, and very sensitive to predict early and long-term response to EGFR-TKI [7,8,22,28], even in patients treated twice. Re-biopsy at the time of progression helps to define molecular changes leading to acquired resistance to EGFR-TKI, to determine new targets for experimental treatments, and to exclude histological transformations in small-cell lung cancers or mesenchymal that origin 14% and 5% of acquired resistance, respectively.

3. Treatments for Refractivity and Dramatic Progression to EGFR-TKI

Few clinical strategies are able to overpass both initial refractivity and primary resistance to EGFR-TKI, which are usually associated with dramatic and symptomatic progressions. Those patients do not respond to EGFR-TKI, and progress in the first months of treatment in a generalized, symptomatic and rapid mode.

Patients without a clinical forecast of EGFR-TKI response should be closely followed-up in order to rapidly detect this initial refractivity, therefore to act accordingly. Wild type tumors, men, heavy smoker patients, non-Asian races, or squamous histologies predict a lower response rate to EGFR-TKI. On the contrary, a large series of 2,105 Caucasian NSCLC patients [2] reported a higher presence of sensitizing *EGFR*-mutations and response rate to EGFR-TKI in women (30% versus 8.2%), elderly patients (22.2% versus 13.9%), never smokers (37.7% versus 5.8%), lung adenocarcinomas and bronchioloalveolar adenocarcinomas (17.3% and 21.3%, respectively).

Initial refractivity is common among wild type patients, translating a lack of sensibility to EGFR-TKIs, and a scarce benefit from TKI-switching or any other EGFR-targeted salvage therapy.

Primary resistance to reversible EGFR-TKI is presented in 20% of Asian and 40% of Caucasian patients [2, 6]. The most renowned mechanism is the T790M mutation changing threonine to methionine in codon 790 of exon 20 of *EGFR*, which could origin secondary resistance too. The T790M related primary resistance tends to associate with a poor response rate to EGFR-TKIs, and a worse outcome [29]. However, the secondary T790M mutations produce 50-60% of acquired resistance to reversible EGFR-TKIs [30-33] and identify a subset of NSCLC with a much indolent behavior [29, 35-39]. Those secondary T790M mutations seem to be more common in non-smoker female patients with lung, pleural, and lymph node metastases that progress in previously known lesions than in patients developing newly metastases (90% versus 10%; p= 0.014) [34].

The irreversible EGFR-TKIs showed an encouraging activity in T790M-mutant *EGFR*-mutant cell lines [40, 41] that, unfortunately, decreases when they are applied to T790-mutant *EGFR*-mutant patients [42, 43]. Afatinib obtains a lower response rate and PFS (2.8 months versus 4.2 months; p< 0.0001) in NSCLC patients with primary rather acquired resistance to reversible EGFR-TKI [43].

4. Treatments for Patients with a Gradual Progression to EGFR-TKI

In contrast to those NSCLC that dramatically progress, most patients with a gradual progression after a prior and prolonged response to EGFR-TKIs are EGFR-mutant, fulfill the Jackman criteria, and present acquired secondary resistance. Besides, gradual progression has been also reported in wild type patients whose response to TKI is probably associated with the presence of uncommon and undetected *EGFR*-mutations. Nevertheless, progression in both wild type or *EGFR*-mutant patient is due to the gradual growing of less sensitive subsets of tumors cells, and respond to many salvage strategies including anti-EGFR therapies.

4.1. EGFR-TKI Maintenance

Patients with a gradual and indolent progression mode have a better outcome, longer PFS and overall survival (OS) than patients with dramatic or early progressions. It allows the TKI maintenance beyond RECIST progression in fit asymptomatic patients with a good tolerance to the drug [20, 44].

Some retrospective Asian series [45-48] reported the benefit from EGFR-TKI maintenance. In the first one [45], the strategy prolonged the PFS of 49 *EGFR*-mutant TKI-treated patients in 10.1 months. In the second one [46], gefitinib maintenance extended the OS of 134 EGFR-mutant patients progressing to gefitinib in 3.2 months. The good performance status, the progression confined to previously known lesions, and more than three months of prior benefit from gefitinib were related to a higher profit of maintenance. In a longer Japanese series [48] with 335 consecutive NSCLC progressing to gefitinib after a prior response, gefitinib re-challenge or maintenance increased the OS (42.4 months versus 25.8 months; p< 0.001). Nishie et al. [47] reviewed other 64 Japanese NSCLC progressing while on EGFR-TKI treatment, and reported a better OS (32.2 months versus 23 months; p= 0.005) in those treated with TKI maintenance than in those switched to chemotherapy beyond progression.

Furthermore, in Caucasian patients, a series of 43 NSCLC progressing while on EGFR-TKI treatment [50], the TKI-maintenance beyond progression increased OS (2 months versus 9 months; p= 0.00002). Besides, data from three prospective trials [49] including 42 *EGFR*-mutant patients progressing to first line erlotinib and treated with erlotinib maintenance with or without local salvage therapy reported that erlotinib maintenance delayed the necessity of an alternate systemic therapy in 45% of the patients for more than three months, and for more than 12 months in 19% of them.

The Asian phase-II ASPIRATION trial will examine the benefit from erlotinib maintenance in patients with a gradual progression to the drug. However, comparison between EGFR-TKI maintenance and observation only is not available yet in this subset of patients.

Despite expending EGFR-TKI to their maximum benefit, EGFR-TKI maintenance beyond progression could be recommended in order to avoid the phenomenon of disease flare. The flare had been reported in endocrine treated breast cancers, and consists of a transient increase of severity and disease extension when the cytostatic therapy is interrupted. The disease flare appears in 20-25% of NSCLC interrupting the EGFR-TKI treatment. The Memorial Sloan-Kettering Cancer Center [51] detected 23% of disease flare in a retrospective series of 61 *EGFR*-mutant NSCLC that discontinued EGFR-TKI after progression. Median time to flare was 8 days (range 3-21), and incidence was higher in patients with a shorter time to TKI-progression, pleural metastases, and brain metastases. The presence of T790M did not increase the percentage of flare.

The rationale for disease flare is heterogeneous composition of NSCLC, whose cells present a wide range of sensibility to EGFR-TKIs. When TKI is interrupted because of the progression in a resistant subset of cells, the remaining sensitive cells suddenly lose the drug control and perform a generalized and sometimes a dramatic growth explosion. In fact, EGFR-TKI reintroduction in patients with disease flare has been demonstrated to normalize the metabolic activity and growing of disease foci in PET/CT [23].

The EGFR-TKI maintenance beyond progression is especially recommended for asymptomatic patients with a slow and gradual failure mode while on TKI treatment. However, the high cost of the drugs, the necessity of a close follow up of the patients so as to prevent a violent change in the pattern of progression, and the potential impossibility of treatment if a patient become symptomatic are eventual disadvantages of this strategy.

4.2. Switch to Conventional Chemotherapy Combined with EGFR-TKI Maintenance

The phase-III INTACT-1, INTACT-2, TRIBUTE, and TALENT trials [52] did not demonstrate any benefit on survival by adding reversible EGFR-TKI to first line chemotherapy in unselected NSCLC. On the other sense, a randomized phase-II trial [53] including 143 *EGFR*-mutant or overexpressed patients did not detected any benefit by adding chemotherapy to first line erlotinib. The PFS was longer with erlotinib alone than combining erlotinib with carboplatin and paclitaxel (18.2 months versus 4.9 months).

Nevertheless, adding conventional chemotherapy to EGFR-TKI maintenance has been explored in patients progressing to EGFR-TKI. In erlotinib-resistant tumor xenografts, the continuous EGFR-inhibition by erlotinib enhances the activity of chemotherapy [56], and combination *in vivo* theoretically maintains the TKI effect over sensitive cells, avoid the disease flare, and eliminate resistant subsets of cells with chemotherapy [54, 55].

In vivo, Goldberg et al. [57] retrospectively explored the benefit of combining chemotherapy with erlotinib in a cohort of 78 *EGFR*-mutant TKI-progressing NSCLCs. The combined treatment obtained a higher response rate than chemotherapy alone (41% versus 18%; p= 0.08), but no significant benefits on PFS and OS. However, in a German retrospective case-control study with 41 erlotinib-progressing NSCLC with a prior benefit from the drug [50], the combined therapy increased OS from the first erlotinib-progression (14.5 months versus 2 months; HR 0.154) and the whole median OS (54.5 months versus 28.3 months; HR 0.474) when compared to chemotherapy alone in both wild type and *EGFR*-mutant patients.

Pemetrexed, an anti-folato cytotoxic drug, has been reported to obtain encouraging results added to erlotinib or gefitinib beyond EGFR-TKI progression. In a series of 27 *EGFR*-mutant NSCLC [58], pemetrexed plus EGFR-TKI achieved a response rate of 26%, a median PFS of 7 months, and an OS of 11.4 months. The administration of pemetrexed could be especially effective in patients with acquired resistance to EGFR-TKI due to *MET*-amplifications [59-64]. Gefitinib down-regulates thymidylate synthase in *MET*-amplified NSCLC cells, and pemetrexed is more effective in tumors with a low level of thymidylate synthase.

Ongoing prospective trials will clarify the role of EGFR-TKI maintenance added to chemotherapy as salvage therapy for TKI-progression. The phase-III LUX-Lung-5 trial [43] will report data from patients progressing to afatinib after a prior response and randomized to receive weekly paclitaxel plus afatinib or single-agent chemotherapy. The phase-III IMPRESS trial will compare the efficacy and safety of gefitinib associated with cisplatin and pemetrexed versus chemotherapy alone in *EGFR*-mutant patients progressing to gefitinib. The PREFER trial which will randomize 180 *EGFR*-mutant patients progressing to first line erlotinib to receive carboplatin plus pemetrexed followed by pemetrexed-maintenance with or without erlotinib-maintenance.

Pulses of EGFR-TKIs inserted along the cycle of chemotherapy could be an alternative to maintain the TKI beyond progression. This kind of combination has obtained promising results as first line treatment for advanced NSCLC. Kanda et al. [65] reported an encouraging PFS of 19.2 months, and 83% 2-years OS in *EGFR*-mutant patients by introducing gefitinib during cisplatin plus docetaxel regimens. The FASTACT-II trial [66] randomized 451 NSCLC to receive first line treatment with six cycles of cisplatin/carboplatin plus gemcitabine and pulses of erlotinib or placebo, followed by erlotinib or placebo-maintenance. The presence of erlotinib in the treatment increased both PFS (16.8 months versus 6.9 months; HR 0.25; $p< 0.001$) and OS (31.4 months versus 20.6 months; HR 0.48; $p< 0.01$) in *EGFR*-mutant patients.

As salvage therapy for patients progressing to chemotherapy, a Japanese phase-I trial [67] intercalated erlotinib on days 2 to 16 of tri-weekly cycles of pemetrexed in 12 nonsquamous NSCLC progressing to chemotherapy. Treatment was well tolerated, response rate was 25%, and disease control was 66%. A subsequent phase-II trial [68] combining tri-weekly pemetrexed on day 1 plus erlotinib on days 2 to 16 in 27 non-squamous advanced wild type NSCLC progressing on or after receiving first-line chemotherapy obtained 11.1% response rate, 63% disease control rate, 2.8 months PFS, and 15.8 months OS. Moreover, the phase-II NVALT-10 trial [69] randomized 231 advanced NSCLCs progressing on or after first-line chemotherapy to receive continuous erlotinib or erlotinib for 15 days intercalated in four cycles of docetaxel (squamous) or pemetrexed (non-squamous NSCLC), and followed by erlotinib-maintenance. Both, PFS (6.1 months versus 4.9 months; HR 0.78; $p= 0.09$), and OS (7.8 months versus 5.5 months; HR 0.67; $p= 0.02$) increased in the combination arm.

On the other hand, Yoshimura et al. [70] analyzed the combination of tri-weekly pemetrexed on day 1 plus gefitinib or erlotinib maintenance on days 2-16 as salvage therapy for 27 *EGFR*-mutant patients progressing while on EGFR-TKI treatment. The combination achieved 25.9% response rate, 77.8% disease control, 7 months PFS, and 11.4 months OS.

4.3. Switch to Conventional Chemotherapy and EGFR-TKI Holidays

The EGFR-TKI withdrawal by itself could recover the sensitiveness to erlotinib or gefitinib of a small number of patients with acquired resistance to the drugs [71]. The Dana-Farber Cancer Institute [73] reported a series of 14 *EGFR*-mutant NSCLC that received adjuvant EGFR-TKI for a median of 17 months and recurred after stopping EGFR-TKI. The re-treatment with EGFR-TKI obtained 73% response rate. Moreover, the retreatment with erlotinib after 11 months of drug-free interval obtained 80% disease control rate, and 4.4 months PFS in a series of 19 progressing to erlotinib patients [74].

These EGFR-TKI "holidays" can be profited to switch to conventional chemotherapy, the first strategy explored for EGFR-TKI progression and cessation [71, 72], and could provides eventual advantages: 1) Chemotherapy can erase growing subsets of TKI-resistant cells and restore the predominance of sensitive subsets; 2) *EGFR*-mutant patients seem to obtain a higher benefit from chemotherapy [6]; 3) Chemotherapy could revert acquired resistance to EGFR-TKI and, finally; 4) the benefit of EGFR-TKI withdrawal is also observed when TKI are reintroduced.

Chemotherapy obtains 28% response rate in EGFR-mutant patients progressing while on EGFR-TKI. In the French phase-II 0504 trial [75], fit elderly patients with advanced NSCLC who were treated with docetaxel plus gemcitabine after progression to first line erlotinib achieved 7.5 months PFS, 9.4 months OS, and 36.2% 1-year OS. Other French trial, the multicenter IFCT-0401 [76], explored the efficacy of chemotherapy in 47 advanced lepidic adenocarcinomas progressing to first line gefitinib. Twenty-nine received doublets of platinum plus taxane, nine received platinum plus gemcitabine, three received gemcitabine alone, and two received pemetrexed alone. Response rate to chemotherapy was 21%, disease control reached 56%, and median PFS was 3 months, with a higher benefit in patients treated with taxanes or pemetrexed. Finally, in a retrospective review of 61 Asian *EGFR*-mutant patients progressing while on gefitinib [77], the switch to cisplatin plus gemcitabine obtained a higher response rate and OS (27.1 months versus 10 months; p=0.035) than the switch to erlotinib.

This TKI "holidays" with chemotherapy could also recover sensitivity to EGFR-TKI. For instance, in a Korean phase-II trial [73] with 23 patients progressing to gefitinib after a prior benefit from the drug, salvage therapy consisted of chemotherapy and gefitinib re-introduction after progression to chemotherapy. The response rate to gefitinib was 21.7%, together with 65.2% of disease control. Over 50% of patients harbored sensitizing *EGFR*-mutations, taking into account that most of them were women, never-smokers, or lung adenocarcinomas. Additionally, in a retrospectively series from the VU University [78] with 14 advanced NSCLC progressing after a long-term benefit from EGFR-TKI, the subsequent treatment with standard chemotherapy and erlotinib at renewed progression obtained 36% response rate, 86% disease control, and 6.5 months PFS.

4.4. Switch to a New EGFR-TKI

The incoming of an acquired resistance to a EGFR-TKI in NSCLC does not always preclude an absolute refractivity to any other EGFR-TKI. In a series [79] with 8 EGFR-mutant lung adenocarcinomas progressing to the experimental EGFR and -HER2 inhibitor XL647, 60% of the patients remained sensitive to erlotinib.

The switch from a reversible EGFR-TKI to another has been reported to be effective in a limited percentage of patients [71, 80, 81]. A retrospective series of 104 Japanese NSCLC [82] reported benefit from erlotinib in wild type and EGFR-mutant patient progressing to gefitinib.

Four series [83-86] including 273 gefitinib-progressing NSCLC reported scarce but significant responses by switching to erlotinib in patients with a prior long benefit from gefitinib. Disease control ranged from 9% to 22%, and the estimated OS was 11.8 months. Most progressions to salvage erlotinib were detected in the first two months of treatment. A good performance status, *EGFR*-mutation, long benefit from gefitinib, and insertion of cytotoxic chemotherapies between gefitinib and erlotinib were predictive factors for disease control and PFS advantage. Patients with those characteristics obtained 72% disease control rate, and 3.4 months PFS. On the other hand, 15 erlotinib-progressing NSCLC treated with gefitinib [87] obtained 40% disease control in patients with a prior benefit from erlotinib. Time to progression to gefitinib reached 3.7 months, and OS was 7.4 months. None of the patient refractory to erlotinib responded to gefitinib. Thus, the option to switch from a reversible EGFR-TKI to another one after progression should be reserved for those patients with a clear prior benefit from TKI. Tang et al. [88] have recently reported a series of 120 NSCLC treated twice with EGFR-TKIs. Over 40% were treated twice with the same EGFR-TKI (25% gefitinib and 15.8% erlotinib), and 59.2% were switched to another TKI (45.8% from gefitinib to erlotinib and 13.4% from erlotinib to gefitinb). The benefit was similar in the four groups, and 1-year OS reached 32.5%. Disease control rate was 52.2%, PFS grew to 2.3 months, and OS became 8 months. Prior benefit from EGFR-TKI, longer than six months PFS with first EGFR-TKI (HR 0.611; p= 0.0076), and longer than four months interval between the two treatments (HR 0.529; p= 0.0088), predicted the benefit from the second administration.

The new generation of irreversible EGFR-TKIs could be more effective over uncommon EGFR-mutations and NSCLC with acquired resistance to reversible EGFR-TKI. In preclinical models, irreversible EGFR-TKIs present an encouraging activity against *EGFR*-mutant cells harboring T790M-mutation [40, 41, 89].

Afatinib (BIBW-2992; Boehringer Ingelheim) is an oral irreversible TKI that binds and blocks EGFR, HER2, HER4, and all the relevant dimers of the ErbB family [89-91]. Afatinib has been approved for the first-line treatment of advanced NSCLC with sensitizing *EGFR*-mutations on exon 19 and exon 21. In vitro, afatinib is able to bind both wild type and *EGFR*-mutant cell lines, including those with T790M or T854a-mutations [89, 91-03] with a higher effect than reversible EGFR-TKI [89, 91]. The afatinib activity in T790M-mutant NSCLC is also presented in diverse in vivo lung cancer models [94].

Eleven patients with primary T790M-mutations were included in the phase-III LUX-Lung-3 trial [43, 90, 95] comparing first-line afatinib versus cisplatin plus pemetrexed in 345 advanced *EGFR*-mutant lung adenocarcinomas. Disease control in T790M-mutant patients was higher and encouraging in the afatinib arm (72.7% versus 18.1%). In the phase-III LUX-

Lung-1 trial [38], 585 advanced lung adenocarcinomas that had progressed to one or two lines of chemotherapy, and at least after 12 weeks of erlotinib or gefitinib, were treated with afatinib or best supportive care. Afatinib significantly improved PFS (3.3 months versus 1.1 months; HR 0.38; p< 0.0001) in the whole population, but not in wild type patients. However, those with acquired resistance to EGFR-TKI obtained a higher benefit on PFS from afatinib (4.4 months versus 0.99 months; HR 0.37).

The Japanese phase-II LUX-LUNG-4 trial [46, 96, 97] analyzed the activity of afatinib over patients with acquired resistance to reversible EGFR-TKI. Sixty-two advanced lung adenocarcinomas progressing after more than 12 weeks of prior erlotinib (11.3%), gefitinib (79%), or both (9.7%) were treated with afatinib. Over 72% of patients were *EGFR*-mutant and 82% of them fulfilled the Jackman criteria of acquired resistance to EGFR-TKI. Acquired T790M-mutation was reported in 3.2% patients. The response rate of afatinib was 8.2%, and disease control reached 65.4%. Most responses to afatinib were observed within 8 weeks from the initiation of the treatment and presented a mean duration of 24.4 weeks. Median PFS was 4.4 months, and median OS was 19 months. Patients with the Jackman criteria approached a median PFS of 4.4 months, 5.9% response rate and 68.6% disease control rate. Disease was stabilized for nine months in one of two patients with acquired T790M-mutations.

Furthermore, in the phase-III LUX-Lung-3 trial [43, 90, 95], 345 advanced *EGFR*-mutant lung adenocarcinomas were treated with first-line afatinib or six cycles of cisplatin plus pemetrexed without maintenance therapy. They included 72% Asian people, 68% never-smokers, and 65% female patients with exon 19 deletions (49%) or L858R point mutations (40%). Median PFS was significantly higher in the afatinib arm (11.1 months versus 6.7 months, respectively; HR 0.49; p= 0.001). The percentage of patients harboring uncommon *EGFR*-mutations was 12% only, and they seemed to take a lower benefit on PFS from afatinib (13.6 months versus 6.9 months; HR 0.41; p= 0.001). Disease control in eleven T790M-mutant patients was higher with afatinib than with chemotherapy (72.7% versus 18.1%), although such small simple did not allow drawing any conclusions.

Likewise, afatinib has been reported active in the treatment of NSCLC patients with uncommon *EGFR*-mutations. In the phase-II LUX-LUNG-2 trial [98, 99], 129 advanced *EGFR*-mutant lung adenocarcinomas were treated with first or second line afatinib, perhaps after a first line of chemotherapy. Response rate lowered from 61% to 39% in those patients with uncommon *EGFR*-mutations. The phase-III LUX-Lung-5 trial [43] also analyzed the efficacy of afatinib in patients progressing to chemotherapy and reversible EGFR-TKI. Correspondingly, response rate in the whole population was 7.6%. The improvement on PFS was higher in patients with acquired resistance to EGFR-TKI than in those with primary resistance (4.2 months versus 2.8 months, respectively; p< 0.0001).

Yang et al. [100, 101] recently reported data from the LUX-Lung-2, 3 and 6 trials regarding the activity of afatinib in patients with uncommon EGFR-mutations. Over 400 patients harboring exon 19 deletions, 308 with L858R-mutations, and 100 with uncommon *EGFR*-mutations were treated with afatinib. Uncommon *EGFR*-mutations included 14 T790M-mutations, 23 exon 20 insertions, and 38 with other *EGFR*-mutations. The response rate became lower in patients with primary T790M-mutations and exon 20 insertions than in the rest of uncommon EGFR-mutations (14%, 8.7%, and 71.1%, respectively), although disease control in patients with resistance-mutations rose to the encouraging rate of 65%. Moreover, PFS and OS lowered in patients with primary T790M-mutation and exon 20 insertions than in the rest of patients with uncommon EGFR-mutations (2.9 months, 2.7 months, and 10.7 months, respectively; and 14.9 months, 9.4 months, and 18.6 months, respectively). The activity of afatinib in those uncommon *EGFR*-mutations less sensitive to erlotinib or gefitinib emerged as extremely high, and ranged from 50% to 100% response rate, 8.2 months to 14.7 months PFS, and 16.9 months to not reached OS.

Data from combinations of afatinib plus docetaxel and pemetrexed in pulsed and continuous doses [102, 103] suggesting that those regimens could be useful salvage therapies warrant further prospective investigations. Besides, the efficacy of any other EGFR-TKI in patients progressing to reversible EGFR-TKI need to be confirmed. Dacomitinib, an EGFR, HER2, and HER4 inhibitor, could be more effective than gefitinib eliminating tumor cells harboring T790M-mutations [41], and more active than erlotinib improving PFS in wild type and *EGFR*-mutant patients [103]. Some data regarding icotinib withdrawal and retreatment after progression to icotinib has been reported [84, 105].

4.5. Not-Exactly Conventional Therapies

Cetuximab (Erbitux®) is a murine monoclonal antibody against the outer portion of EGFR, approved for colorectal, head and neck cancers, and explored for the treatment of advanced NSCLC [54, 55, 106]. A series from the Massachusetts General Hospital [106] analyzed the effect of cetuximab in 18 NSCLC patients heavily pretreated with chemotherapy and EGFR-TKIs. Only three patients were *EGFR*-mutant. Disease was stabilized in 28% of patients. Median PFS was 1.8 months, and median OS was 7.5 months.

In vitro, the vertical EGFR-inhibition combining erlotinib and cetuximab is reported to increase apoptosis in T790M-mutant NSCLC cells lines [108]. *In vivo*, the combination of erlotinib plus cetuximab does not seem to be so active [109].

In vitro and in murine models [110, 111], the combination of afatinib plus cetuximab induces the regression of erlotinib-resistant NSCLC cells. *In vivo*, early data suggest that the combination of afatinib plus cetuximab is tolerable and active in patients with acquired resistance to EGFR-TKI [112]. A phase-I/II trial [113] including 100 *EGFR*-mutant heavily pretreated NSCLC, the combination of afatinib plus cetuximab obtained 32% response rate and 4.6 months PFS in spite of the T790M status. The response rate did not significantly differ from T790M-mutant patients to the rest of them (38% versus 47%).

Intermittent, high-dose and concurrent afatinib plus cetuximab [109] are being explored to overcome T790M-resistance. An ongoing ECOG trial is analyzing the efficacy of afatinib with or without cetuximab in EGFR-mutant patients progressing to first line reversible EGFR-TKI, while a SWOG trial will analyze the effect of afatinib with or without cetuximab as first line treatment for EGFR-mutant patients.

HER2 mutations are found in 1-4% of lung adenocarcinomas [94, 114]. They tend to present the same phenotype as *EGFR*-mutant NSCLCs. A French work [94] reported *HER2*-mutations in 1.7% of 3800 NSCLC. Those patients had a median age of 60 years. *HER2*-mutations were most common among women (69%), never-smokers (52.3%), and lung adenocarcinomas (100%). Specific anti-HER2 treatments were administered in 22 patients. The response rate was 50%, and the disease control rate 82%. The disease control rate was 93% in 15 patients treated with trastuzumab-based therapies. The disease control rate in three patients treated with afatinib was 100%. The PFS in patients treated with anti-HER2 therapies was 5.1 months, and median OS was 22.9 months. A phase-II trial also reported the activity of afatinib in the treatment of *HER2*-mutant patients after failure to other EGFR- and/or HER2-targeted therapies [114]. The M. D. Anderson Cancer Center has reported *HER2*-mutant NSCLC regressions by combining dual anti-HER2 and VEGF targeted therapies [50].

HER2-amplification is found in 1% of NSCLC. However, this percentage rises to 12% in patients with acquired resistance to EGFR-TKI [115]. The combination of afatinib and cetuximab has been reported to significantly inhibit the HER2 phosphorylation in preclinical models, but no clinical evidence of afatinib activity in HER2-overexpressed NSCLC has been acquainted. There have only been case reports regarding the treatment with afatinib or trastuzumab in this kind of patients.

Ziv-Aflibercept (Zaltrap, Sanofi U.S., Inc.) is a recombinant fusion protein that blocks the activity of the vascular endothelial growth factor A and the placental growth factor. Aflibercept in combination with irinotecan plus 5-Fluoruracil and folinid acid has been approved to treat metastatic colorectal cancers after oxaliplatin-failure. An open-label, multicenter trial [116] analyzed the efficacy of Ziv-Aflibercept in 89 platinum- and erlotinib-resistant lung adenocarcinomas. Response rate was 2%, median PFS 2.7 months, and OS 6.2 months. Six- and 12-month OS rates were 54 and 29%, respectively.

5. Treatment for Solitary or Oligo-Metastatic Progressions

In spite of the generalized disease progression in the whole tumor spread, EGFR-TKI treated patients could suffer: 1) Newly metastatic lesions meanwhile the previously known lesions remain controlled by the therapy, or; 2) a disease progression limited to some previously known tumor sites whereas the rest of them remains under control. These locally confined oligo-progressions are rare in the beginning of the treatment with EGFR-TKI, being more common after a certain period of time. The rational for them is: 1) the histological heterogeneity of NSCLC that are composed of different cell populations. Any subset of cells has a different sensibility to EGFR-TKI depending on the presence of sensitizing *EGFR*-mutations, resistance *EGFR*-mutations, and alterations in the *EGFR*-related pathways [18, 117], and they express a different metastatic potential. Hence, every metastatic site presents a different behavior. Over 27% of discordance in the *EGFR* status has been reported between primary and metastatic NSCLC [118-120]; 2) Molecular changes leading to EGFR-TKI resistance [29] could be developed in a limited number of metastases and they evolve in a different way. The apparition of disease flare days after EGFR-TKI discontinuation in over 20% of patients [51] implies the persistent therapeutic effect of the drug over many metastatic sites while disease is progressing at other locations as a consequence of acquired resistance; 3) Oligo progression defined as newly metastatic lesions could be explained by the existence of sanctuary areas, such as the brain, where EGFR-TKI are less effective. This phenomenon widely explored while on the treatment with monoclonal antibodies against HER2 in breast cancer eventually occurs while on EGFR-TKI treatments.

Frequency and implications of these solitary or oligo-progressions to EGFR-TKI in NSCLC are not clearly defined [17, 19]. The percentage of oligo-progressions ranges from 7.69% to 24.22% among EGFR-TKI failures [6, 13, 17, 19], which increases if only prior

EGFR-TKI responders are considered [13], and may further increase if only newly metastatic progression are taken into account in controlled patients [16, 19].

It is not clear if the outcome of oligo-progressive patients differs too much from the outcome of those with generalized-progression to EGFR-TKI. Yang et al. [6] reported that both PFS (9.2 months versus 12.9 months; p= 0.007) and OS (23.1 months versus 39.4 months; p< 0.001) worsened in patients with local-progression compared to those with gradual-progression, while another series [13] reported that PFS gradually increased from less than 3 months in initially refractory patients to 11.2 months in those with generalized-progression, and to 20.7 months in those with oligo-progression to EGFR-TKI. The OS increased from 13.4 month in patients with generalized-progression to 49.8 months in those with oligo-progression only.

The small size of these series interjects caution, but results could be explained by an eventual better prognosis of oligo-progression by itself, the applying of salvage therapies, and/or the EGFR-TKI maintenance in patients with localized progression.

Surgery or radical radiotherapy could salvage those oligo-progressions, allowing the EGFR-TKI maintenance beyond progression in selected patients. Both techniques have been commonly used to erase oligo-metastases in breast and colorectal cancer, and are claimed to be able to cure a considerable percentage of NSCLC with adrenal or brain metastases [121].

5.1. Treatment of Newly Brain Metastatic Lesions While on EGFR-TKI Effective Therapy

Over 30% of *EGFR*-mutant patients develop brain metastases [122]. The cumulative risk of brain progressions among *EGFR*-mutant gefitinib or erlotinib-treated NSCLC [123] is 19% at the time of diagnosis, and 28% while on the treatment, with a 1- and 2-year actuarial risk of brain progression of 7% and 19%, respectively. These newly brain metastases appearing while on the EGFR-TKI therapy seem to have a lower presence of acquired T790M mutations [124]. The EGFR-TKI concentration in cerebrospinal fluid tends to be inadequately low [16, 125-127], and the onset of newly brain lesions in EGFR-TKI-treated NSCLC does not always preclude a systemic failure to the drugs. It sets an example of feasibility of local salvage therapies.

The combination of palliative radiation and EGFR-TKI treatment in *EGFR*-mutant patients with newly brain metastases inclines towards obtaining a favorable response and 6-12 months PFS [16, 128-130]. The M. D. Anderson Cancer Center [131] analyzed the benefit from whole-brain radiation plus erlotinib in 40 NSCLC developing newly brain metastases. Treatment was well tolerated and reached an overall response rate of 86%, and a median survival of 11.8 months.

Therefore, OS seems to be higher in *EGFR*-mutant patients (9.3 months versus 19.1 months). In 17 advanced NSCLC developing newly solitary brain metastases while on EGFR-TKI treatment [16], brain radiation and EGFR-TKI-maintenance obtained 76% brain control rate, 2.6 months PFS, and almost six months extra-cranial PFS.

5.2. Treatment of Extra-Cranial Oligo-Progression While on EGFR-TKI therapy

In a series [2] of 10 *EGFR*-mutant EGFR-TKI treated NSCLC and oligo-progression, adrenalectomy and radiation were reported feasible and effective salvage therapies, allowing the EGFR-TKI maintenance. They obtained a benefit on PFS of 6.2 months that seemed to be higher when patients with extra-cranial progression only were analyzed (7.1 versus 4 months, p= 0.26).

In extra-cranial oligo-progression, surgery resection is feasible and effective to prolong PFS and improve quality of life in selected EGFR-TKI treated patients [132]. The Memorial Sloan-Kettering Cancer Center [12] reported 27 *EGFR*-mutant TKI-treated patients with newly extra-cranial oligo-progression and treated with local salvage therapies plus EGFR-TKI-maintenance. They obtained a median time to progression of 19 months. Furthermore, Oxnard et al. [49] gathered data from three prospective trials including 42 *EGFR*-mutant Caucasian patients progressing to first line erlotinib. Over 21% were treated with local salvage therapies plus erlotinib maintenance. Median PFS was 13 months. As a result, treatment after progression delayed more than three months an alternate systemic therapy in 45% of patients, and more than 12 months in 19% of patients.

A series [17] of 23 non-squamous TKI-treated NSCLCs developing lung oligo-progression reported the efficacy of lung salvage radiotherapy and TKI-maintenance. They obtained an overall response rate of 84%, and a median PFS of 16 months. Another retrospective series [19] of 10 TKI-treated NSCLC with bony oligo-progression reported a median benefit on PFS of 2.9 months by applying salvage radiation and EGFR-TKI maintenance. Finally, the report of four NSCLC with bony and lung oligo-progressions while on long-term erlotinib treatments [13] showed 100% response rate, and 41-140% benefit on PFS with erlotinib-maintenance and salvage radiation, even when the salvage strategy was applied twice. All those series report an excellent tolerance by applying local salvage therapies and TKI-maintenance, and a clear improvement on PFS. Prospective trials are warranted to evaluate the real value of those strategies in front of systemic approaches.

Conclusion

Selected patients with NSCLC clearly benefit from EGFR-TKI. However, even those with a long profit from the drug, finally progress in a mean time of 12-14 months and physicians need to be trained in order to manage any failure and to be able to use the maximum advantage from EGFR-TKI. In virtue of data absence from either randomized prospective trials, treatments are required to be customized for each patient, likewise clinical skills have to be sharpened.

Acknowledgments

The author would like to thank Svetozara Georgieva Hristova for her collaboration and convenient suggestions about language review and style.

References

[1] Ferlay J, Shin HR, Bray F, Forman D, Mathers C, Parkin DM. Estimates of worldwide burden of cancer in 2008: Globocan 2008. *Int. J. Cancer.* 2010; 127 (12): 2893-917.

[2] Rosell R, Moran T, Queralt C, et al. Screening for epidermal growth factor receptor mutations in lung cancer. *N. Engl. J. Med.* 2009; 361 (10): 958–67.

[3] Jackman D, Pao W, Riely GJ, et al. Clinical definition of acquired resistance to epidermal growth factor receptor tyrosine kinase inhibitors in non-small cell lung cacner. *J. Clin. Oncol.* 2010; 28: 357-60.

[4] Shepherd FA, Rodrigues Pereira J, Ciuleanu T, et al. Erlotinib in previously treated non-small-cell lung cancer. *N. Engl. J. Med.* 2005; 353 (2): 123-32.

[5] Thatcher N, Chang A, Parikh P, et al. Gefitinib plus best supportive care in previously treated patients with refractory advanced non-small-cell lung cancer: results from a randomised, placebo-controlled, multicentre study (Iressa Survival Evaluation in Lung Cancer). *Lancet.* 2005; 366 (9496): 1527-37.

[6] Rosell R, Carcereny E, Gervais R, et al. Erlotinib versus standard chemotherapy as first-line treatment for European patients with advanced EGFR mutation-positive non-small-cell lung cancer (EURTAC): a multicentre, open-label, randomised phase 3 trial. *Lancet Oncol.* 2012; 13 (3): 239-46.

[7] Mok TS, Wu YL, Thongprasert S, et al. Gefitinib or carboplatin-paclitaxel in pulmonary adenocarcinoma. *N. Engl. J. Med.* 2009; 361 (10): 947-57.

[8] Costa DB, Kobayashi S, Tenen DG, et al. Pooled analysis of the prospective trials of gefitinib monotherapy for EGFR-mutant non-small cell lung cancers. *Lung Cancer.* 2007; 58: 95-103.

[9] Miller VA, Riely GJ, Zakowski MF, et al. Molecular characteristics of bronchioloalveolar carcinoma and adenocarcinoma, bronchioloalveolar carcinoma subtype, predict response to erlotinib. *J. Clin. Oncol.* 2008; 26: 1472-8.

[10] Jackman DM, Miller VA, Cioffredi LA, et al. Impact of epidermal growth factor receptor and KRAS mutations on clinical outcomes in previously untreated non-small cell lung cancer patients: Results of an online tumor registry of clinical trials. *Clin. Cancer Res.* 2009; 15: 5267-73.

[11] Yang J-CH, Schuler M, Yamamoto N, et al. LUX-lung 3: a randomized open- label phase III study of afatinib versus pemetrexed and cisplatin as first-line treatment for patients with advanced adenocarcinoma of the lung harboring EGFR-activating mutations. *J. Clin. Oncol.* 2012: 30 (LBA 7500).

[12] Mitsudomi T, Morita S, Yatabe Y, et al. Gefitnib versus cisplatin plus docetaxel in patients with non-small cell lung cancer harboring mutations of the epidermal growth factor receptor (WJTOG3405): an open label, randomized phase 3 trial. *Lancet Oncol.* 2010; 11: 121–83.

[13] Zhou C, Wu YL, Chen G, et al. Erlotinib versus chemotherapy as first line treatment for patients with advanced EGFR mutation-positive non-small cell lung cancer (OPTIMAL, CTONG-0802): a multicentre, open-label, randomised phase 3 study. *Lancer Oncol.* 2011; 12: 735–42.

[14] Inoue A, Kobayashi K, Maemondo M, et al. Updated overall survival results from a randomized phase III trial comparing gefitinib with carboplatin- paclitaxel for chemo-

naïve non-small cell lung cancer with sensitive EGFR mutations (NEJ002). *Ann. Oncol.* 2013; 24: 54–9.

[15] Paz-Ares L, Soulieres D, Melezinek I, et al. Clinical outcomes in non- small-cell lung cancer patients with EGFR mutations: pooled analysis. *J. Cell Mol. Med.* 2010; 14 (1–2): 51–69.

[16] Massarelli E, Johnson FM, Erickson HS, et al. Uncommon Epidermal Growth Factor Receptor mutations in non-small cell lung cancer and their mechanisms of EGFR tyrosine kinase inhibitors sensitivity and resistance. *Lung Cancer.* 2013; 80 (3): 235-41.

[17] De Pas T, Toffalorio F, Manzotti M, et al. Activity of Epidermal Growth Factor Receptor-Tyrosine Kinase Inhibitors in Patients with Non-small Cell Lung Cancer Harboring Rare Epidermal Growth Factor Receptor Mutations. *J. Thorac. Oncol.* 2011; 6 (11): 1895-901.

[18] Wu JY, Yu CJ, Chang YC, et al. Effectiveness of tyrosine kinase inhibitors on uncommon epidermal growth factor receptor mutations of unknown clinical significance in non-small cell lung cancer. *Clin. Cancer Res.* 2011; 17 (11): 3812-21.

[19] Borget I, Cadranel J, Pignon JP, et al. Cost-effectiveness of three strategies for second-line erlotinib initiation in nonsmall-cell lung cancer: the ERMETIC study part 3. *Eur. Respir. J.* 2012; 39 (1): 172-9.

[20] Yang JJ, Chen HJ, Yan HH, et al. Clinical modes of EGFR tyrosine kinase inhibitor failure and subsequent management in advanced non-small cell lung cancer. *Lung Cancer.* 2013; 79: 33-9.

[21] Marquez-Medina D, Chachoua A, Martin-Marco A, Desai AM, Garcia-Reglero V, Salud-Salvia A, Muggia F. Continued erlotinib maintenance and salvage radiation *Clin. Transl. Oncol.* 2013; 15 (11): 959-64.

[22] Benz MR, Herrmann K, Walter F, et al. 18F-FDG PET/CT for Monitoring Treatment Responses to the Epidermal Growth Factor Receptor Inhibitor Erlotinib. *J. Nucl. Med.* 2011; 52: 1684-9.

[23] Scheffler M, Kobe C, Zander T, et al. Monitoring reversible and irreversible EGFR inhibition with erlotinib and afatinib in a patient with EGFR-mutated non-small cell lung cancer (NSCLC) using sequential [(18)F]fluorothymidine (FLT-)PET. *Lung Cancer.* 2012; 77 (3): 617-20.

[24] Weickhardt AJ, Scheier B, Burke JM, et al. Local ablative therapy of oligoprogressive disease prolongs disease control by tyrosine kinase inhibitors in oncogene-addicted non-small-cell lung cancer. *J. Thorac. Oncol.* 2012; 7 (12): 1807-14.

[25] Yu HA, Sima CS, De la Cruz Drilon AE, et al. Local therapy as a treatment strategy in EGFR-mutant advanced lung cancers that have developed acquired resistance to EGFR tyrosine kinase inhibitors. *J. Clin. Oncol.* 2012; 30 (suppl): 7527.

[26] Brower V. Radiologists urge FDA to accept PET-based tumor response criteria in clinical trials. *J. Natl. Cancer Inst.* 2011; 103: 622-4.

[27] Bengtsson T, Hicks RJ, Peterson A, Port RE. 18F-FDG PET as a Surrogate Biomarker in Non-Small Cell Lung Cancer Treated with Erlotinib: Newly Identified Lesions Are More Informative Than Standardized Uptake Value. *J. Nucl. Med.* 2012; 53 (4): 530-7.

[28] Riely GJ, Kris MG, Zhao B, et al. Prospective assessment of discontinuation and reinitiation of erlotinib or gefitinib in patients with acquired resistance to erlotinib or gefitinib followed by the addition of everolimus. *Clin. Cancer Res.* 2007; 13: 5150-5.

[29] Rosell R, Molina MA, Costa C, et al. Pre-treatment EGFR T790M mutation and BRCA1 mRNA expression in erlotinib-treated advanced non-small-cell lung cancer patients with EGFR mutations. *Clin. Cancer Res.* 2011; 17 (5): 1160-8.

[30] Kobayashi S, Boggon TJ, Dayaram T, et al. EGFR mutation and resistance of non-small-cell lung cancer to gefitinib. *N. Engl. J. Med.* 2005; 352: 786-792.

[31] Pao W, Miller VA, Politi KA, et al. Acquired resistance of lung adenocarcinomas to gefitinib or erlotinib is associated with a second mutation in the EGFR kinase domain. *PLoS Med.* 2005; 2: e73.

[32] Sequist LV, Waltman BA, Dias-Santagata D, et al. Genotypic and histological evolution of lung cancers acquiring resistance to EGFR inhibitors. *Sci. Transl. Med.* 2011; 3: 75ra26.

[33] Arcila ME, Oxnard GR, Nafa K, et al. Rebiopsy of lung cancer patients with acquired resistance to EGFR inhibitors and enhanced detection of the T790M mutation using a locked nucleic acid-based assay. *Clin. Cancer Res.* 2011; 17 (5): 1169–80.

[34] Oxnard GR, Arcila ME, Sima CS et al. Acquired resistance to EGFR tyrosine kinase inhibitor in *EGFR*-mutant lung cancer: distinct natural history of patients with tumors harboring the T790M mutation. *Clin. Cancer Res.* 2011; 17: 1616-22.

[35] Maheswaran S, Sequist LV, Nagrath S, et al. Detection of mutations in EGFR in circulating lung cancer cells. *N. Engl. J. Med.* 2008; 359: 366-77.

[36] Gazdar AF. Activating and resistance mutations of EGFR in non-small-cell lung cancer: Role in clinical response to EGFR tyrosine kinase inhibitors. *Oncogene.* 2009; 28: S24-S31 (suppl 1).

[37] Su KY, Chen HY, Li KC, et al. Pretreatment epidermal growth factor receptor (EGFR) T790M mutation predicts shorter EGFR tyrosine kinase inhibitor response duration in patients with non–small- cell lung cancer. *J. Clin. Oncol.* 2012; 30: 433-40.

[38] Miller VA, Hirsh V, Cadranel J, et al. Afatinib versus placebo for patients with advanced, metastatic non-small-cell lung cancer after failure of erlotinib, gefitinib, or both, and one or two lines of chemotherapy (LUX-Lung 1): A phase 2b/3 ran- domised trial. *Lancet Oncol.* 2012; 13: 528-38.

[39] Chmielecki J, Foo J, Oxnard GR, et al. Optimizing of dosing for *EGFR*-mutant non-small cell lung cancer with evolutionary cancer modelling. *Sci. Transl. Med.* 2011; 3: 90ra59.

[40] Kwak EL, Sordella R, Bell DW, et al. Irreversible inhibitors of the EGF receptor may circumvent acquired resistance to gefitinib. *Proc. Natl. Acad. Sci. U S A.* 2005; 102: 7665-70.

[41] Engelman JA, Zejnullahu K, Gale CM, et al. PF00299804, an irreversible pan-ERBB inhibitor, is effective in lung cancer models with EGFR and ERBB2 mutations that are resistant to gefitinib. *Cancer Res.* 2007; 67: 11924-32.

[42] Sequist LV, Besse B, Lynch TJ, et al. Neratinib, an irreversible pan-ErbB receptor tyrosine kinase inhibitor: results of a phase II trial in patients with advanced non-small-cell lung cancer. *J. Clin. Oncol.* 2010; 28: 3076-83.

[43] Schuler MH, Planchard D, Yang JC, et al. Interim analysis of afatinib monotherapy in patients with metastatic NSCLC progressing after chemotherapy and erlotinib/gefi-tinib (E/G) in a trial of afatinib plus paclitaxel versus investigator's choice chemotherapy following progression on afatinib monotherapy. *J. Clin. oncol.* 2012; 30: abstr 7557.

[44] Hirsch FR, Jänne PA, Eberhardt WE, et al. Epidermal growth factor receptor inhibition in lung cancer. Status 2012. *J. Thoracic. Oncol.* 2013; 8: 373-84.
[45] Nishino M, Cardarella S, Dahlberg SE, et al. Radiographic assessment and therapeutic decisions at RECIST progression in EGFR-mutant NSCLC treated with EGFR tyrosine-kinase inhibitors. *Lung Cancer.* 2013; 79: 283-8.
[46] Asami K, Akuma T, Hirashima T, et al. Continued treatment with gefitinib beyond progressive disease benefits patients with activating EGFR mutations. *Lung Cancer.* 2013; 79: 276-82.
[47] Nishie K, Kawaguchi T, Tamiya A, et al. Epidermal growth *J. Thorac. Oncol.* 2012; 7 (11): 1722-7.
[48] Nishino K, Imamura F, Morita S, Mori M, et al. A retrospective analysis of 335 Japanese lung cancer patients who responded to initial gefitinib treatment. *Lung Cancer.* 2013; 82 (2): 299-304.
[49] Oxnard GR, Lo P, Jackman DM, et al. Delay of chemotherapy through use of post-progression erlotinib in patients with *EGFR*-mutant lung cancer. *J. Clin. Oncol.* 2012; 30 (Abstr 7547).
[50] Faehling M, Eckert R, Kamp T, et al. EGFR tyrosine kinase inhibitor treatment beyond progression in long-term Caucasian responders to erlotinib in advanced non-small cell lung cancer: A case-control study of overall survival. *Lung Cancer.* 2013; 80 (3): 306-12.
[51] Chaft JE, Oxnard GR, Sima CS, Kris MG, Miller VA, Riely GJ. Disease flare after tyrosine kinase inhibitor discontinuation in patients with EGFR-mutant lung cancer and acquired resistance to erlotinib or gefitinib. *Clin. Cancer Res.* 2011; 17 (19): 6298-303.
[52] Eberhard DA, Johnson BE, Amler LC, et al. Mutations in the epidermal growth *J. Clin. Oncol.* 2005; 23 (25): 5900-9.
[53] Hirsch FR, Kabbinavar F, Eisen T, et al. A Randomized, Phase II, Biomarker-Selected Study Comparing Erlotinib to Erlotinib Intercalated With Chemotherapy in First-Line Therapy for Advanced Non-Small-Cell Lung Cancer. *J. Clin. Oncol.* 2011; 29 (26): 3567-73.
[54] Horiike A, Kudo K, Miyauchi E, Ohyanagi F, Kasahara K, Horai T, Nishio M. Phase I study of irinotecan and gefitinib in patients with gefitinib treatment failure for non-small cell lung cancer. *Br. J. Cancer.* 2011; 105 (8): 1131-6.
[55] Takeuchi S, Wang W, Li Q, et al. Dual Inhibition of Met Kinase and Angiogenesis to Overcome HGF-Induced EGFR-TKI Resistance in EGFR Mutant Lung Cancer. *Am. J. Pathol.* 2012; 181 (3): 1034-43.
[56] Iwai T, Moriya Y, Shirane M, et al. Continuous inhibition of epidermal growth factor receptor phosphorylation by erlotinib enhances antitumor activity of chemotherapy in erlotinib-resistant tumor xenografts. *Oncol. Rep.* 2012; 27: 923-8.
[57] Goldberg SB, Oxnard GR, Digumarthy S, et al. Chemotherapy with erlotinib or chemotherapy alone in advanced NSCLC and acquired resistance to EGFR tyrosine kinase inhibitors. *J. Clin. Oncol.* 2012; 30 (Abstr 7524).
[58] Yoshimura N, Okishio K, Mitsuoka S, et al. Prospective assessment of continuation of erlotinib or gefitinib in patients with acquired resistance to erlotinib or gefitinib followed by the addition of pemetrexed. *J. Thorac. Oncol.* 2013; 8: 96-101.

[59] Robinson KW, Sandler AB. The role of MET receptor tyrosine kinase in non-small cell lung cancer and clinical development of targeted anti-MET agents. *The Oncologist.* 2013; 18: 115-22.

[60] Engelman JA, Zejnullahu K, Mitsudomi T, et al. MET amplification leads to gefitinib resistance in lung cancer by activating ERBB3 signalling. Science. 2007; 316: 1039-43.

[61] Bean J, Brennan C, Shih JY, et al. MET amplification occurs with or without T790M mutation in *EGFR*-mutant lung cancer tumors with acquired resistance to gefitinib or erlotinib. *Proc. Natl. Acad. Sci. USA.* 2007; 104: 20932-7.

[62] Shan B, Yao TP, Nguyen HT, et al. requirement of HDAC6 for transforming growth factor-beta-1-induced epithelial-mesenchymal transition. *J. Biol. Chem.* 2008; 283: 21065-73.

[63] Shimizu T, Nakanishi Y, Nakagawa Y, et al. Association between expression of thymidylate synthase, dihidrofolate reductase and glycinamide ribonucleotide formyltransferase and efficacy of pemetrexed in advanced non-small cell lung cancer. *Anticancer Res.* 2012; 32: 4589-96.

[64] Okabe T, Okamoto I, Tsukioka S, et al. Addition of S-1 to the epidermal growth factor receptor inhibitor gefitinib overcomes gefitinib resistance in non-small cell lung cancer cell lines with MET amplification. *Clin. Cancer Res.* 2009; 15: 907-13.

[65] Kanda S, Ohe Y, Horinouchi H, et al. Phase II study of gefitinib and inserted cisplatin plus docetaxel as a first-line treatment for advanced non-small cell lung cancer harboring an epidermal growth factor receptor activating mutation. *J. Clin. Oncol.* 31, 2013 (suppl; abstr 8064).

[66] Leung L, Mok T, Loong H. Combining chemotherapy with epidermal growth factor receptor inhibition in advanced non-small cell lung cancer. *Ther. Adv. Med. Oncol.* 2012; 4 (4): 173–81.

[67] Minami S, Kijima T, Takahashi R, et al. Combination chemotherapy with intermittent erlotinib and pemetrexed for pretreated patients with advanced non-small cell lung cancer: a phase I dose-finding study. *BMC Cancer.* 2012; 12: 296.

[68] Minami S, Kijima T, Hamaguchi M, Nakatani T, et al. Phase II study of pemetrexed plus intermittent erlotinib combination therapy for pretreated advanced non-squamous non-small cell lung cancer with documentation of epidermal growth factor receptor mutation status. *Lung Cancer.* 2013; 82 (2): 271-5.

[69] Aerts JG, Codrington H, Lankheet NA, et al. A randomized phase II study comparing erlotinib versus erlotinib with alternating chemotherapy in relapsed non-small-cell lung cancer patients: the NVALT-10 study. *Ann. Oncol.* 2013; 24 (11): 2860-5.

[70] Yoshimura N, Okishio K, Mitsuoka S, et al. Prospective assessment of continuation of erlotinib or gefitinib in patients with acquired resistance to erlotinib or gefitinib followed by the addition of pemetrexed. *J. Thorac. Oncol.* 2013; 8: 96-101.

[71] Watanabe S, Tanaka J, Ota T, et al. Clinical responses to EGFR-tyrosine kinase inhibitor retreatment in non-small cell lung cancer patients who benefited from prior effective gefitinib therapy: a retrospective analysis. *BMC Cancer.* 2011; 11: 1.

[72] Oh IJ, Ban HJ, Kim KS, Kim YC. Retreatment of gefitinib in patients with non-small-cell lung cancer who previously controlled to gefitinib: A single-arm, open-label, phase II study. *Lung Cancer.* 2012; 77 (1): 121-7.

[73] Oxnard GR, Janjigian YY, Arcila ME, et al. Maintained sensitivity to EGFR tyrosine kinase inhibitors in EGFR-mutant lung cancer recurring after adjuvant erlotinib or gefitinib. *Clin. Cancer Res.* 2011; 17 (19): 6322-8.

[74] Heon S, Nishino M, Goldberg S, et al. Response to EGFR tyrosine kinase inhibitor retreatment after a drug-free interval in EGFR-mutant advanced non-small cell lung cancer with acquired resistance. *J. Clin. Oncol.* 2012, 30 (suppl; abstr 7525).

[75] Lecaer H, Barlesi F, Corre R, et al. A multicentre phase II randomised trial of weekly docetaxel/gemcitabine followed by erlotinib on progression, vs the reverse sequence, in elderly patients with advanced non small-cell lung cancer selected with a comprehensive geriatric assessment (the GFPC 0504 study). *Br. J. Cancer.* 2011; 105 (8): 1123-30.

[76] Duruisseaux M, Baudrin L, Quoix E, et al. Chemotherapy effectiveness after first-line gefitinib treatment for advanced lepidic predominant adenocarcinoma (formerly advanced bronchioloalveolar carcinoma): exploratory analysis of the IFCT-0401 trial. *J. Thorac. Oncol.* 2012; 7 (9): 1423-31.

[77] Wu JY, Shih JY, Yang CH, et al. Second-line treatments after first-line gefitinib therapy in advanced nonsmall cell lung cancer. *Int. J. Cancer.* 2010; 126: 247-55.

[78] Becker A, Crombag L, Heideman DA, et al. Retreatment with erlotinib: Regain of TKI sensitivity following a drug holiday for patients with NSCLC who initially responded to EGFR-TKI treatment. *Eur. J. Cancer.* 2011; 47: 2603-6.

[79] Chmielecki J, Pietanza MC, Aftab D, et al. EGFR-mutant lung adenocarcinomas treated first-line with the novel EGFR inhibitor, XL647, can subsequently retain moderate sensitivity to erlotinib. *J. Thorac. Oncol.* 2012. 7: 434-42.

[80] Hata A, Katakami N, Yoshioka H, et al. Erlotinib after gefitinib failure in relapsed non-small cell lung cancer: Clinical benefit with optimal patient selection. *Lung Cancer.* 2011; 74 (2): 268-73.

[81] Vasile E, Tibaldi C, Chella A, et al. Erlotinib after failure of gefitinib in patients with advanced non-small cell lung cancer previously responding to gefitinib. *J. Thorac. Oncol.* 2008; 3: 912-4.

[82] Koyama N, Uchida Y. Clinical Significance of Erlotinib Monotherapy for Gefitinib-resistant Non-small Cell Lung Cancer with EGFR Mutations. *Anticancer Res.* 2013; 33: 5083-9.

[83] Kaira K, Naito T, Takahashi T, et al. Pooled analysis of the reports of erlotinib after failure if gefitinib for non-small cell lung cancer. *Lung Cancer.* 2010; 68: 99-104.

[84] Ohashi K, Maruvka YE, Michor F, Pao W. Epidermal growth *J. Clin. Oncol.* 2013; 31 (8): 1070-80.

[85] Costa DB, Nguyen KS, Cho BC, et al. Effects of erlotinib in EGFR mutated non-small cell lung cancers with resistance to gefitinib. *Clin. Cancer Res.* 2008; 14: 7060-7.

[86] Lee DH, Kim SW, Suh C, et al. Phase II study of erlotinib as a salvage treatment for non-small-cell lung cancer patients after failure of gefitinib treatment. *Ann. Oncol.* 2008; 19 (12): 2039-42.

[87] Grossi F, Rijavec E, Dal Bello MG, et al. The administration of gefitinib in patients with advanced non-small-cell lung cancer after the failure of erlotinib. *Cancer Chemother. Pharmacol.* 2012; 69 (6): 1407-12.

[88] TANG C, Gao H, Li X, et al. Different treatment orders achieved similar clinical results: a retrospective study for retreatment of epidermal growth factor receptor

tyrosine kinase inhibitors in 120 patients with non-small-cell lung cancer. *J. Cancer Res. Clin. Oncol.* 2014.

[89] Li D, Ambrogio L, Shimamura T, et al.: BIBW2992, an irreversible EGFR/HER2 inhibitor highly effective in preclinical lung cancer models. *Oncogene.* 2008; 27: 4702-11.

[90] Sequist LV, Yang J, Yamamoto N, et al. Phase III Study of Afatinib or Cisplatin Plus Pemetrexed in Patients With Metastatic Lung Adenocarcinoma With Epidermal Growth Factor Receptor Mutations. *J. Clin. Oncol.* 2013.

[91] Solca F, Dahl C, Zoephel A, et al.: Target binding properties and cellular activity of afatinib (BIBW 2992), an irreversible ErbB family blocker. *J. Pharmacol. Exp. Ther.* 2012; 343: 342-50.

[92] Bean J, Riely GJ, Balak M, Marks JL, Ladanyi M, Miller VA, Pao W. Acquired resistance to epidermal growth factor receptor kinase inhibitors associated with a novel T854A mutation in a patient with EGFR-mutant lung adenocarcinoma. *Clin. Cancer. Res.* 2008; 14 (22): 7519-25.

[93] Ninomiya T, Takigawa N, Ichihara E, et al. Afatinib prolongs survival compared with gefitinib in an epidermal growth factor receptor-driven lung cancer model. *Mol. Cancer Ther.* 2013; 12 (5): 589-97.

[94] Mazieres J, Peters S, Lepage B, et al. Lung Cancer That Harbors an HER2 Mutation: Epidemiologic Characteristics and Therapeutic Perspectives. *J. Clin. Oncol.* 2013; 31 (16): 1997-2003.

[95] Yang JC, Hirsh V, Schuler M, et al. Symptom control and quality of life in LUX-Lung 3: A phase III study of afatinib or cisplatin/pemetrexed in patients with advanced lung adenocarcinoma with EGFR mutations. *J. Clin. oncol.* 2013; 31 (27): 3342-50.

[96] Murakami H, Tamura T, Takahashi T, et al. Phase I study of continuous afatinib (BIBW 2992) in patients with advanced non-small cell lung cancer after prior chemotherapy/erlotinib/gefitinib (LUX-Lung 4). *Cancer Chemother. pharmacol.* 2012; 69 (4): 891-9.

[97] Katakami N, Atagi S, Goto K, et al. LUX-Lung 4: A phase II trial of afatinib in patients with advanced non-small-cell lung cancer who progressed during prior treatment with erlotinib, gefitinib, or both. *J. Clin. oncol.* 2013; 31 (27): 3335-41.

[98] Yang JC, Shih JY, Su WC, et al.: Afatinib for patients with lung adenocarcinoma and epidermal growth factor receptor mutations (LUX-Lung 2): A phase 2 trial. *Lancet Oncol.* 2012; 13: 539-48.

[99] Yang JC, Shih JY, Su WC, et al. Afatinib for patients with lung adenocarcinoma and epidermal growth factor receptor mutations (LUX-Lung 2): a phase 2 trial. *Lancet oncol.* 2012; 13 (5): 539-48.

[100] Wu YL, Zhou C, Hu CP, et al. LUX-Lung 6: A randomized, open-label, phase III study of afatinib (A) versus gemcitabine/cisplatin (GC) as first-line treatment for Asian patients (pts) with EGFR mutation-positive (EGFR M+) advanced adenocarcinoma of the lung. *J. Clin. Oncol.* 2013; 31: abstr. 8016.

[101] Yang JC, Sequist LV, Geater SL, et al. Activity of afatinib in uncommon epidermal growth factor receptor (EGFR) mutations: Finding from three trials of afatinib in EGFR mutation-positive lung cancer. 15th World Conference on Lung Cancer. Sydney, 2013.

[102] Awada AH, Dumez H, Hendlisz A, et al. Phase I study of pulsatile 3-day administration of afatinib (BIBW 2992) in combination with docetaxel in advanced solid tumors. Invest new Drugs 2013; 31 (3): 734-41.

[103] Chu QS, Sangha RS, Hotte SJ, et al. A phase I, dose-escalation trial of continuous and pulsed-dose afatinib (A) combined with pemetrexed (P) in patients (pts) with advanced solid tumors: Final analysis. *J. Clin. Oncol.* 2013; 31: abstr 2523.

[104] Ramalingam SS, Blackhall F, Krzakowski M, et al. Randomized phase II study of dacomitinib (PF-00299804), an irreversible pan-human epidermal growth factor receptor inhibitor, versus erlotinib in patients with advanced non- small-cell lung cancer. *J. Clin. oncol.* 2012; 30 (27): 3337-44.

[105] Sun, Zheng Y. Retreatment with icotinib in a patient with metastatic lung adenocarcinoma. *Tumori.* 2013; 99 (3): 124e-6e.

[106] Carillio G, Montanino A, Costanzo R, et al. Cetuximab in non-small-cell lung cancer *Expert. Rev. Anticancer. Ther.* 2012; 12 (2): 163-75.

[107] Neal JW, Heist RS, Fidias P, et al. Cetuximab Monotherapy in Patients with Advanced Non-small Cell Lung Cancer After Prior Epidermal Growth Factor Receptor Tyrosine Kinase Inhibitor Therapy. *J. Thorac. Oncol.* 2010; 5: 1855-8.

[108] Wang M, Zhao J, Zhang LM, et al. Combined Erlotinib and Cetuximab overcome the acquired resistance to epidermal growth factor receptors tyrosine kinase inhibitor in non-small-cell lung cancer. *J. Cancer Res. Clin. Oncol.* 2012; 138 (12): 2069-77.

[109] Janjigian YY, Azzoli CG, Krug LM, et al. Phase I/II of cetuximab and erlotinib in patients with lung adenocarcinoma and acquired resistance to erlotinib. *Clin. Cancer Res.* 2011; 17: 2521-7.

[110] Regales L, Gong Y Shen R, et al. Dual targeting of EGFR can overcome a major drug resistance in mouse model of *EGFR*-mutant lung cancer. *J. Clin. Invest.* 2009; 119: 3000-10.

[111] Wang M, Zhao J, Zhang LM, et al. Combined erlotinib and cetuximab overcome the acquired resistance to epidermal growth factor receptos tyrosine kinase inhibitor in non-small-cell lung cancer. *J. Cancer Res. Clin. Oncol.* 2012; 138: 2069-77.

[112] Janjigian YY, Groen HJ, Horn L, et al. Activity and tolerability of afatinib (BIBW 2992) and cetuximab in NSCLC patients with acquired resistance to erlotinib or gefitinib. *J. Clin. Oncol.* 2011; 29 (suppl); abstr. 7525.

[113] Janjigian YY, Smit EF, Horn L, et al. Activity of afatinib / cetuximab in patients with EGFR-mutant non-small cell lung cancer and acquired resistance to EGFR inhibitors. ESMO 2012 (abstract 12270).

[114] De Greve J, Teugels E, Geers C, et al. Clinical activity of afatinib (BIBW 2992) in patients with lung adenocarcinoma with mutations in the kinase domain of HER2/neu. *Lung Cancer.* 2012; 76: 123-7.

[115] Takezawa K, Pirazzoli V, Arcila ME, et al. HER2 amplification: a potential mechanism of acquired resistance to EGFR inhibitor in *EGFR*-mutant lung cancers that lack the second-site EGFRT790M mutation. *Cancer Discover.* 2012; 2: 922-33.

[116] Leighl NB, Raez LE, Besse B, et al. A multicenter, phase 2 study of vascular endothelial growth factor trap Aflibercept) in platinum- and erlotinib-resistant adenocarcinoma of the lung. *J. Thorac. Oncol.* 2010; 5: 1054-9.

[117] Cappuzzo F, Jänne PA, Skokan M, et al. MET increased gene copy number and primary resistance to gefitinib therapy in non-small-cell lung cancer patients. *Ann Oncol.* 2009; 20 (2): 298-304.
[118] Gow CH, Chang YL, Hsu YC, et al. Comparison of epidermal growth factor receptor mutations between primary and corresponding metastatic tumors in tyrosine kinase inhibitor-naive non-small-cell lung cancer. *Ann. Oncol.* 2009; 20 (4): 696-702.
[119] Kalikaki A, Koutsopoulos A, Trypaki M, et al. Comparison of EGFR and K-RAS gene status between primary tumours and corresponding metastases in NSCLC. *Br. J. Cancer. 2008*; 99 (6): 923-9.
[120] Bozzetti C, Tiseo M, Lagrasta C, et al. Comparison between epidermal growth factor receptor (EGFR) gene expression in primary non-small cell lung cancer (NSCLC) and in fine-needle aspirates from distant metastatic sites. *J. Thorac. Oncol.* 2008; 3 (1): 18-22.
[121] Salah S, Tanvetyanon T, Abbasi S. Metastatectomy for extra-cranial extra-adrenal non-small cell lung cancer solitary metastases: Systematic review and analysis of reported cases. *Lung Cancer.* 2012; 75 (1): 9-14.
[122] Omuro AM, Kris MG, Miller VA, et al. High incidence of disease recurrence in the brain and leptomeninges in patients with non-small cell lung carcinoma after response to gefitinib. *Cancer* 2005; 103: 2344-8.
[123] Heon S, Yeap BY, Britt GJ, et al. Development of Central Nervous System Metastases in Patients with Advanced Non-Small Cell Lung Cancer and Somatic EGFR Mutations Treated with Gefitinib or Erlotinib. *Clin. Cancer Res.* 2010; 16 (23): 5873-82.
[124] Porta R, Massuti B, Paz-Ares L, et al. Brain metastases from lung cancer responding to erlotinib: the importance of EGFR mutation. *Eur. Respir. J.* 2011; 37 (3): 624-31.
[125] Grommes C, Oxnard GR, Kris MG, et al. Pulsatile high-dose weekly erlotinib for CNS metastases from EGFR mutant non-small cell lung cancer. *Neuro Oncol.* 2011; 13: 1364-9.
[126] Zhao J, Chen M, Zhong W, et al. Cerebroespinal fluid concentrations of gefitinib in patients with lung adenocarcinoma. *Clin. Lung Cancer.* 2013; 14: 188-93.
[127] Togashi Y, Masago K, Fukudo M, et al. efficacy of increased-dose erlotinib for central nervous system metastases in non-small cell lung cancer patients with epidermal growth factor receptor mutation. *Cancer Chemother. Pharmacol.* 2011; 68: 1089-2.
[128] Jamal-Hanjani M, Spicer J. Epidermal growth factor receptor tyrosine kinase inhibitors in the treatment of epidermal growth factor receptor-mutant non-small cell lung cancer metastatic to the brain. *Clin. Cancer Res.* 2012; 18: 938-44.
[129] Park SJ, Kim HT, Lee DH, et al. Efficacy of epidermal growth factor receptor tyrosine kinase inhibitors for brain metastasis in non-small cell lung cancer patients harboring either exon 19 or 21 mutation. *Lung Cancer.* 2012; 77 (3): 556-60.
[130] Hata A, Ktakami N, Yoshioka H, et al. Rebiopsy of non-small cell lung cancer patients with acquired resistance to EGFR-TKI: Comparison between T790M mutation-positive nad –negative populations. *J. Clin. Oncol.* 2012; 30: 487s (suppl) abstr. 7528.
[131] Welsh JW, Komaki R, Amini A, et al. Phase II trial of erlotinib plus concurrent whole-brain radiation therapy for patients with brain metastases from non-small-cell lung cancer. *J. Clin. Oncol.* 2013; 31: 895-2.

[132] Liu M, Jiang G, He W, Zhang P, Song N. Surgical resection of locally advanced pulmonary adenocarcinoma after gefitinib therapy. *Ann. Thorac. Surg*. 2011; 92: e11-2.

In: Fighting Lung Cancer through the HER Family ...
Editor: Diego Márquez-Medina
ISBN: 978-1-63321-092-9

Chapter 15

Other Malignancies I. Breast Cancer

***E. Aguirre, M.D.*[1]*, S. Morales, M.D.*[1] *and A. Llombart, M.D., Ph.D.*[2]**

[1]Medical Oncology Department, Arnau de Vilanova University, Hospital of Lleida, Spain

[2]Medical Oncology Department, Arnau de Vilanova University, Hospital of Valencia, Spain

Abstract

The Human Epidermal Growth Factor Receptor 2 (HER2) is overexpressed and/or amplified in 17-23% of female breast cancers, and it is associated with a decreased disease-free and overall survival. The development of monoclonal antibodies as well as small tyrosine kinase inhibitors against the outer and inner portions of the cell membrane growth factor receptors, in particular of the HER family, has been one of the most successful strategies in the era of targeted therapies. The combination of some of these agents with chemotherapy has demonstrated a remarkable activity, being able to modify the natural course of HER2-positive breast cancer phenotype. Unfortunately, not all HER2-positive tumors benefit from targeted agents, and almost all the patients with advanced disease eventually became resistant. Several mechanisms of resistance to anti-HER2 agents have been explored. Preclinical and clinical experiences confirm that the combination of targeted agents with different mechanism of action results in a more comprehensive blockade that may lead to dramatic gains in survival. At present, the dual blockade is a standard therapeutic option in advanced disease, and it is being intensively explored in early stages.

1. Introduction

The human epidermal growth factor receptor (HER) family includes four receptors: The epidermal growth factor receptor (EGFR) or HER1, and the HER2, HER3 and HER4 receptors. All those receptors are composed of an extracellular ligand-binding domain, a transmembrane domain, and an intracellular tyrosine kinase domain (with the exception of

HER3), and they are involved in the regulation of proliferation and survival of epithelial cells. Several ligands have been recognized to bind HER1, HER3 and HER4, but no ligand for HER2 has been identified. The evidence suggests that HER2 is the preferred dimerization partner for the activation of any other HER receptors. Homo- or heterodimerization of HER results in the phosphorylation of some residues in the intracellular domain of the receptor, the recruitment of signaling molecules from the cytoplasm, and the subsequent activation of different signaling pathways that lead to growth, differentiation, migration, adhesion, apoptosis and angiogenesis processes [1].

HER2 is overexpressed and/or amplified in 17-23% of breast cancers, and it has been associated with a worse disease-free (DFS) and overall survival (OS) [2]. HER2-overexpression has been also associated with an increased risk of central nervous system (CNS) metastases [3-5].

The HER2-overexpression is detected by standardized immunochemistry (IHC) 3+, and the *HER2*-amplification is detected by fluorescent in situ hybridization. Both two predict a clinical benefit from anti-HER2 drugs [6-7].

2. Trastuzumab

Trastuzumab (Herceptin®) is a recombinant, monoclonal IgG1-class humanized murine antibody directed against HER2 [8]. Trastuzumab is able to generate different mechanisms of antitumor activity: activation of antibody-dependent cellular cytotoxicity, blockage of proteolytic cleavage of the HER2 extracellular domain, inhibition of intracellular signal transduction, inhibition of tumor-induced angiogenesis, or inhibition of DNA repair mechanisms have been identified [9].

2.1. Trastuzumab in Metastatic Breast Cancer

a) Single Agent

Trastuzumab is moderately active in *HER2*-positive metastatic breast cancer (MBC) patients; with response rate (RR) ranging from 15 to 26%, clinical benefit (CBR) ranging from 36% to 48%, and a median duration of response of 9 months. I

b) Combination with Chemotherapy

The registration study by Slamon et al. [10] randomized 469 women with *HER2*-positive (defined as either IHC 2+ or 3+) MBC to receive a first-line treatment chemotherapy regimen (doxorubicin plus cyclophosphamide or paclitaxel) with or without trastuzumab. The addition of trastuzumab significantly increased the RR (32% versus 50%), the median duration of response (6 months versus 9 months), and the OS (20 months versus 25 months). The OS gain is remarkable as 65% of patients receiving chemotherapy alone were eventually crossed over to trastuzumab. The combination of anthracycline and trastuzumab was associated with an unacceptable rate of cardiac toxicity and the combination of trastuzumab with anthracyclines is currently not recommended in the clinical practice Accordingly to this data, the US Food and Drug Administration (FDA) approved trastuzumab for the treatment of

HER2-positive MBC in 1998. Two subsequent studies evaluating the addition of trastuzumab to first-line chemotherapy with docetaxel and paclitaxel, respectively [11, 12], confirmed the efficacy of the taxane/trastuzumab combination in *HER2*-positive patients (IHC3+). Since then, this combination has been considered the standard of care and the control arm for subsequent clinical trials in *HER2*-positive MBC.

The activity of trastuzumab in combination with capecitabine [13-15], gemcitabine [16], platinum salts [17], or vinorelbine [18] has been confirmed in multiple phase II-III studies. In the TRAVIOTA study, 81 *HER2*-positive MBC patients were randomly to receive trastuzumab plus weekly vinorelbine or taxane therapy. The efficacy of both regimens was similar, although safety differences in favor of vinorelbine were observed. Most recently, the phase III HERNATA trial [19] compared docetaxel plus trastuzumab versus vinorelbine plus trastuzumab as first line therapy for 284 MBC. There were no significant differences in RR (59.3% in both groups), time to progression (TTP) (12 months versus 15 months; HR 0.94; p= 0.67), or OS. However, more patients in the docetaxel arm discontinued therapy due to toxicity (p< 0.001). The authors concluded that vinorelbine plus trastuzumab might be considered as an alternative standard regimen in the first line setting [20].

c) Combinations with Endocrine Therapy

Different studies confirm a significant inverse correlation between the HER2 and the estrogen receptor expression [21]. Preclinical studies suggest an interaction between these two pathways and, moreover, a higher HER2 expression has been associated with the resistance to tamoxifen. Two clinical trials explored the activity of trastuzumab in combination with hormonotherapy as a first line treatment for ER-positive, HER2-positive MBC. In the TAnDEM study [22], trastuzumab plus anastrozole was superior to single agent anastrozole in tems of PFS (5 months versus 2 months), and RR (20% versus 7%). In addition, the eLEcTRA study [23] comparing trastuzumab plus letrozole versus letrozole reported an increased median PFS (14 months versus 3 months), and RR (27% versus 13%) for the combination arm.

d) Timing and Duration of Trastuzumab Therapy

The optimal timing and duration of trastuzumab treatment have been addressed in several studies. Two phase III trials [24, 25] explored the convenience of the combination or sequencing strategies with chemotherapy and trastuzumab in the first line. Although one trial did not find any difference in PFS, the second one was prematurely stopped when the interim analysis showed a dramatic increase in PFS (4 months versus 15 months; HR 4.24; p< 0.01), and OS (HR 2.72; p= 0.04) in favor of the combination arm instead of delaying trastuzumab therapy.

Reintroducing trastuzumab on progression to trastuzumab is a reasonable, effective, and safe approach that was initially supported by retrospective series [26]. In a phase III study [27], 156 *HER2*-positive MBCs progressing to first line trastuzumab-containing treatment were randomized to receive second line capecitabine with or without trastuzumab. The maintenance of trastuzumab plus capecitabine was superior in terms of RR (48% versus 27%; p= 0.012), PFS (8 months versus 6 months; HR 0.69; p= 0.034), and a trend to improve the OS (26 months versus 20 months; HR 0.76; p= 0.26) [28].

Several studies have reported an increased risk of CNS metastases [5, 29, 30] in trastuzumab-treated patients. However, this phenomenon seems to be more related to a higher risk of CNS metastases for *HER2* positive patients [3, 4] as well as to the prolonged survival [29] of trastuzumab-treated patients.

Data from institutional series comparing the outcome of women treated in the pre-trastuzumab and the post-trastuzumab era indicate that trastuzumab has changed the natural history of *HER2*-positive MBC with an important gain in OS [20].

2.2. Trastuzumab in Early Stage Breast Cancer

a) The Neoadjuvant Setting

The addition of trastuzumab to conventional chemotherapy significantly increases the rate of pathological complete response (pCR), reduces the risk of recurrence, and improves the OS in the neoadjuvant setting [31]. In single-arm phase II studies, the rate of pCR to neoadjuvant trastuzumab ranged from 12-76%. Four randomized phase II and III clinical trials [32-35] have investigated the addition of trastuzumab to neoadjuvant chemotherapy, reporting an increase in the pCR rate (26-65% versus 19-27%) for trastuzumab independently of the chemotherapy regimen used.

In the NeOAdjuvant Herceptin study [36], 228 patients with *HER2*-positive locally advanced breast cancer were randomized to receive sequential anthracycline–taxane-based chemotherapy with or without trastuzumab. The addition of trastuzumab led to increase the pCR rate from 22% to 43% (p= 0.0007). Similar results were communicated in the phase III GeparQuattro study [37], in which the combination of trastuzumab and sequential anthracycline–taxane chemotherapy increased the pCR rate from 16% to 32%.

A vast investigation program for metastatic and early HER2-positive breast cancer is ongoing including combinations of trastuzumab with other anti-EGFR therapies [38-42].

b) The Adjuvant Setting

In the adjuvant setting [29], several independent randomized studies have demonstrated that the addition of trastuzumab to chemotherapy improves the DFS by 38% and the OS by 34%, and substantially reduces the risk of local and distant recurrence by 42% and 40%, respectively.

Accordingly, the FDA approved trastuzumab in combination with standard chemotherapy for the adjuvant setting in 2006. The standard duration of adjuvant trastuzumab therapy is 1 year [43]. Neither shorter treatments (six months) nor extended therapies (two years) have achieved better results than the conventional one-year treatment.

Trastuzumab is a well-tolerated drug, although it has been associated with a small but significant increase in the risk of symptomatic cardiac failure (up to 4% at 4 years), particularly in patients that were previously treated with anthracycline-based chemotherapy [36].

Asymptomatic reductions in the left ventricular ejection fraction are relatively common [44] and require the trastuzumab discontinuation in 8-10% of patients. The final underlying mechanism of trastuzumab-related cardiotoxicity has not been fully cleared, and mechanisms involving the expression of HER2 on cardiac myocytes during embryogenesis have been proposed [45]. Contrarily to the anthracicline one, the trastuzumab-related cardiotoxicity uses to be less severe and readily reversible [46].

3. Pertuzumab

Pertuzumab (Perjeta®) is a monoclonal antibody that binds to subdomain II of the HER2 extracellular domain and prevents HER2 from dimerizing with other ligand-activated HER2 receptors, mostly HER3 [47]. As trastuzumab, pertuzumab stimulates antibody-dependent, cell-mediated cytotoxicity [48].

In preclinical studies, the combination of pertuzumab and trastuzumab had synergistic antitumor activity in *HER2*-positive breast cancer xenograft models, even after progression to trastuzumab [48].

In a study with 29 *HER2*-positive MBC progressing on trastuzumab-based therapy, single-agent pertuzumab showed a modest activity (RR 3.4%, and CBR 10.3%). Subsequently, Trastuzumab was added to pertuzumab at disease progression in 17 patients, yielding an overall RR of 17.6% and a CBR of 41.2%. Furthermore, a longer PFS was registered in those patients receiving the combined treatment than in those receiving pertuzumab alone (17 weeks versus 7 weeks), suggesting that the pertuzumab monotherapy has a modest activity that improved with the dual blockade [49].

The dual combination was assessed by Baselga et al. [50] in 66 *HER2* positive MBC patients progressing to a prior trastuzumab-based therapy. The regimen was active and obtained 24% RR, and 50% CBR, with a median PFS of 5.5 months. The combination of anti-HER2 therapies was generally well tolerated. The most common adverse event was diarrhea in 64% patients, and the risk of cardiotoxicity did not increase [27, 51, 52].

These encouraging results led to the launch of the CLinical Evaluation Of Pertuzumab And TRAstuzumab (CLEOPATRA) trial [53]. In this is phase III trial, 808 *HER2*-positive MBC were randomized to receive placebo plus trastuzumab plus docetaxel (control group) or pertuzumab plus trastuzumab plus docetaxel (pertuzumab group) as a first line therapy. Prior trastuzumab in the adjuvant or neoadjuvant setting was permitted if disease-free interval was longer than 12 months.

Primary endpoint was achieved reporting a median PFS of 12.4 months in the control group versus 18.5 months in the pertuzumab group (HR 0.62; 95 % CI 0.51-0.75; p< 0.001). With a median follow-up of 30 months and 267 registered events, the median OS (37.6 months versus not reached; HR 0.66, 95% CI 0.52-0.84; p= 0.0008) was higher in the pertuzumab group and did not increase the rate of heart dysfunction. The benefit was similar in previously trastuzumab-treated and trastuzumab naïve patients. The FDA approved the combination of pertuzumab plus trastuzumab plus docetaxel for the first line treatment of *HER2*-positive MBC in 2012.

A vast clinical research program is currently exploring the dual blockage of trastuzumab and pertuzumab in the metastatic and early stage breast cancer settings. Two neoadjuvant phase II trials (NeoSphere and TRYPHAENA) explored the combination of Pertuzumab and trastuzumab with or without chemotherapy.

The four-arm randomized phase II NeoSphere study [42], randomized 417 patients to receive the combination of pertuzumab and trastuzumab with or without docetaxel, and single-agent trastuzumab or pertuzumab in combination with docetaxel during 12 weeks prior to surgery as a neoadjuvant treatment. The patients also received four cycles of anthracycline-based chemotherapy after surgery. The pCR rate was significantly higher in the pertuzumab plus trastuzumab plus docetaxel arm than in the trastuzumab plus docetaxel, pertuzumab plus docetaxel, and pertuzumab plus trastuzumab arms (45.8% versus 29% versus 24% versus 16.8%, respectively). The presence of 17% pCR in the trastuzumab plus pertuzumab arm clearly suggested the existence of a subset of patients where chemotherapy could be avoided.

The TRYPHAENA trial randomized 225 *HER2*-positive stage II and III breast cancers to receive concurrent or sequential pertuzumab-trastuzumab with an anthracycline or non-anthracycline containing regimen. The pCR rate was similar across the three arms of the study (57 to 66%) [54].

Moreover, five randomized neoadjuvant trials [38-42] have compared other anti-HER2 targeted agents alone or combined with trastuzumab. he presence of 17% pCR in the trastuzumab plus pertuzumab arm clearly suggested the existence of a subset of patients where chemotherapy could be avoided.

4. Trastuzumab-DM1

Antibody-toxin conjugates have been developed in order to increase the potency of antibody-directed therapy, and the fungal toxin maytansine DM1 has been linked to anti-HER2 antibodies.

In a phase II study, trastuzumab-DM1 (T-DM1) showed robust activity [55] in 112 heavily pretreated trastuzumab-resistant *HER2*-positive MBC, recording an objective RR of almost 26% and a median PFS of 4.6 months. Another phase II study in heavily pretreated MBC, T-DM1 showed an overall RR of 33%, and a CBR of 48%, with a median PFS of 7 months [56].

A randomized phase II trial in the first line setting [57] compared trastuzumab-DM1 versus trastuzumab plus docetaxel in 137 *HER2*-positive MBC patients. The RR was similar in both arms (64% versus 58%), although the PFS was significantly longer in the T-DM1 group (14 months versus 9 months; HR 0.59; p= 0.035). The trastuzumab-docetaxel group was associated with more grade III or higher adverse events (89.4% versus 46.4%).

Results from the phase III EMILIA trial has been recently published. This study randomized 978 *HER2*-positive MBC patients to receive T-DM1 monotherapy or the combination of capecitabine plus lapatinib in patients progressing to trastuzumab [58]. T-DM1 was well tolerated and significantly improved both the PFS (10 months versus 6 months; HR 0.65, 95% CI 0.55-0.77; p< 0.0001) and the OS (not reached versus 23 months; HR 0.62, 95% CI 0.48-0.81; p= 0.0005) [59].

The most common grade 3/4 adverse events for T-DM1 were thrombocytopenia (12.9%), increased AST (4.3%), and increased ALT (2.9%). The TH3RESA trial, evaluating the efficacy of T-DM1 beyond the second line of treatment has recently shown similar benefit rates in terms of PFS and OS.

A phase Ib/II trial explored the combination of T-DM1 and pertuzumab in trastuzumab-treated *HER2*-positive MBC [60] and reported a RR of 41% and 42% in first and second line of treatment, respectively, without any substantial increment of toxicity.

Different clinical trials are currently evaluating T-DM1 in the adjuvant, neoadjuvant, and metastatic setting. The MARIANNE trial will assess the safety and tolerability of T-DM1 in combination with pertuzumab or placebo versus trastuzumab plus docetaxel in the first line of treatment.

5. Lapatinib

Lapatinib (Tyverb®) is a dual and reversible tyrosine kinase inhibitor of both HER1 and HER2. A phase II study [61] explored the efficacy of lapatinib as first-line therapy for patients with *HER2*-positive MBC and reported a RR of 24%. Other phase II trial treating 100 *HER2*-positive MBC (after prior anthracycline, taxane and trastuzumab therapy) with lapatinib monotherapy reported a RR of 19% [62]. In contrast, a very low clinical activity of lapatinib (RR <2%) was reported in other phase II trial including 140 *HER2*-positive heavily pretreated MBC patients [63].

The combination of lapatinib and capecitabine [64, 65] has been compared with capecitabine alone in a phase III study including 321 heavily pretreated (anthracycline, taxane, and trastuzumab) *HER2* positive MBC. The median PFS (8.4 months versus 4.4 months) and OS (75 weeks versus 64.7 weeks) were higher in the combination arm, with no worsening in the toxic and cardiac profile. The most common adverse events in the combination arm were diarrhea (60%), hand foot syndrome (49%), rash (27%), nausea (44%), vomiting (26%), and fatigue (18%). The benefit on PFS by adding lapatinib to capecitabine seems similar to the benefit of continuing trastuzumab in combination with capecitabine.

Lapatinib has been combined with paclitaxel in a second phase III study [66] randomizing patients with MBC to receive triweekly paclitaxel with or without lapatinib. In the subgroup of 86 *HER2* positive patients, the addition of lapatinib was associated with a longer TTP (36.4 weeks versus 25.1 weeks; HR 0.53, 95% CI 0.31-0.89; p= 0.005).

A phase III study comparing letrozole plus lapatinib versus letrozole [67, 68] in 219 patients with ER-positive *HER2*-positive MBC has shown that the addition of lapatinib increased the median PFS (8 months versus 3 months) and the CBR (48% versus 29%). suboptimal dose of fulvestrant.

Lapatinib, as a small molecule, easily cross the blood-brain barrier and achieves therapeutic concentrations in CNS that may provide a clinical benefit for patients with CNS metastases. The phase II LANDSCAPE study [69] treated 43 *HER2* positive patients with CNS metastases with lapatinib plus capecitabine before the whole-brain radiotherapy. The CNS RR was 67%, and the median TTP was 6 months.

The combination of trastuzumab and lapatinib has been explored in a phase I study [70] including 50 trastuzumab-progressing *HER2*-positive MBC, and provided an encouraging clinical activity. A phase II study [71] of trastuzumab and lapatinib reported a RR of 42% and 25%, and a CBR of 47% and 40% in the first and second-third line of treatment, respectively. A phase III study comparing trastuzumab and lapatinib with lapatinib alone in 296 heavily pretreated trastuzumab-progressing MBC patients [51] demonstrated a synergistic effect between both compounds. The CBR (25% versus 12%; p= 0.01), the PFS (12 weeks versus 8 weeks; HR 0.73, 95% CI 0.57-0.93; p= 0.008), and the OS (HR 0.65, 95% CI 0.46-0.94; p= 0.009) were higher in the combination arm, and provided a survival benefit of 4.5 months [72].

Lapatinib in combination with capecitabine was FDA-approved for *HER2*-positive MBC previously exposed to an anthracycline, a taxane, and trastuzumab in 2007. Subsequently, in 2010, the FDA granted approval to lapatinib plus letrozole for the treatment of postmenopausal women with hormone receptor-positive *HER2*-positive tumors.

A vast investigation program for metastatic and early HER2-positive breast cancer is ongoing. Five randomized neoadjuvant trials have compared lapatinib with or without trastuzumab versus trastuzumab-containing regimens [38-42]. In the NeoALTTO trial, 450 patients were randomized to receive paclitaxel with lapatinib, trastuzumab, or the combination of them as a neoadjuvant therapy. The breast and axilla pCR rate was significantly higher in the combination arm than in the trastuzumab arm (46.8% versus 27.6%; p= 0.0007). However, no significant differences were observed between the lapatinib and the trastuzumab arm (20% versus 27.6%). Almost a third of the patients from the lapatinib arm did not complete the therapy due to diarrhea and/or liver enzyme alterations. The GeparQuintto study evaluated the value of adding trastuzumab or lapatinib to anthracycline-/taxane-based chemotherapy. The pCR rate was higher in the trastuzumab arm (30.3% versus 22.7%; OR 0.68; p= 0.04). Dose reductions were more common in the lapatinib arm. Two smaller neoadjuvant studies have compared different combinations of trastuzumab, lapatinib or both with conventional chemotherapy. Holmes et al. [40] reported high pCR rates in the trastuzumab, lapatinib, and combined arms (54% versus 45% versus 74%, respectively), that decreased to 25% versus 26% versus 47%, respectively in the CHER-LOB study [41].

6. Neratinib

Neratinib (HKI-272), an orally administered small molecule, is an irreversible panHER tyrosine kinase inhibitor. In the BT474 cell line, Neratinib repressed the phosphorylation of the mitogen activated protein kinase and the serine-threonine kinase signal pathways, whereas trastuzumab failed to inhibit the HER2 phosphorylation and downstream signaling. In tumor xenografts overexpressing HER2, neratinib has been reported to reduce the tumor growth in a dose-dependent manner [73].

A phase II trial explored the neratinib monotherapy in 136 MBC patients. Twenty four per cent of trastuzumab-treated patients and 56% of the trastuzumab naïve ones responded to neratinib with a PFS of 22 and 39 weeks, respectively [74].

A phase I/II study treated 22 previously trastuzumab and taxane-treated MBC with the combination of neratinib and capecitabine [75] and reported a RR of 50%.. The most common adverse event was diarrhea. Another a phase Ib/II study [76] explored the combination of neratinib plus paclitaxel in 38 MBC progressing to a prior anti-HER2 therapy. The RR was 68%. Grade III diarrhea occurred in 28% of patients. The combination of trastuzumab and neratinib has been evaluated in a phase I/II study [77] including 33 *HER2*-positive trastuzumab-progressing MBC, obtaining a RR of 27% and a median PFS of 5 months.

7. Other Agents Targeting the HER2 Pathway

7.1. mTOR Inhibitors

Eventual mechanisms of resistance to trastuzumab include the loss of expression in tumor suppressor PTEN and/or the activation of the PI3K/AKT-signaling proteins. The inhibitors of the mammalian target of rapamycin (mTOR), a downstream component of the PTEN/PI3K pathway, are being currently investigated in order to bypass those acquired resistances. In a pooled analysis of two small studies, the combination of everolimus and trastuzumab [78] obtained RR of 15%, and a PFS of 4.1 months in trastuzumab-pretreated patients.

In a phase I study, the combination of everolimus plus trastuzumab and paclitaxel [79] yielded a RR of 44% in heavily pretreated patients. Another phase I study [80] adding trastuzumab and everolimus to vinorelbine obtained a RR of 19.1%. The combination of everolimus, trastuzumab is being evaluating with paclitaxel in the first-line setting of treatment, and with vinorelbine in the second/third-line setting. Preliminary data of the combination of everolimus plus trastuzumab plus vinorelbine in the BOLERO-3 trial has been reported.

7.2. Afatinib

Afatinib is an irreversible inhibitor of EGFR and HER2. Preliminary data reported a promising activity for afatinib monotherapy after trastuzumab-failure in 41 *HER2*-positive MBC [81], including 10% RR and 46% CBR. The addition of afatinib to letrozole in 28 estrogen-positive patients progressing to letrozole obtained an small rate of tumor stabilization [82].

The LUX-Breast 1 trial [83] is a phase III study comparing the efficacy and safety of afatinib plus vinorelbine versus trastuzumab plus vinorelbine in *HER2*-positive MBC patients progressing on or after trastuzumab-based treatments. The LUX-Breast 3 trial [84] is a randomized phase II study of afatinib with or without vinorelbine versus the investigator's choice of treatment in patients with *HER2*-positive MBC with brain metastases after trastuzumab or lapatinib-based therapy. The most common side effect of afatinib was diarrhea.

7.3. HSP90 Inhibitors

The maturation and conformational stabilization of the HER2 protein is dependent on the chaperone heat shock protein 90 (HSP90). The HSP90 inhibition is an eventual therapeutic strategy for *HER2*-positive MBC. The development of tanespimycin (17-allylamino-17-demethoxygeldanamycin), one of the most promising agents of this group, has been suspended. However, several phase I and II trials are currently evaluating other HSP90 inhibitors in combination with anti-HER2 therapies [85].

7.4. Ertumaxomab

Ertumaxomab is a trifunctional, bispecific antibody against HER2 and CD3 that selectively binds the Fcϒ type I/III receptors, and interacts between tumor cells, T-cells, macrophages and dendritic cells. A phase I study including 15 *HER2*-positive MBC treated with ertumaxomab reported 20% RR and 33% CBR [86].

7.5. ARRY-380

ARRY-380 selectively binds and inhibits the phosphorylation of HER2. Preliminary data from a phase I study in patients with solid tumors reported a CBR of 43% in heavily pretreated *HER2*-positive MBC [87].

7.6. EGFR Inhibitors

Results from a phase I/II trial of the combination of trastuzumab and gefitinib, an EGFR tyrosine kinase inhibitor, in *HER2*-positive MBC has been disappointed [88]. A phase I/II study of trastuzumab plus erlotinib, another EGFR tyrosine kinase inhibitor, in 12 chemotherapy and trastuzumab naïve MBC reported a RR of 33% and a median TTP of 9 months [89].

References

[1] Nahta R., Esteva F. J. Herceptin: mechanisms of action and resistance. *Cancer Lett.,* 2006; 232: 123e38.

[2] Slamon D. J., Clark G. M., Wong S. G., Levin W. J., Ullrich A., McGuire W. L. Human breast cancer: correlation of relapse and survival with amplification of the HER-2/neu oncogene. *Science,* 1987; 235 (4785): 177-82.

[3] Sanna G., Franceschelli L., Rotmensz N., et al. Brain metastases in patients with advanced breast cancer. *Anticancer Res.,* 2007; 27: 2865-9.

[4] Heitz F., Harter P., Lueck H. J., et al. Triple-negative and HER2-overexpressing breast cancers exhibit an elevated risk and an earlier occurrence of cerebral metastases. *Eur. J. Cancer*, 2009; 45: 2792-8.

[5] Musolino A., Ciccolallo L., Panebianco M., et al. Multifactorial central nervous system recurrence susceptibility in patients with HER2-positive breast cancer: epidemiological and clinical data from a population-based cancer registry study. *Cancer,* 2011; 117: 1837-46.

[6] Wolff A. C., Hammond M. E., Schwartz J. N., et al. American Society of Clinical Oncology/College of American Pathologists guideline recommendations for human epidermal growth receptor 2 testing in breast cancer. *J. Clin. Oncol.*, 2007; 25: 118-45.

[7] Seidman A. D., Berry D., Cirrincione C., et al. Randomized phase III trial of weekly compared with every-3-weeks paclitaxelfor metastatic breast cancer, with trastuzumab for all HER-2 non overexpressors: final results of Cancer and Leukaemia Group B Protocol 9840. *J. Clin. Oncol.*, 2008; 26: 1642-9.

[8] Rosen L. S., Ashurst H. L., Chap L. Targeting signal transduction pathways in metastatic breast cancer: a comprehensive review. *Oncologist,* 2010; 15: 216-35.

[9] Spector N. L., Blackwell K. L. Understanding the mechanisms behind trastuzumab therapy for human epidermal growth factor receptor 2-positive breast cancer. *J. Clin. Oncol.*, 2009; 27 (34): 5838-47.

[10] Slamon D. J., Leyland-Jones B., Shak S., et al. Use of chemotherapy plus monoclonal antibody against HER2 for metastatic breast cancer that overexpresses HER2. *N. Engl. J. Med.*, 2001; 344: 783-92.

[11] Marty M., Cognetti F., Maraninchi D., et al. Randomized phase II trial of the efficacy and safety of trastuzumab combined with docetaxel in patients with human epidermal growth factor receptor 2-positive metastatic breast cancer administered as first-line treatment: the M77001 study group. *J. Clin. Oncol.*, 2005; 23: 4265-74.

[12] Gasparini G., Gion M., Mariani L., et al. Randomized phase II trial of weekly paclitaxel alone versus trastuzumab plus weekly paclitaxel as first-line therapy of patients with Her-2 positive advanced breast cancer. *Breast Cancer Res. Treat.*, 2007; 101: 355-65.

[13] Bartsch R., Wenzel C., Altorjai G., et al. Capecitabine and trastuzumab in heavily pretreated metastatic breast cancer. *J. Clin. Oncol.,* 2007; 25: 3853-8.

[14] Schaller G., Fuchs I., Gonsch T., et al. Phase II study of capecitabine plus trastuzumab in human epidermal growth factor receptor 2 overexpressing metastatic breast cancer pretreated with anthracyclines or taxanes. *J. Clin. Oncol.*, 2007; 25: 3246-50.

[15] Yamamoto D., Iwase S., Kitamura K., Odagiri H., Yamamoto C., Nagumo Y. A phase II study of trastuzumab and capecitabine for patients with HER2-overexpressing metastatic breast cancer: Japan Breast Cancer Research Network (JBCRN) 00 Trial. *Cancer Chemother. Pharmacol.*, 2008; 61:509-14.

[16] O'Shaughnessy J. A., Vukelja S., Marsland T., Kimmel G., Ratnam S., Pippen J. E. Phase II study of trastuzumab plus gemcitabine in chemotherapypretreated patients with metastatic breast cancer. *Clin. Breast Cancer*, 2004; 5: 142-7.

[17] Pegram M. D., Lipton A., Hayes D. F., et al. Phase II study of receptor-enhanced chemosensitivity using recombinant humanized anti-p185HER2/neu monoclonal antibody plus cisplatin in patients with HER2/neu-overexpressing metastatic breast cancer refractory to chemotherapy treatment. *J. Clin. Oncol.*, 1998; 16: 2659-71.

[18] Burstein H. J., Keshaviah A., Baron A. D., et al. Trastuzumab plus vinorelbine or taxane chemotherapy for HER2-overexpressing metastatic breast cancer: the trastuzumab and vinorelbine or taxane study. *Cancer,* 2007; 110: 965-72.

[19] Andersson M., Lidbrink E., Bjerre K., et al. Phase III randomized study comparing docetaxel plus trastuzumab with vinorelbine plus trastuzumab as first-line therapy of metastatic or locally advanced human epidermal growth factor receptor 2-positive breast cancer: the HERNATA study. J. Clin. Oncol., 2011; 29: 264-71.

[20] Dawood S., Broglio K., Buzdar A. U., Hortobagyi G. N., Giordano S. H. Prognosis of women with metastatic breast cancer by HER2 status and trastuzumab treatment: an institutional-based review. *J. Clin. Oncol.*, 2010; 28: 92-8.

[21] Shou J., Massarweh S., Osborne C. K., et al. Mechanisms of tamoxifen resistance: increased estrogen receptor-HER2/neu crosstalk in ER/HER2-positive breast cancer. *Natl. Cancer Inst.*, 2004; 96: 926-35.

[22] Kaufman B., Mackey J. R., Clemens M. R., et al. Trastuzumab plus anastrozole versus anastrozole alone for the treatment of postmenopausal women with human epidermal growth factor receptor 2-positive, hormone receptor-positive metastatic breast cancer: results from the randomized phase III TAnDEM study. *J. Clin. Oncol.*, 2009; 27: 5529-37.

[23] Huober J., Fasching P. A., Barsoum M., et al. Higher efficacy of letrozole in combination with trastuzumab compared to letrozole monotherapy as first-line

treatment in patients with HER2- positive, hormone-receptor-positive metastatic breast cancer e results of the eLEcTRA trial. *Breast,* 2012; 21: 27-33.
[24] Hamberg P., Bos M. M., Braun H. J., et al. Randomized phase II study comparing efficacy and safety of combinationtherapy trastuzumab and docetaxel vs. sequential therapy of trastuzumab followed by docetaxel alone at progression as first-line chemotherapy in patients with HER2þ metastatic breast cancer: HERTAX trial. *Clin. Breast Cancer,* 2011; 11: 103-13.
[25] Inoue K., Nakagami K., Mizutani M., et al. Randomized phase III trial of trastuzumab monotherapy followed by trastuzumab plus docetaxel versus trastuzumab plus docetaxel as first-line therapy in patients with HER2-positive metastatic breast cancer: the JO17360 Trial Group. *Breast Cancer Res. Treat.*, 2010; 119: 127-36.
[26] Tripathy D., Slamon D. J., Cobleigh M., et al. Safety of treatment of metastatic breast cancer with trastuzumab beyond disease progression. *J. Clin. Oncol.*, 2004; 22: 1063-70.
[27] von Minckwitz G., du Bois A., Schmidt M., et al. Trastuzumab beyond progression in human epidermal growth factor receptor 2-positive advanced breast cancer: a German Breast Group 26/Breast International Group 03-05 Study. *J. Clin. Oncol.*, 2009; 27: 1999-2006.
[28] Mannocci A., De Feo E., de Waure C., et al. Use of trastuzumab in HER2-positive metastatic breast cancer beyond disease progression: a systematic review of published studies. *Tumors,* 2010; 96 (3): 385-91.
[29] Dahabreh I. J., Linardou H., Siannis F., et al. Trastuzumab in the adjuvant treatment of early-stage breast cancer: a systematic review and meta-analysis of randomized controlled trials. *Oncologist,* 2008; 13: 620-30.
[30] Montagna E., Cancello G., D'Agostino D., et al. Central nervous system metastases in a cohort of metastatic breast cancer patients treated with trastuzumab. *Cancer Chemother. Pharmacol.*, 2009; 63: 275-80.
[31] Petrelli F., Borgonovo K., Cabiddu M., et al. Neoadjuvant chemotherapy and concomitant trastuzumab in breast cancer: a pooled analysis of two randomized trials. *Anticancer Drugs*, 2010; 22: 128-35.
[32] Buzdar A. U., Ibrahim N. K., Francis D., et al. Significantly higher pathologic complete remission rate after neoadjuvant therapy with trastuzumab, paclitaxel, and epirubicin chemotherapy: results of a randomized trial in human epidermal growth factor receptor 2-positive operable breast cancer. *J. Clin. Oncol.*, 2005; 23: 3676-85.
[33] Gianni L., Eiermann W., Semiglazov V., et al. Neoadjuvant chemotherapy with trastuzumab followed by adjuvant trastuzumab versus neoadjuvant chemotherapy alone, in patients with HER2-positive locally advanced breast cancer (the NOAH trial): a randomized controlled superiority trial with a parallel HER2-negative cohort. *Lancet,* 2010; 375:377-84.
[34] Pierga J. Y., Delaloge S., Espié M., et al. A multicenter randomized phase II study of sequential epirubicin/cyclophosphamide followed by docetaxel with or without celecoxib or trastuzumab according to HER2 status, as primary chemotherapy for localized invasive breast cancer patients. *Breast Cancer Res. Treat.*, 2010; 122: 429-37.
[35] Steger G., Greil R., Jakesz R., et al. Final results of ABCSG-24, a randomized phase III study comparing epirubicin, docetaxel, and capecitabine (EDC) to epirubicin and docetaxel (ED) as neoadjuvant treatment for early breast cancer and comparing

ED/EDC plus trastuzumab (T) to ED/EDC as neoadjuvant treatment for early HER-2 positive breast cancer. *Cancer Res.,* 2009; 69 (S24): S64s abstr. 1081.

[36] Perez E. A., Suman V. J., Davidson N. E., et al. Sequential verus concurrent trastuzumab in adjuvant chemotherapy for breast cancer. *J. Clin. Oncol.,* 2011; 29: 4491-7.

[37] Untch M., Rezai M., Loibl S., Fasching P. A., Huober J., Tesch H., et al. Neoadjuvant treatment with trastuzumab in HER2-positive breast cancer: results from the GeparQuattro study. *J. Clin. Oncol.*, 2010; 28: 2024-31.

[38] Baselga J., Bradbury I., Eidtmann H., et al. Lapatinib with trastuzumab for HER2-positive early breast cancer (NeoALTTO): a randomized, open-label, multicentre, phase 3 trial. *Lancet,* 2012; 379: 633-40.

[39] Untch M., Loibl S., Bischoff J., et al. Lapatinib versus trastuzumab in combination with neoadjuvant anthracycline-taxane-based chemotherapy (GeparQuinto, GBG 44): a randomized phase 3 trial. *Lancet Oncol.,* 2012;13:135–44.

[40] Holmes F. A., Nagarwala Y. M., Espina V. A., et al. Correlation of molecular effects and pathologic complete response to preoperative lapatinib and trastuzumab, separately and combined prior to neoadjuvant breast cancer chemotherapy. *J. Clin. Oncol.*, 2011; 29 (S15): 46s abstr. 506.

[41] Guarneri V., Frassoldati A., Bottini A., et al. Preoperative chemotherapy plus trastuzumab, lapatinib, or both in human epidermal growth factor receptor 2-positive operable breast cancer: results of the randomized phase II CHER-LOB study. *J. Clin. Oncol.*, 2012; 30: 1989-95.

[42] Gianni L., Pienkowski T., Im Y. H., et al. Efficacy and safety of neoadjuvant pertuzumab and trastuzumab in women with locally advanced, inflammatory, or early HER2-positive breast cancer (NeoSphere): a randomized multicentre, open-label, phase 2 trial. *Lancet Oncol.*, 2012; 13: 25-32.

[43] Hudis C. A. Trastuzumab-mechanism of action and use in clinical practice. *N. Engl. J. Med.,* 2007; 357 (1): 39-51.

[44] Perez E. A., Suman V. J., Davidson N. E., et al. Cardiac safety analysis of doxorubicin and cyclophosphamide followed by paclitaxel with or without trastuzumab in the North Central Cancer Treatment Group N9831 Adjuvant Breast Cancer Trial. *J. Clin. Oncol.,* 2008; 26: 1231-8.

[45] Ozcelik C., Erdmann B., Pilz B., et al. Conditional mutation of the ErbB2 (HER2) receptor in cardiomyocytes leads to dilated cardiomyopathy. *Proc. Natl. Acad. Sci. USA,* 2002; 99:8880–8885.

[46] Morris P. G., Hudis C. A. Trastuzumab-related cardiotoxicity following anthracycline-based adjuvant chemotherapy: how worried should we be? *J. Clin. Oncol.*, 2010; 28: 3407-10.

[47] Bernard-Marty C., Lebrun F., Awarda A., Piccart M. J. Monoclonal antibody-based targeted therapy in breast cancer: current status and future directions. *Drugs,* 2006; 66: 1577-91.

[48] Scheuer W., Friess T., Burtscher H., Bossenmaier B., Endl J., Hasmann M. Strongly enhanced antitumor activity of trastuzumab and pertuzumab combination treatment on HER2-positive human xenograft tumor models. *Cancer Res.*, 2009; 69 (24): 9330-6.

[49] Cortes J., Fumoleau P., Bianchi G. V., et al. Pertuzumab monotherapy after trastuzumab-based treatment and subsequent reintroduction of trastuzumab: activity and

tolerability in patients with advanced human epidermal growth factor receptor 2-positive breast cancer. *J. Clin. Oncol.*, 2012; 30: 1594-600.

[50] Baselga J., Gelmon K. A., Verma S., et al. Phase II trial of pertuzumab and trastuzumab in patients with human epidermal growth factor receptor 2-positive metastatic breast cancer that progressed during prior trastuzumab therapy. *J. Clin. Oncol.*, 2010; 28 (7): 1738-44.

[51] Blackwell K., Burstein H., Storniolo A., et al. Randomized study of lapatinib alone or in combination with trastuzumab in women with ErbB2-positive, trastuzumab-refractory metastatic breast cancer. *J. Clin. Oncol.*, 2010; 28 (7): 1124-30.

[52] Gianni L., Lladó A., Bianchi G., et al. Open-label, phase II, multicenter, randomized study of the efficacy and safety of two dose levels of pertuzumab, a human epidermal growth factor receptor 2 dimerization inhibitor, in patients with human epidermal growth factor receptor 2-negative metastatic breast cancer. *J. Clin. Oncol.*, 2010; 28: 1131-7.

[53] Swain S. M., Kim S. B., Cortés J., et al. Pertuzumab, trastuzumab, and docetaxel for HER2-positive metastatic breast cancer (CLEOPATRA study): overall survival results from a randomized, double-blind, placebo-controlled, phase 3 study. *Lancet Oncol.*, 2013; 14 (6): 461-71.

[54] Schneeweiss A. C. S., Hickish T., Harvey V., et al. Neoadjuvant pertuzumab and trastuzumab concurrent or sequential with an anthracycline-containing or k9oconcurrent with an anthracycline-free standard regimen: a randomized phase II study (TRYPHAENA). *Cancer Res.*, 2011; 71 (Suppl. 24): 112s.

[55] Burris 3rd H. A., Rugo H. S., Vukelja S. J., et al. Phase II study of the antibody drug conjugate trastuzumab-DM1 for the treatment of human epidermal growth factor receptor 2 (HER2)-positive breast cancer after prior HER2-directed therapy. *J. Clin. Oncol.*, 2011; 29: 398-405.

[56] Krop I. E., Lorusso P., Miller K. D., et al. A Phase II study of trastuzumab emtansine in patients with human epidermal growth factor receptor 2 -positive metastatic breast cancer who were previously treated with trastuzumab, lapatinib, an anthracycline, a taxane, and capecitabine. *J. Clin. Oncol.*, 2012; 30 (26): 3234-41.

[57] Hurvitz S. A., Dirix L., Kocsis J., Gianni L., Lu M. J., Vinholes J. Trastuzumab emtansine (T-DM1) versus trastuzumab þ docetaxel in previously untreated HER2-positive metastatic breast cancer (MBC): primary results of a randomized, Multicenter, open-label phase II study (TDM4450g/BO21976). *ESMO*, 2011, Abstr. 5001.

[58] Blackwell K. L., Miles D., Gianni L., et al. Primary results from EMILIA, a phase III study of trastuzumab emtansine (T-DM1) versus capecitabine (X) and lapatinib (L) in HER2-positive locally advanced or metastatic breast cancer (MBC) previously treated with trastuzumab (T) and a taxane. *J. Clin. Oncol.*, 2012; 30 (26): 3234-41.

[59] Verma S., Miles D., Gianni L., et al. Trastuzumab emtansine for HER2-positive advanced breast cancer. *N. Engl. J. Med.*, 2012; 367 (19): 1783-91.

[60] Diéras V., Harbeck N., Albain K., et al. Phase Ib/II trial of T-DM1 with pertuzumab for patients with HER2-positive locally advanced or metastatic breast cancer. *Cancer Res.*, 2010; 70 (Suppl.): abstr. P3-14-01.

[61] Gomez H. L., Doval D. C., Chavez M. A., et al. Efficacy and safety of lapatinib as first-line therapy for ErbB2-amplified locally advanced or metastatic breast cancer. *J. Clin. Oncol.*, 2008; 26: 2999-3005.

[62] Toi M., Iwata H., Fujiwara Y., et al. Lapatinib monotherapy in patients with relapsed, advanced, or metastatic breast cancer: efficacy, safety, and biomarker results from Japanese patients phase II studies. *Br. J. Cancer*, 2009; 101: 1676-82.

[63] Burstein H. J., Storniolo A. M., Franco S., et al. A phase II study of lapatinib monotherapy in chemotherapy-refractory HER2-positive and HER2-negative advanced or metastatic breast cancer. *Ann. Oncol.*, 2008; 19: 1068-74.

[64] Geyer C. E., Forster J., Lindquist D., et al. Lapatinib plus capecitabine for HER2-positive advanced breast cancer. *N. Engl. J. Med.*, 2006; 355: 2733-43.

[65] Cameron D., Casey M., Press M., et al. A phase III randomized comparison of lapatinib plus capecitabine versus capecitabine alone in women with advanced breast cancer that has progressed on trastuzumab: updated efficacy and biomarker analyses. *Breast Cancer Res. Treat.*, 2008; 112: 533-43.

[66] Di Leo A., Gomez H. L., Aziz Z., et al. Phase III, double-blind, randomized study comparing lapatinib plus paclitaxel with placebo plus paclitaxel as first-line treatment for metastatic breast cancer. *J. Clin. Oncol.*, 2008; 26: 5544-52.

[67] Johnston S., Pippen Jr. J., Pivot X., et al. Lapatinib combined with letrozole and placebo as first-line therapy for postmenopausal hormone receptor-positive metastatic breast cancer. *J. Clin. Oncol.*, 2009; 27: 5538-46.

[68] Burstein H. J., Barry W. T., Cirrincione C., et al. Fulvestrant with or without lapatinib as therapy for hormone receptor positive advanced breast cancer: a double-blinded, placebo-controlled, randomized phase III study. *Cancer Res.*, 2010; 70 (Suppl.) abstr. PD05-01.

[69] Bachelot T. D., Romieu G., Campone M., et al. LANDSCAPE: an FNCLCC phase II study with lapatinib (L) and capecitabine (C) in patients with brain metastases (BM) from HER2-positive (þ) metastatic breast cancer (MBC) before whole-brain radiotherapy (WBR). *J. Clin. Oncol.*, 2011; 29 (Suppl.) abstr. 509.

[70] Storniolo A. M., Pegram M. D., Overmoyer B., et al. A phase I, dose escalation and pharmacokinetic study of lapatinib in combination with trastuzumab in patients with advanced ErbB2-positive breast cancer. *J. Clin. Oncol.*, 2008; 26 (20): 3317-23.

[71] Lin N. U., Mayer I. A., Najita J. S., et al. TBCRC 003: phase II trial of trastuzumab (T) and lapatinib (L) in patients (pts) with HER2þ metastatic breast cancer (MBC). *J. Clin. Oncol.*, 2011; 29 (Suppl.): abstr. 527.

[72] Esteva F. J., Franco S., Hagan M. K., et al. Updated efficacy and safety assessment of first-line therapy with lapatinib, trastuzumab, and paclitaxel in HER2þ metastatic breast cancer. *J. Clin. Oncol.*, 2010; 28 (15S): abstr. 1046.

[73] Rabindran S. K., Discafani C. M., Rosfjord E. C., et al. Antitumor activity of HKI-272, an orally active, irreversible inhibitor of the HER-2 tyrosine kinase. *Clin. Cancer Res.*, 2004; 64 (11): 3958-65.

[74] Burstein H. J., Sun Y., Dirix L. Y., et al. Neratinib, an irreversible ErbB receptor tyrosine kinase inhibitor, in patients with advanced ErbB2-positive breast cancer. *J. Clin. Oncol.*, 2010; 28: 1301-7.

[75] Saura C., Garcia-Saenz J. A., Xu B., et al. Safety and efficacy of neratinib in combination with capecitabine in patients with ErbB2-positive breast cancer. *Cancer Res.*, 2011; 71 (24 Suppl.): abstr. P1-12-09.

[76] Chow L., Gupta S., Hershman D. L., et al. Efficacy and safety of neratinib (HKI-272) in combination with paclitaxel in Her2 + metastatic breast cancer. *San Antonio Breast Cancer Symp.*, 2010; 14-04.
[77] Swaby R., Blackwell K., Jiang Z., et al. Neratinib in combination with trastuzumab for the treatment of advanced breast cancer: a phase I/II study. *J. Clin. Oncol.*, 2009; 27 (15S): abstr. 1004.
[78] Morrow P. K., Wulf G. M., Ensor J., et al. Phase I/II study of trastuzumab in combination with everolimus (RAD001) in patients with HER2-overexpressing metastatic breast cancer who progressed on trastuzumab-based therapy. *J. Clin. Oncol.*, 2011; 29: 3126-32.
[79] Andre F., Campone M., O'Regan R., et al. Phase I study of everolimus plus weekly paclitaxel and trastuzumab in patients with metastatic breast cancer pretreated with trastuzumab. *J. Clin. Oncol.*, 2010; 28: 5110-5.
[80] Jerusalem G., Fasolo A., Dieras V., et al. Phase I trial of oral mTOR inhibitor everolimus in combination with trastuzumab and vinorelbine in pre-treated patients with HER2-overexpressing metastatic breast cancer. *Breast Cancer Res. Treat.*, 2011; 125: 447-55.
[81] Lin N. U., Winer E. P., Wheatley D., et al. A phase II study of afatinib (BIBW 2992), an irreversible ErbB family blocker, in patients with HER2-positive metastatic breast cancer progressing after trastuzumab. *Breast Cancer Res. Treat.*, 2012; ;133 (3): 1057-65.
[82] Gunzer K., de Mont-Serrat H., Uttenreuther-Fischer M. M., Misset J. Addition of BIBW 2992, an irreversible inhibitor of EGFR/HER1 and HER2, to letrozole in estrogen receptor (ER)-positive metastatic breast cancer (mBC) progressingon letrozole monotherapy. *J. Clin. Oncol.*, 2010; 28 (15s): abstr 1072.
[83] Hickish T., Lin N., Carey L., et al. Use of BIBW 2992, a novel irreversible EGFR/HER2 tyrosine kinase inhibitor (TKI), to treat patients with HER2-positive metastatic breast cancer after failure of treatment with trastuzumab. *J. Clin. Oncol.*, 2009; 27 (Suppl.): 15s, abstr. 1023.
[84] Harbeck N., Huang C.-S., Im Y.-H., et al. LUX-breast 1: Randomized, phase III trial of afatinib and vinorelbine versus trastuzumab and vinorelbine in patients with HER2-overexpressing metastatic breast cancer (MBC) failing one prior trastuzumab treatment. *J. Clin. Oncol.*, 2012; 30 (Suppl.): abstr. TPS649.
[85] Modi S., Stopeck A. T., Gordon M. S., et al. Combination of trastuzumab and tanespimycin (17-AAG, KOS-953) is safe and active in trastuzumab-refractory HER-2 overexpressing breast cancer: a phase I dose-escalation study. *J. Clin. Oncol.*, 2007; 25: 5410-7.
[86] Kiewe P., Hasmüller S., Kahlert S., et al. Phase I trial of the trifunctional anti-HER2 x anti-CD3 antibody ertumaxomab in metastatic breast cancer. *Clin. Cancer Res.*, 2006; 12: 3085-91.
[87] Moulder S. L., Baetz T., D'Aloisio S., et al. A phase 1 study to assess the safety, tolerability and PK of ARRY-380-an oral HER2 inhibitor. *Cancer Res.*, 2010; 70 (Suppl.): abstr. P3-14-07.
[88] Arteaga C. L., O'neill A., Moulder S. L., et al. A phase I-II study of combined blockade of the ErbB receptor network with trastuzumab and gefitinib in patients with HER2 (ErbB2)-overexpressing metastatic breast cancer. *Clin. Cancer Res.*, 2008; 14: 6277-83.

[89] Britten C. D., Finn R. S., Bosserman L. D., et al. A phase I/II trial of trastuzumab plus erlotinib in metastatic HER2-positive breast cancer: a dual ErbB targeted approach. *Clin. Breast Cancer*, 2009; 9: 16-22.

In: Fighting Lung Cancer through the HER Family … ISBN: 978-1-63321-092-9
Editor: Diego Márquez-Medina

Chapter 16

Other Malignancies II. Gynaecological and Head and Neck Cancer

Yolanda García García, M.D., Estefania García Pérez, M.D. and Julio Ocaña Rojas, M.D.
Medical Oncology Department, University
Hospital Parc Taulí of Sabadell, Spain

Abstract

Anticancer target drugs against the human epidermal growth factor (HER) family of surface receptors (EGFR, HER2, HER3 and HER4) were included in the pharmaceutical repertoire during the last decade of the XX century.

This chapter reviews recent advances in the treatment of gynaecological and head and neck malignancies involving anti-HER therapies. The role of monoclonal antibodies and tyrosine kinase inhibitors is exhaustively discussed.

1. Gynaecological Cancer

Improvements in surgery, chemotherapy and radiotherapy have improved the outcome of patients with gynaecological cancers. However, a survival plateau seems to have been reached in the past few years, and the urgent need for more effective treatments has prompted researchers to investigate new target therapies. Targeted therapies against the epidermal growth factor receptor (EGFR) in gynaecological cancers will be resumed below.

1.1. Ovarian Cancer

EGFR is overexpressed in 50-70% of advanced epithelial ovarian cancers, and has been correlated with a poor survival. Interfering with EGFR pathways is a main line of investigation in ovarian cancer, although it commonly shows little efficacy in clinical trials.

Pertuzumab, which inhibits dimerization of HER2 with EGFR, HER3 and HER4, is the most studied anti-EGFR drug in ovarian cancer. The anti-HER2 monoclonal antibody (mAB) trastuzumab inhibits the growth of HER2-overexpressing ovarian, lung, breast, and prostate tumour cells [1]. However, the mechanism of action of pertuzumab is not dependent on HER2-overexpression. A phase I trial reported an overall response rate (RR) of 5% by administering pertuzumab to patients with ovarian cancer [2]. Bookman et al. conducted a phase II trial of patients with platinum-resistant ovarian cancer treated with gemcitabine and pertuzumab. The combination obtained a very limited clinical activity in the global population.

However, a pre-planned subgroup analysis conducted as a secondary objective explored different *HER3* mRNA groups and showed an eventual benefit from pertuzumab in patients with low *HER3* RNA levels [3].

Conversely, another phase II randomized trial that treated ovarian-sensitive patients with platinum-based chemotherapy with or without pertuzumab did not find significant differences in efficacy between the combined arm and chemotherapy alone. Likewise, no differences were found in an exploratory biomarker analysis of *HER3* levels [4]. The ongoing phase III PENELOPE trial will test the activity of pertuzumab combined with chemotherapy in platinum-resistant ovarian cancer patients with low *HER3* RNA level (NCT01684878).

Trastuzumab, a highly active anti-HER2 mAB in *HER2* FISH-positive breast cancers, has been tested on ovarian cancer with HER2 overexpression by immunohistochemistry.

Bookman et al. conducted a phase II study in highly pre-treated refractory ovarian cancer patients. HER2 was overexpressed in 11% of samples tested, and trastuzumab monotherapy obtained only 7.3% overall RR.

Preclinical data showed an eventual additive antitumour effect by combining erlotinib, an EGFR tyrosine kinase inhibitor (EGFR-TKI), and chemotherapeutic agents such as carboplatin [5]. Several trials, mainly phase II studies, included patients managed with different treatment strategies. Erlotinib monotherapy showed 5% overall RR in 34 patients overexpressing EGFR [6]. The combination of erlotinib and carboplatin was explored in a phase II study including 50 patients with sensitive and resistant disease.

Overall RR was 57% in 33 platinum-sensitive patients and 7% in platinum-resistant patients. Erlotinib did not add any significant benefit over chemotherapy in such subgroups of patients [7]. A similar minimum activity has been observed with gefitinib, which obtains a scarce overall RR of 3% [8].

1.2. Uterine Cancer

Anti-EGFR therapies have mostly been explored in cervical carcinoma that presents EGFR overexpression in 85% of tumours. Recurrent/metastatic cervical cancer carries a very poor prognosis. Conventional chemotherapy with cisplatin combined with either topotecan or paclitaxel is the standard treatment and obtains a median survival of 9-10 months [9, 10]. Recent data from the GOG-240 trial reported a benefit on overall survival (OS) when chemotherapy is combined with the antiangiogenic mAB bevacizumab [11].

Anti-EGFR treatments do not provide a significant benefit in cervical cancer. Cetuximab monotherapy did not obtain objective response in previously treated cervical carcinoma [12].

The addition of cetuximab to either chemotherapy or chemoradiation did not improve the efficacy of the treatment and clearly increased the toxic profile [12-14].

EGFR-TKIs obtained the same disappointing results in monotherapy or combination. Lapatinib alone or combined with pazopanib, and oral antiangiogenic TKI did not seem to achieve meaningful results [15].

Type II endometrial carcinoma carries the poorest prognosis of all endometrial carcinomas, and HER2 overexpression is commonly present [16]. Trastuzumab has been reported to obtain response in endometrial cancer. Nevertheless, a phase II trial administering trastuzumab to endometrial carcinomas with *HER2* overexpression or amplification did not show any benefit [17, 18]. Ongoing studies will test the activity of anti-HER2 treatments in type II endometrial carcinomas, mostly papillary-serous carcinomas.

2. Squamous Cell Carcinoma of Head and Neck

The rising global burden of squamous cell carcinoma of head and neck (SCCHN) and the fact that the vast majority of cases are diagnosed at locally advanced stages has prompted researchers to develop optimal treatment strategies for these patients. The adoption of both induction chemotherapy and concurrent chemoradiotherapy (CTRT) has contributed to increase survival, achieve local and distant disease control and improve organ preservation rates. Yet the recurrence rate remains high and short-term prognosis poor. EGFR is overexpressed in 90% of the SCCHN cells and is correlated with poor survival outcome and poor response to conventional treatment strategies. For this reason, over the past years, efforts have been directed toward a better understanding of the molecular biology of SCCHN, focusing on the investigation on the EGFR pathway and the treatment with either monoclonal antibodies or tyrosine-kinase inhibitors. The results yielded are promising.

Moreover, human papilloma virus (HPV) infection has been added to the known risk factors for the development of SCCHN. HPV infection is more frequent in oropharyngeal tumours and seems to be a different entity that carries a better prognosis and better treatment response. An eventual association between HPV status and response to anti-EGFR treatment is being investigated, opening the door to new therapeutic strategies.

SCCHN accounts for 3-5% of newly diagnosed cancers every year and 2% of cancer deaths, with a global incidence of more than 600,000 new cases/year, and represents the sixth most frequent cancer worldwide [19, 20]. SCCHN is mostly diagnosed as a locally advanced disease (III and IV stages), and 2-year OS is less than 50%. Despite the best treatment strategy, 60% SCCHN will recur either locally or with distant metastasis, with a global OS rate between 6-9 months [21-24]. EGFR overexpression by immunochemistry is observed in 80-90% of SCCHN. Several studies have shown a correlation between *EGFR* overexpression or amplification and a worse prognosis, with lower OS and disease-free survival (DFS) rates, and an increased resistance to treatment [25-29]. Two molecular-driven therapies have been evaluated in the treatment of SCCHN: anti-EGFR mAB against the extracellular domain of the receptor, which blocks the ligand union and the dimerization; and EGFR-TKI against the intracellular domain of the receptor, which inhibits its phosphorylation and the downstream signal cascade. Both strategies seem promising. However, SCCHN eventually progresses due to resistance mechanisms such as the formation of homodimer and heterodimer within the HER receptor family, and the activation of downstream signalling pathways from another family member (i.e., HER2 or HER4 if EGFR is inactivated).

A specific mutation in the *EGFR* gene, a deletion of the exon 2-7 encoded in chromosome 7 named the *EGFR* vIII variant, associates a defect in the extracellular domain that lacks the ligand union site and constitutively activates the receptor in the absence of ligand. This variant is detected in 40% of all SCCHN and may account for the resistance to anti-EGFR mAB [26]. The *EGFRvIII* mutation promotes proliferation and tumour growth and has been shown to confer resistance to chemotherapy, radiotherapy and to cetuximab treatment in *in vitro* and *in vivo* studies [30, 31].

HPV infection is a risk factor for development in about 20-30% of the head and neck cancers in which HPV-DNA is detected, with higher rates of detection in oropharyngeal carcinomas (40.66%). The presence of high-risk HPV-DNA infections (commonly HPV-16) correlates with the expression of viral oncogenes E6 and E7 that interfere with suppressor genes such as retinoblastoma and p53 gene, overexpressing p16-INK4A. Immunochemistry detected that p16 is associated with HPV-positive status, and low expression of EGFR has been shown to correlate with expression of p16 and may be associated with high response to EGFR-TKI and to a good prognosis. This hypothesis of the interaction between HPV and EGFR pathway is being explored [32-35].

3. Anti-EGFR mAB in SCCHN

3.1. Cetuximab

Cetuximab is a chimeric human monoclonal IgG1 directed against the extracellular domain of the EGFR. Cetuximab has a dual mechanism of action. It prevents the ligand-receptor attachment and presents an antibody-dependent cytotoxicity.

Cetuximab is the only anti-EGFR targeted drug approved for the treatment of SCCHN, combined with radiotherapy in locally advanced stage, and combined with platinum-based chemotherapy in recurrent/metastatic (R/M) stage [20, 36, 37].

A) Cetuximab in Locally Advanced SCCHN

In 2000, Bonner et al. reported that cetuximab combined with radiotherapy produced low cellular proliferation rates compared to radiotherapy alone [38]. Robert et al. evaluated the activity of cetuximab in a phase I trial combined with conventional or hyperfractionated radiotherapy in locally advanced SCCHN. It demonstrated activity in all the patients (13 complete and 2 partial responses), and the recommended dose was established at 400-500/m^2 loading dose, and 250 mg/m^2 weekly dose [39]. Based on the results of this previous study, a phase III pivotal multinational trial conducted by Bonner et al. was published in 2006, leading to the approval of cetuximab combined with radiotherapy in locally advanced SCCHN. A total of 424 locally advanced oropharyngeal, hypopharyngeal or laryngeal SCCHN, stages III and IV were randomized to either conventional radiotherapy or weekly cetuximab combined with radiotherapy concurrently on the phase I established doses. They allowed three different high-dose radiotherapy schemes at investigator choice (70Gy administered in 35 daily fractions, 72-76.8Gy in 60-64 bid fractions or a concurrent boost of 72Gy in 42 fractions). The results favoured the cetuximab arm in the primary objective, locoregional control with a median of 24.4 months versus 14.9 months (HR 0.68; p=0.005), and in median OS (49 months versus 29.3 moths; HR 0.73; p= 0.018). Regarding toxicity, 4 patients discontinued cetuximab treatment due to hypersensitivity reactions and 8 due to acneiform rash grade 3. Acneiform rash occurred in 87% of patients, mostly grades 1-2. Excluding rash, pruritus and infusional reactions (higher in the cetuximab arm), adverse effects were similar in all the arms. Consequently, the authors concluded that cetuximab does not increase radiotherapy-induced toxicity [40]. A 5-year results update reported OS rates of 45.6% versus 35 % in favour of cetuximab treatment, and also higher survival rates in patients with grade 2-4 rash than those with grade 0-1 (68.8 months versus 25.6 months; HR 0.49; p= 0.002).

A subgroup analysis favoured patients receiving the concurrent boost radiotherapy arm [41], but the analysis was not pre-planned.

A phase II study conducted in 91 oropharyngeal tumours was published in 2012, evaluating the efficacy of 12-week maintenance cetuximab treatment after the completion of cetuximab and concurrent radiotherapy treatment. The primary objective, 1-year locoregional control, was 59% versus 47% favouring cetuximab maintenance, but this benefit was lost at two years' follow-up, which suggests that maintenance of EGFR blockade is not enough to eliminate residual disease [42].

After gathering the results of the Bonner phase III study and the synergistic effects of the addition of cetuximab to cisplatin observed in preclinical studies, the next step was the evaluation of cetuximab to standard platinum-based chemoradiotherapy regimens. The phase II EGOG-3303 trial evaluated the response rate and toxicity in 61 platinum-based chemoradiotherapy plus cetuximab-treated patients. Only 5% of progressive disease with an overall RR of 48% was observed. The addition of cetuximab was associated to higher incidence of mucositis or acneiform rash ≥ grade 3 [43]. A phase III RTOG-0522 study was performed in 895 locally advanced SCCHN stage III and IV patients, performance status 0-1. They were randomized to receive radiotherapy (72 Gy in 42 fractions for 6 weeks) with cisplatin $100mg/m^2$ administered on days 1 and 22, with or without weekly cetuximab. After 2-4 years' follow-up, no differences in DFS (63% cetuximab arm versus 64%; p= 0.66), OS (83% versus 80%; p=0.66), or locoregional control (24.5% versus 19.8%; p= 0.92) were observed. No differences in grade 3-4 adverse events other than cutaneous toxicity (40% versus 17%) and mucositis (45% versus 35%) higher in cetuximab arm were observed. A hypothesis to explain the negative results of the addition of cetuximab to cisplatin-based chemoradiotherapy is the negative impact of HPV in cetuximab response or a possible confounding factor in the control arm [44]. In the phase II study conducted by Argiris et al., the authors tested the possibility of enhancing the radio-sensitizing effects of cisplatin with cetuximab. Thirty-nine PS0-1 patients were treated with induction chemotherapy (Docetaxel $75mg/m^2$ D1 + Cisplatin $75mg/m^2$ D1 + cetuximab $250mg/m^2$ D1, 8, 15 after a loading dose of $400mg/m^2/21$ d x 3 courses-TPE), followed by concurrent radiotherapy and weekly cisplatin $30mg/m^2$ + weekly Cetuximab-TPX, and cetuximab weekly maintenance for 6 months. Overall RR was 86% for TPE and 100% after XPD. Three year DFS and OS were 70% and 74%, respectively.

The most frequent grade 3-4 toxicity in the TPE arm was neu-tropenia 77% (10% febrile neutropenia) and oral mucositis 54%, dysphagia 48%, and hypo-magnesaemia 39% in TPX treatment. HPV positivity was determined by in situ hybridization and by immunochemistry detection of p16, and *EGFR* amplification by FISH. No differences in terms of DFS, OS were detected by HPV or *EGFR* status [45, 46].

The RTOG-1016 trial is being conducted to test whether HPV status promotes different treatment effects in cisplatin- and cetuximab-treated patients.

Patients with locally advanced HPV positive SCCHN are randomized to concurrent radiotherapy plus triweekly cisplatin (100 mg/m^2 x 2 cycles) or weekly cetuximab concurrent to radiotherapy. The primary end point is OS rates at 5 years.

Finally, the TREMPLIN study is a phase II trial in 149 treatment naïve hypopharyngeal or laryngeal squamous carcinomas, ($T_{2\text{-}3}N_{0\text{-}3}$) surgery candidates. They received induction chemotherapy with 3 cycles of TPF and surgery (total laryngectomy) was performed in patients with < 50% response (N= 23). Patients whose tumours responded ≥50% were randomized to radiotherapy (70 Gy in 35 fractions) and concurrent cisplatin 100 mg/m^2 D1, 22, 43 (N= 60) or the same radiotherapy scheme plus weekly cetuximab. The results showed better compliance to treatment in the cetuximab arm (71% versus 43%). No differences were observed in the primary objective of the study, larynx preservation at 3 months, which was 95% in the CTRT arm and 93% in the bioRT arm. Secondary objectives such as laryngeal function at 18 months and survival at 18 and 36 months showed no differences.

Local recurrences were higher in the bioRT arm at 18 and 36 months compared to CTRT (14.3% versus 8.3% at 18 months and 21.4% versus 13.3% at 36 months), but surgical salvage treatment was more feasible in the bioRT arm and local recurrence at the end of the comprehensive treatment was similar (10.7% versus 13.3%). Two-year laryngoesophageal dysfunction-free survival was 71% in the cetuximab arm and 79% in the cisplatin arm.

Toxicity other than infusional reactions (5 vs. 0%) and rash (57 vs. 26%), more frequent in cetuximab arms, was higher in the cisplatin arm (renal, haematological and performance status deterioration). There were no differences in grade 3-4 mucositis between arms [47].

To resume, evidence of better treatment results of the addition of cetuximab to a CTRT standard is insufficient, and toxicity is increased.

Furthermore, no randomized phase III study comparing standard cisplatin-based CTRT versus Cetuximab-based bioRT have been performed to date.

B) Cetuximab in R/M SCCHN

Standard treatment of R/M disease is a doublet platinum-based chemotherapy. The most active regimens are the combination of platinum with either 5-FU or taxanes. Response rates of 40% with median DFS of 3-4 months and median OS of 6-9 months are achieved. But after first-line CT, median OS falls to 3-4 months. The need for more of effective treatments in M/R SCCHN has prompted researchers to explore anti-EGFR therapies [48].

The value of cetuximab in platinum-refractory patients was tested in several phase II studies. In a phase II study, Basel et al. included 96 patients with cetuximab combined with either cisplatin or carboplatin.

Results showed an overall RR of 10% and a disease control rate (DCR) of 53% [49]. Trigo et al. conducted a phase II trial involving 103 platinum-refractory patients treated with cetuximab alone. An overall RR of 16.5% and a DCR of 53.4% were noted [50].

Once cetuximab activity was demonstrated in prior phase I and II studies, Burtness et al. conducted a phase III study in 117 patients with R/M SCCHN. Patients were randomized to receive cisplatin 100 mg/m2/4weeks with either weekly cetuximab, 200 ml/m^2 w1, and 125 ml/m^2 thereafter (arm A, N= 57) or placebo (arm B, N= 60). Grade 3-4 toxicities were 90% versus 73% (Arm A versus Arm B), mostly cisplatin-related toxicities (vomiting, haematological toxicity, hyponatraemia and asthenia). Cetuximab-related toxicities were hypomagnesaemia (14% versus 0%), rash (77% versus 24%) and hypersensitivity reactions (6% versus 2%).

There were no significant statistical differences in both disease-free survival (4.2 months versus 2.7 months; HR 0.78; p= 0.09) and median OS (9.2 months versus 8 months; p= 0.21). An exploratory analysis showed differences in overall RR in patients with any grade skin rash versus none (33% versus 7%; p= 0.08) [51].

Vermorken et al. published the EXTREME study in 2008. A total of 442 R/M SCCHN patients were randomized to first-line treatment with cisplatin 100 mg/m^2 or carboplatin AUC 5, at investigator choice, combined with 5-FU 1000mg/m^2/day in continuous infusion of 4 days with or without weekly cetuximab at 250 mg/m^2 weekly dose with a first loading dose of 400 mg/m^2 for 6 weeks. Maintenance treatment with cetuximab was allowed in stabilized and responding patients until unacceptable toxicity or progressive disease. A median of 5 cycles was administered in the cetuximab arm and a median of 4 in the CT alone arm. The primary endpoint of the study, OS, was 10.1 months versus 4 months (p= 0.04) favoured the cetuximab arm. The cetuximab arm was favoured for secondary endpoints such as DFS (5.6 months versus 3.3 months; p< 0.001) and overall RR (36 versus 20%; p<0.001). Local control and time to treatment failure also favoured the cetuximab arm. No correlation was present with rash and efficacy parameters. Regarding safety, no significant differences in grade 3-4 effects were detected but more sepsis (9 versus 1; p= 0.02), hypomagnesaemia (11 versus 3; p= 0.05), hypersensitivity reactions (3%) and skin toxicity (9%). Twenty per cent of patients discontinued treatment in both arms and there were no cetuximab-related deaths [23].

In the ERBITAX study, Hitt et al. tested the efficacy of weekly cetuximab combined with weekly paclitaxel 80 mg/m^2 on 46 R/M SCCHM unfit for platinum treatment. Sixty-one percent of patients had a Karnofsky index of 70-80%, 47% had locoregional recurrence with no distant metastasis and 43% had previous curative intention treatment (33% with platinum-based CT). Overall RR was 54% (22% complete response, 32% partial response), with 80% DCR. Median PFS was 4.2 months and median OS 8.1 months.

A positive correlation was found between rash and no previous CT treatment, with a higher response rate but no differences in OS. Main grade 3-4 toxicities were skin rash (24%), asthenia (17%) and neutropenia (13%) [52].

In the GORTEC 2008-03 study, a phase II in first line treatment trial, 54 patients, PS 0-1, less than 70 years-old received treatment with docetaxel 70mg/m^2 and cisplatin 75 mg/m^2 triweekly x 4 cycles, combined with weekly cetuximab at 250 mg/m^2 with a loading dose of 400 mg/m^2. Maintenance with biweekly 500mg/m^2 cetuximab was allowed until disease progression or unacceptable toxicity was noted, regardless of which occurred first.

G-CSF supportive treatment with lenogastrim was administered during CT treatment.

One toxic death secondary to sepsis was reported. The overall RR at 12 weeks, primary objective of the study, was 54% with a PFS of 7.1 months, and a median OS of 15.3 months. One-year OS was 58.8% [53].

Only scarce data is available on second-line R/M SCCHN cetuximab-treated patients arising from phase II studies. Data showed an overall RR of 10-13% with the addition of cetuximab to cisplatin, and a DCR of 50% for treatment with cetuximab monotherapy, with an increase of 2.5 months in OS [49, 54, 55].

C) EGFR As a Predictive Factor to Cetuximab Treatment

It remains unclear whether EGFR functionality and expression, tested by different techniques, is a predictive marker for cetuximab treatment response in SCCHN, and substudies performed in the main trials of cetuximab treatment yield conflicting results.

Burtness et al. retrospectively determined EGFR expression by immunochemistry techniques in a 0 to 3 scale in 86 patients. No differences in the high levels of EGFR expression (3+ in ≥80% cells) were found when treatment arms (cetuximab-treated versus non-cetuximab arm) were compared. Higher overall RR in the cetuximab arm was noted (26% versus 9%; p= 0.029), but when analyzed by EGFR expression (high versus low/ moderate), this difference was only sustained in the low/moderate group expression (40% versus 11.5%; p= 0.027) and was negative in the high expression group (11.8% versus 5.9%).

The authors comment on the possibility that the cetuximab dose was too low to saturate all the receptors in the high expression group [51].

In the EXTREME study, the authors prospectively analyzed the immunohistochemistry expression of EGFR in 411 out of 442 included patients. An immunohistochemistry scale of 1-300 was used to determine EGFR expression. Scores ≥220 were considered high expression. They found a positive effect for all the cetuximab-treated patients and no correlation with EGFR score levels, although their data suggest that EGFR high levels may confer resistance to chemotherapy in head and neck cancer cells.

Similar data have been reported in other neoplasms. The CRYSTAL study on colorectal cancer demonstrated that the addition of cetuximab to chemotherapy correlated with a benefit in OS with no association found depending on levels of EGFR.

Longer OS had been reported in the FLEX study in non-small cell lung cancer patients with high levels of EGFR measured by immunohistochemistry score and treated with platinum-based chemotherapy plus cetuximab compared to chemotherapy alone [56, 57].

Finally, in the ERBITAX trial, *EGFR* gene amplification determined by FISH was performed in 29 patients and EGFR expression determined by immunohistochemistry was performed in 33 patients. Neither EGFR amplification nor EGFR expression correlated with RR, rash toxicity, PFS or median OS [52].

The data presently available does not support testing EGFR as a predictive marker of benefit in cetuximab-treated patients.

3.2. Other mAB

A) Panitumumab

Panitumumab is a fully human IgG2 mAB that binds to the extracellular domain of EGFR, prevents union to ligand and receptor activation, and has antibody-dependent cellular cytotoxicity [58]. The first data of the activity of panitumumab came from a phase I study in combination with chemotherapy (carboplatin and paclitaxel on a weekly basis) and concurrent radiotherapy performed in 19 patients.

The most frequent adverse events were xerostomia, mucositis, dermatitis, acneiform rash and oral cavity pain, with no significant increase of toxicity due to CTRT and progressively increased panitumumab dose. An overall RR of 95% was noted, and all patients presented a partial response [59].

The SPECTRUM study is a phase III trial that included 657 first-line treatment R/M SCCHN patients, randomized to cisplatin 100 mg/m^2 plus 5-FU 1000 mg/m^2/day x 4 days with or without panitumumab 9 mg/kg. All drugs were administered triweekly with a maximum of 6 cycles. Maintenance treatment with panitumumab was allowed in the experi-mental arm until unacceptable toxicity or disease progression.

Table 1. Trials and results with cetuximab in R/M SCCHN

	Burtness. p-III 1st line R/M	EXTREME p-III 1st line R/M	ERBITAX p-II 1st line R/M	GORTEC p-II 1st line R/M	Vermorken p-II 2nd line R/M
N	117	442	46	54	103
Treatment	CDDP + Cet Vs. CDDP	CDDP + 5-FU + Cet Vs. CDDP + 5-FU	Paclitaxel + Cet	CDDP + DCX + Cet	p.1: Cet p.2 (after PD): Cet + CDDP
RR	26% vs. 10% (p= 0.03)	36% vs. 20% (p< 0.001)	54%	54%	p.1: 13% p.2: 0%
DCR					p.1: 46% p.2: 26%
PFS	4.2 months vs. 2.7 months (p= 0.09)	5.6 months vs. 3.3 months. (p< 0.001)	4.2 months	7 months	p.1: 70 days p.2: 50 days
OS	9.2 months vs. 8 months (p= 0.21)	10.1 months vs. 7.4 months (p= 0.04)	8.1 months	15.3 months	178 days

CDDP (cisplatin), 5-FU (5-Fluorouracil), Cet (Cetuximab), DCX (Docetaxel), p.1 (1st part of study treatment), p.2 (2nd part of study treatment).

Patients were stratified by previous curative intent treatment, primary tumour site and performance status (all of them 0 or 1). Switch to carboplatin AUC 5 was allowed if nephrotoxicity (creatinine clearance <50 mL/min) or neurotoxicity ≥ grade 2 developed. Ninety-five patients continued on panitumumab treatment and a switch to carboplatin was made in 21% of panitumumab patients and 26% in the control arm. No significant differences in the primary endpoint, median overall survival were detected, 11.1 months in the panitumumab arm and 9 months in the control arm. Differences were observed in secondary endpoints and progression-free survival and response rate favouring the experimental arm in PFS (5.8 months versus 4.6 months; p= 0.0036) and overall RR (36% versus 20%; p= 0.0065).

Grade 3-4 toxicity was higher in the experimental arm: Skin/ocular toxicity (19% versus 2%), hypomagnesaemia (12% versus 4%), hypokalaemia (10% versus 7%), dehydration (5% versus 2%) and diarrhoea (5% versus 1%). A total of 22 toxic deaths were reported (14 panitumumab arm), 5 of which were considered panitumumab-related.

Although this is a negative study with no differences in the primary endpoint, it should be noted that median overall survival in the control arm is higher than foreseen in other studies.

This may be the result of an inclusion bias of Asian patients who carried a better overall survival.

HPV status was retrospectively analyzed by immunohistochemistry of p16 to assess HPV status as a predictive marker of benefit of panitumumab. P16 was determined in 443 patients: 22% positive and 78% negative with similar proportion between treatment arms: 24% in the panitumumab arm and 22% in the control arm, mostly in oropharyngeal tumours.

OS was longer in p16-negative patients in the control arm (11.7 months versus 8.6 months; p= 0.01), but not in p16-positive cases. In the control arm, p16-positive patients had a higher non-significant OS.

B) Zalutumumab

Zalutumumab is a fully human IgG1k mAB that, as seen in preclinical models, acts through a competitive inhibition of the union the ligands TGF-Alpha and EGF to the extra-cellular domain of EGFR, precludes the activation of the receptor and also has antibody mediated cellular cytotoxicity [60].

In a phase I/II trial conducted by Bastholt et al. including 28 patients, no dose limiting toxicity was observed up to 8mg/kg [61] with a clinical benefit in 39% of the patients (7% overall RR) and skin rash was the most frequent toxicity.

Machiels et al. published the ZALUTE phase III trial in 2011. A total of 286 R/M SCCHN who had previously been treated with one or more treatment lines, with progressive disease less than 6 months of previous platinum treatment, were included.

Patients were randomized in a 2:1 ratio to zalutumumab plus best supportive care (experi-mental arm) or best supportive care and optional methotrexate treatment. Patients were stratified by perfor-mance status and prior anti-EGFR treatment was not allowed.

Zalutumumab was administered at a dose of 8mg/kg, and 4 mg/kg/weekly for 2 weeks. Incremental doses were allowed up to a maximum of 16 mg/kg in the absence of toxicity.

Treatment was maintained until unacceptable toxicity or progressive disease. It was a negative trial, with no significant differences in median overall survival as primary endpoint (6.7 months versus 5.2 months; p= 0.064). Grade 3-4 toxicity, mainly rash, anaemia and infections, was higher in the experimental arm.

C) Nimotuzumab

Nimotuzumab is a humanized mAB that recognizes the EGFR external domain and has demonstrated anti-proliferative, pro-apoptotic, radio-sensitizing, and anti-angiogenic proper-ties *in vivo* and *in vitro*. Several phase II trials tested the activity of this mab in SCCHN patients. Rodriguez et al. randomized 106 locally advanced SCCHN patients to radiotherapy with either nimotuzumab 200 mg/weekly/6 weeks or placebo.

The results obtained favoured the experimental arm in terms of overall RR, primary endpoint, (59.5% versus 34.2%, p= 0.028) and median OS (14 months versus 8.83 months; p= 0.0237). EGFR expression was analyzed in 55 tumour sections. EGFR-positive patients on nimotuzumab treatment showed a significantly better overall survival than placebo-treated patients (16.5 months versus 7.2 months; p= 0.0038). EGFR-negative patients showed no differences in survival. Toxicity was not increased by the addition of nimotuzumab. No cases of skin rash were noted as was presumed by the in vitro data of the absence of effects of nimotuzumab in skin EGFR [62]. In another phase II study, Babu et al. randomized 92 locally advanced SCCHN, stages III-Iva in a double randomization design study that compared the addition of nimotuzumab to radiation (arm A: RT versus RT plus nimotuzumab) and the addition to CTRT (arm B: platinum-based CT+ RT versus the same CT plus nimotuzumab), there were no differences in the arms of RT versus bioRT (overall RR 73% versus 76%; OS 12 months versus 14.3 months), but nimotu-zumab improved both overall RR and survival when added to platinum-based CTRT (RR 100% versus 70%; OS not reached versus 21.9 months). Nimotuzomab arms did not increase grade 3-4 toxicities [63].

D) Sym004

Sym004 is a first-in-class drug mixture of two chimeric mAB targeting non-overlapping epitopes on the EGFR. In preclinical models, Sym004 exhibits more pronounced inhibition of EGFR mediated signals and is active even when mechanisms of acquired resistance to anti-EGFR appear, such as the increase in the ligand production or the interaction with other EGFR family members.

Diestman et al. conducted a phase I trial to test safety, with a good safety profile.

Toxicity was as expected, rash, hypomagnesaemia and infusional reactions). With a 9 mg/kg/ weekly dose, the maximum tolerated dose was not found [64]. In a multicentre phase II study performed by Machiels et al., 26 advanced and incurable SCCHN patients progressed in <12 weeks after a regimen that included an anti-EGFR mAB with Sym004 12 mg/kg/ weekly until disease progression. Tumour size decreased in 8/20 evaluable patients and stabilized in 14/20. The primary endpoint, DFS, was 82 days, and progression-free rate at 24 weeks was 12%. Skin rash and hypomagnesaemia were the main toxicities [65].

Table 2. Ongoing trials with cetuximab

NCT and status	Sponsor	Phase	Target	Description	1ary outcome
00956007 (recruiting)	RTOG	3	N=700	LA after surgery IMRT+/-Cet	Overall survival
01969877 (recruiting)	Lund University Hospital	3	N=618	LA. 4 arms: RT 68Gy+ Cet RT 73.1Gy+Cet RT 68Gy+CDDPw RT 73.1Gy+CDDPw	Overall survival
00265941 (ongoing, not recruiting)	RTOG	3	N=720	LA RT+CDDP w 1and4 RT+CDDP W 1and4 + Cet	DFS
01855451 (active, not recruiting)	TROG	3	N=200	LA HPV Oropharynx: RT+CDDPw RT+Cet	Toxicity (acuteandlong term side effects
01084083 (ongoing, not recruiting)	ECOG	2	N=83	LA HPV Oropharynx resectable: Induction chemotherapy (Paclitaxel+CDDP+Cet), follow by IMRT (27Fr)+Cet vs IMRT (33Fr)+Cet	2 years PFS
01435252 (recruiting)	University of Zurich	2	N=60	Chemoradiotherapy + Cet, after patients are randomized to consolidation therapy with cetuximab 2w vs. no consolidation therapy	2 year locoregional control rate

Table 2. (Continued)

NCT and status	Sponsor	Phase	Target	Description	1ary outcome
00791141 (completed)	Heinrich-Hein University, Duesseldorf	2	N=80	Adjuvant therapy (high risk of recurrence): 5-FU+CDDP+Cet+RT followed by maintenance therapy with cetuximab every 2 w over 6 months	G.3/4 acut toxicity and 2-year DFS
00765011 (recruiting)	Grupo Español TTCC	2	N=92	Resectable and LA larynx cancer: Induction chemotherapy (TPF) followed by RR+Cet vs. surgery	3 years specific survival free of laringectomy
01884623 (recruiting)	Gustave Roussy, Cancer Campus, Grand Paris	3	N=164	R/M unfit elderly patients, 1st line therapy: Metotrexate vs. Cet	FFS
01437449 (recruiting)	Standford university	2		R/M Docetaxel+CDDP+Cet w.	8 weeks response rate

RTOG (Radiation Therapy Oncology Group), TROG (Trans-Tasman Radiation Oncology Group), ECOG (Eastern Cooperative Oncology Group), Grupo Español TTCC (Grupo Español de Tratamiento de Tumores de Cabeza y Cuello), LA (locally advanced), R/M (recurrent/metastatic), RT (Radiation Therapy), IMRT (Intensity Modulated Radiation Therapy), Cet (Cetuximab), CDDP (Cisplatin), 5-FU (5-Fluorouracil), TPF (Docetaxel+Cisplatin+5-Fluorouracil), DFS (disease free survival), PFS (progression-free survival), FFS (failure-free survival).

4. EGFR-TKI in SCCHN

4.1. Gefitinib and Erlotinib

Gefitinib and erlotinib are two selective reversible EGFR-TKIs. The results obtained with these drugs in SCCHN are disappointing, with overall RR 8-10% in gefitinib-treated patients and 4% with erlotinib, time to progression around 3 months and a median OS of 8 months in M/R SCCHN, in studies comparing these drugs with placebo, methotrexate chemotherapy or even when combined with drugs like docetaxel. When used in locoregional advanced disease, the addition of either gefitinib or erlotinib to platinum-based CTRT did not improve results.

The most frequent adverse events are rash and diarrhoea.

Acneiform rash has been studied as a predictive response factor in several studies, and patients with any grade of cutaneous toxicity presented better statistically significant results.

Stewart et al. presented a phase III randomized study involving 212 patients treated with gefitinib at two different doses (250 mg and 500 mg/ oral/ daily) or methotrexate. The amplification by FISH was present in 40% of the 250 mg gefitinib arm, 41% of the 500 mg gefitinib arm, and 34% of the methotrexate arm.

Table 3. Ongoing trials with other monoclonal antibodies

NCT and status	Sponsor	Phase	Target	Description	1ary outcome
00798655 (recruiting)	Robert Ferris	2	N=43	LA after surgery: Panitumumab 2.5mg/kg w + CDDP w+RT	2 years PFS
00500760 (completed)	Amgen	2	N=153	LA. 2 arms: RT+CDDP 100mg/m2 D1,22,43 vs RT+CDDP 75mg/m2 D1,22,43 +Panitumumab 9mg/kg D1,22,43	2 years locoregional control rate
00707655 (completed)	Genmab	1/2	N=8	LA ineligible for platinum based chemotherapy: Zalutumumab 4m/kg 8w+RT Vs. Zalutumumab 8mg/kg 8w+RT	Adverse events
00702481 (recruiting)	National Cancer Centre, Singapore	2	N=37	LA: Nimotuzumab 200mg/w 8w+ CDDP 100mg/2 w1,4,7 + RT	16 weeks response rate
00957086 (recruiting)	National Cancer Centre, Singapore	2	N=710	Adjuvant Therapy: CDDP+RT+Nimotuzumab Vs. CDDP+RT+Placebo	5 years DFS
02012062 (recruiting)	Fudan University	3	N=320	LA nasopharyngeal carcinoma: Induction chemotherapy (TPF), follow by IMRT+CDDP vs. IMRT+Nimotuzumab	Adverse events
00910117 (completed)	Fudan University	2	N=40	LA: Induction chemotherapy with PF (CDDP+5-FU) + Nimotuzumab	6 weeks overall response rate
01425736 (completed)	Wei Guo	2	N=91	Induction chemotherapy (TPF) with or without Nimotuzumab	4 years DCR
01616849 (recruiting)	Sun Yat-sen University	2	N=39	Untreated metastatic nasopharyngeal carcinoma: CDDP+5-FU+Nimotuzumab	19 months objective response rate

LA (locally advanced), R/M (recurrent/metastatic), RT (Radiation Therapy), IMRT (Intensity Modulated Radiation Therapy), CDDP (Cisplatin), 5-FU (5-Fluorouracil), TPF (Docetaxel + Cisplatin + 5-Fluorouracil), PFS (progression-free survival), DFS (disease-free survival), DCR (disease control rate).

No differences in OS by the *EGFR* status were found, although overall RR was slightly higher in the 500 mg gefitinib dose for *EGFR*-amplified patients (13.8% vs. 4.8%) [66]. Soulières et al. conducted a phase II study testing the activity of erlotinib monotherapy in R/M disease, and even though overexpression of EGFR was positive in 87% of tumour samples, there were no differences in OS, rash toxicity, or intensity of EGFR expression, between groups [67]. Martins et al. performed an exploratory analysis in 50 oropharyngeal tumours with positive HPV status (p-16+), but no differences were found in overall RR or PFS between erlotinib-treated patients versus no treatment.

Table 4. Trials and results with gefitinib and erlotinib

	Martins et al. P.II LA	Grégoire et al. P.II LA	Soulières et al. P.II R/M > ó = 2nd line	Cohen et al. P.II R/M	Stewart et al. P.III R/M (1st line-no fits for platinum or 2nd line- fits for platinum)	Argiris et al. P.III R/M 1st line
N	204	226	115	52	486	270
Scheme	CRT+Erl.150 CRT+Pb	CRT+Gef.250 CRT+Gef.500 CRT+placebo	Erlotinib 150 monotherapy	Gef. 500 monotherapy	Gef. 250 Gef. 500 MTX	DCX+Pb. DCX+Gef. 500
ORR	CRR (1ary e.p): CRT+Erl. 52% vs. CRT+Pb 40% (p=0.08)	p= n.s	4.3%	10.6%	Gef. 250 2.7% Gef. 500 7.6% MTX 3.9% (p= n.s)	DCX.+Pb 6.2% DCX.+Gef 12.5% (p=n.s)
DCR		2-year LDCR (1ary e.p) Concomitant p.: CRT+Gef. 32.7% vs. CRT+Pb. 33.6% (p= n.s) Maintenance p.: CRT+Gef. 28.8% vs. CRT+Pb. 37.4% (p= n.s)		53%		
PFS	p=n.s	p= n.s	9.6 w.	3.4 m.		DCX+Pb 6.2% DCX+Gef 12.5% (p=n.s)
OS		p= n.s	6 m.	8.1 m.	1ary e.p Gef. 250 5.6m. Gef. 500 6m. MTX 6.7m. (p=0.39)	1ary e.p DCX+Pb 6m. DCX+Gef 7.3m. (p=n.s)
Rash and Results	Increase: CRR (p=0.06) and PFS (p=0.03)		Increase: OS (7.4m. vs. 4m.,p=0.045)	Increase: TTP (4.3m.vs. 2.1m., p=0.0002) and OS (11.1m. vs. 5.3m., p=0.001)		

P = n.s (p with non-significance value); 1ary e.p (primary end point); Gef. (Gefitinib); Erl. (Erlotinib); CRT (chemoradiotherapy, CDDP 100mg/m2 D1,22,43 x 3 cycles + RT 70Gy in 35Fr); MTX (Methotrexate); DCX (Docetaxel), Pb. (placebo).

4.2. EGFR/HER2 and Pan-HER Inhibitors

A) Lapatinib

Lapatinib is a dual TKI that interrupts the HER2 and EGFR pathways. Some published data suggest the activation of HER2 as a mechanism of resistance to cetuximab anti-EGFR treatment [68]. Two phase II studies that test lapatinib in locally advanced SCCHN have been carried out, one combined with CTRT and the other as induction monotherapy previous to CTRT treatment. Harrington et al. treated 76 patients with radiotherapy (70 Gy in 35 Fractions for 7 weeks) plus cisplatin 100 mg/m^2/triweekly x 3 courses with either lapatinib 1500 mg/day or placebo. Lapatinib/placebo was maintained until progression. Ninety-seven percent of patients were performance status 0-1 and 82% were stage IV. The hazard ratio for OS was 0.7 and for PFS 0.71. All toxicities were similar but more incidence of grade 3 rash and diarrhoea in the lapatinib arm was reported (3% and 6%) [69]. The other study by del Campo et al. included 107 patients randomized in a 2:1 ratio to lapatinib or placebo for 6 weeks previous to CTRT. Biopsies were obtained at inclusion and after 2 weeks of treatment. Primary endpoint was the apoptotic index determined at two weeks after treatment, but showed no differences (8% versus 9.4%).

Positive results in other secondary endpoints were reported as decrease in the proliferative index, overall RR at 4 weeks and before CTRT begin (17% versus 4%) but no differences at the end of CTRT were found (70% versus 53%). All the responders to lapatinib had EGFR overexpression either measured by FISH or immunochemistry [70].

In R/M disease, we wish to highlight a phase II trial that included 45 patients in two treatment cohorts: arm A, 27 anti-EGFR therapy-naïve patients and arm B, 18 previously pretreated with anti-EGFR agent patients. All patients received lapatinib 1500 mg/day. Most frequent adverse events were diarrhoea (49%) and rash (33%), mostly grade 1-2. No toxic deaths were reported with no complete responses and no differences in PFS (52 days both treatment arms). Results from biopsy specimens revealed a significant decrease in HER2 phosphorylation but not in EGFR phosphorylation after treatment initiation, and authors explained it might be the main reason for the lack of efficacy of lapatinib in SCCHN patients [71].

B) Afatinib (BIBW-2992)

Afatinib is an orally available potent, irreversible TKI that blocks EGFR, HER2 and HER4 activation. Preclinical studies have demonstrated activity against several EGFR mutations, and in EGFRvIII [72].

In a phase I trial in patients with advanced solid tumours, the main dose-limiting toxicities were rash and diarrhoea [73]. Seiwert treated 124 recurrent/metastatic SCCHN patients on second-line treatment after platinum regimen failure. Patients were randomized to afatinib 50mg/day versus weekly cetuximab. Crossover was allowed at progression. Afatinib showed higher activity when compared to cetuximab in the first part of the study (overall RR 18% versus 8%, establish disease 53% versus 50%), but also a higher benefit rate with 33% for afatinib and 19% for cetuximab. Most frequent adverse events were rash, diarrhoea and stomatitis. Grade 3 effects were 47% in the afatinib and 17% in the cetuximab arm. They concluded that there is no cross-resistance between agents and second-line afatinib is more effective when compared to cetuximab but severe toxicity was noted.

Clinical research with afatinib in SCCHN is ongoing, such as a phase III study in patients with recurrent and/or metastatic disease that compares methotrexate versus afatinib after progression to platinum-based therapy (NCT01856478, recruiting).

Afatinib is also being tested in two phase III trials as a maintenance treatment, compared to placebo after CTRT in unresectable locoregionally advanced HNSCC (NCT01345669, recruiting), and after surgery and CTRT (NCT01427478, recruiting).

Another ongoing phase II study aims to identify predictive and pharmacodynamic biomarkers of activity and efficacy of preoperatory afatinib (NCT01415674, recruiting).

C) Dacomitinib (PF-00299804)

An orally active, irreversible, pan-HER TKI, with activity in EGFRvIII mutation and xenograft models resistant to reversible TKI. Siu et al. treated 69 recurrent/metastatic SCCHM patients with dacomitinib 45 mg/day in 21 days cycles in first line, naïve anti-EGFR treatment. A clinical benefit of 74% (11% partial response) with 11% stable disease maintained more than 24 weeks was observed. PFS was 2.8 months, and OS 7.6 months.

Most common adverse events were diarrhoea 13%, asthenia 9%, acneiform rash 7%, and hand-foot syndrome 4%. A further study involving EGFRvIII mutated patients is testing the value of EGFRvIII mutation as predictive factor of response to dacomitinib. Two other trials on dacomitinib are currently ongoing: a phase II study in patients with recurrent/metastatic disease after failure of platinum-containing therapy, to assess the response rate with dacomitinib (NCT01449201, ongoing not recruiting); the other is a phase I study of patients with locally advanced SCCHN who receive dacomitinib and RT versus dacomitinib and CTRT, in two stages: a dose escalation phase and a dose expansion phase (NCT01737008, recruiting).

Conclusion

Neither anti-EGFR nor anti-Her2 therapies present a favourable activity in gynaecological neoplasm, which may be explained by the heterogeneity of different tumours.

Improving the knowledge of the tumour biology, better and trustful markers and individual selection of patients based on molecular features is essential to improve efficacy data on those patients.

Cetuximab has become a paradigm in the treatment of SCCHN, mostly in R/M disease when combined with platinum agents and with taxanes in patients unfit for platinum.

In locally advanced disease, a clear benefit of the radiotherapy and cetuximab over radiotherapy alone has been demonstrated, but further evidence should be provided to replace bioRT over standard CTRT.

Regarding TKI agents, afatinib and dacomitinib show promising activity but further studies are needed. HPV is being studied as a predictive and prognostic factor in SCCHN and in the future may be a factor to improve therapeutic strategy in the treatment of SCCHN.

References

[1] Langdon, S. P., Faratian, D., Nagumo, Y., Mullen, P., Harrison, D. J. Pertuzumab for the treatment of ovarian cancer. *Expert Opin. Biol. Ther.* 2010; 10 (7): 1113-20.

[2] Gordon, M. S., Matei, D., Aghajanian, C., et al. Clinical activity of pertuzumab (rhu MAb 2C4), a HER dimerization inhibitor, in advanced ovarian cancer: potential predictive relationship with tumor HER2 activation status. *J. Clin. Oncol.* 2006; 24 (26): 4324-32.

[3] Makhija, S., Amler, L. C., Glenn, D., et al. Clinical activity of gemcitabine plus pertuzumab in platinum-resistant ovarian cancer, fallopian tube cancer, or primary peritoneal cancer. *J. Clin. Oncol.* 2010; 28 (7): 1215-23.

[4] Kaye, S. B., Poole, C. J., Danska-Bidzinska, A., et al. A randomized phase II study evaluating the combination of carboplatin-based chemotherapy with pertuzumab versus carboplatin-based therapy alone in patients with relapsed, platinum-sensitive ovarian cancer. *Ann. Oncol.* 2013; 24 (1): 145-52.

[5] Akita, R. W., Sliwkowski, M. X. Preclinical studies with Erlotinib (Tarceva). *Semin. Oncol.* 2003; 30 (3 Suppl. 7): 15-24.

[6] Gordon, A. N., Finkler, N., Edwards, R. P., et al. Efficacy and safety of erlotinib HCl, an epidermal growth factor receptor (HER1/EGFR) tyrosine kinase inhibitor, in patients with advanced ovarian carcinoma: results from a phase II multicenter study. *Int. J. Gynecol. Cancer.* 2005; 15 (5): 785-92.

[7] Hirte, H., Oza, A., Swenerton, K., et al. A phase II study of erlotinib (OSI-774) given in combination with carboplatin in patients with recurrent epithelial ovarian cancer (NCIC CTG IND.149). *Gynecol. Oncol.* 2010; 118 (3): 308-12.

[8] Schilder, R. J., Sill, M. W., Chen, X., et al. Phase II study of gefitinib in patients with relapsed or persistent ovarian or primary peritoneal carcinoma and evaluation of epidermal growth factor receptor mutations and immunohistochemical expression: a Gynecologic Oncology Group Study. *Clin. Cancer Res.* 2005; 11 (15): 5539-48.

[9] Long H. J., 3rd, Bundy, B. N., Grendys, E. C. Jr, et al. Randomized phase III trial of cisplatin with or without topotecan in carcinoma of the uterine cervix: a Gynecologic Oncology Group Study. *J. Clin. Oncol.* 2005; 23 (21): 4626-33.

[10] Monk, B. J., Sill, M. W., McMeekin, D. S., et al. Phase III trial of four cisplatin-containing doublet combinations in stage IVB, recurrent, or persistent cervical carcinoma: a Gynecologic Oncology Group study. *J. Clin. Oncol.* 2009; 27 (28): 4649-55.

[11] Tewari, K. S., Sill, M. W., Long H. J. 3rd, et al. Improved survival with bevacizumab in advanced cervical cancer. *N. Engl. J. Med.* 2014; 370 (8): 734-43.

[12] Santin, A. D., Sill, M. W., McMeekin, D. S., et al. Phase II trial of cetuximab in the treatment of persistent or recurrent squamous or non-squamous cell carcinoma of the cervix: a Gynecologic Oncology Group study. *Gynecol. Oncol.* 2011; 122 (3): 495-500.

[13] Kurtz, J. E., Hardy-Bessard, A. C., Deslandres, M., et al. Cetuximab, topotecan and cisplatin for the treatment of advanced cervical cancer: A phase II GINECO trial. *Gynecol. Oncol.* 2009; 113 (1): 16-20.

[14] Moore, K. N., Sill, M. W., Miller, D. S., McCourt, C., De Geest, K., Rose, P. G., et al. A phase I trial of tailored radiation therapy with concomitant cetuximab and cisplatin in

the treatment of patients with cervical cancer: A gynecologic oncology group study. *Gynecol. Oncol.* 2012; 127 (3): 456-61.

[15] Monk, B. J., Mas Lopez, L., Zarba, J. J., et al. Phase II, open-label study of pazopanib or lapatinib monotherapy compared with pazopanib plus lapatinib combination therapy in patients with advanced and recurrent cervical cancer. *J. Clin. Oncol.* 2010; 28 (22): 3562-9.

[16] Prat, J., Gallardo, A., Cuatrecasas, M., Catasus, L. Endometrial carcinoma: pathology and genetics. *Pathology.* 2007; 39 (1): 72-87.

[17] Fleming, G. F., Sill, M. W., Darcy, K. M., et al. Phase II trial of trastuzumab in women with advanced or recurrent, HER2-positive endometrial carcinoma: a Gynecologic Oncology Group study. *Gynecol. Oncol.* 2010; 116 (1): 15-20.

[18] Santin, A. D., Bellone, S., Roman, J. J., McKenney, J. K., Pecorelli, S. Trastuzumab treatment in patients with advanced or recurrent endometrial carcinoma overexpressing HER2/neu. *Int. J. Gynaecol. Obstet.* 2008; 102 (2): 128-31.

[19] Ferlay, J., Shin, H. R., Bray, F., Forman, D., Mathers, C., Parkin, D. M. Estimates of worldwide burden of cancer in 2008: GLOBOCAN 2008. *Int. J. Cancer.* 2010; 127 (12): 2893-917.

[20] Specenier, P., Vermorken, J. B. Biologic therapy in head and neck cancer: a road with hurdles. *ISRN Oncol.* 2012; 2012: 163752.

[21] Adelstein, D. J., Li, Y., Adams, G. L., et al. An intergroup phase III comparison of standard radiation therapy and two schedules of concurrent chemoradiotherapy in patients with unresectable squamous cell head and neck cancer. *J. Clin. Oncol.* 2003; 21 (1): 92-8.

[22] Forastiere, A. A., Goepfert, H., Maor, M., et al. Concurrent chemotherapy and radiotherapy for organ preservation in advanced laryngeal cancer. *N. Engl. J. Med.* 2003; 349 (22): 2091-8.

[23] Vermorken, J. B., Mesia, R., Rivera, F., et al. Platinum-based chemotherapy plus cetuximab in head and neck cancer. *N. Engl. J. Med.* 2008; 359 (11): 1116-27.

[24] Vokes, E. E., Weichselbaum, R. R., Lippman, S. M., Hong, W. K. Head and neck cancer. *N. Engl. J. Med.* 1993; 328 (3): 184-94.

[25] Ang, K. K., Andratschke, N. H., Milas, L. Epidermal growth factor receptor and response of head-and-neck carcinoma to therapy. *Int. J. Radiat. Oncol. Biol. Phys.* 2004; 58 (3): 959-65.

[26] Chung, C. H., Zhang, Q., Hammond, E. M., et al. Integrating epidermal growth factor receptor assay with clinical parameters improves risk classification for relapse and survival in head-and-neck squamous cell carcinoma. *Int. J. Radiat. Oncol. Biol. Phys.* 2011; 81 (2): 331-8.

[27] Grandis, J. R., Tweardy, D. J. Elevated levels of transforming growth factor alpha and epidermal growth factor receptor messenger RNA are early markers of carcinogenesis in head and neck cancer. *Cancer Res.* 1993; 53 (15): 3579-84.

[28] Pomerantz, R. G., Grandis, J. R. The role of epidermal growth factor receptor in head and neck squamous cell carcinoma. *Curr. Oncol. Rep.* 2003; 5 (2): 140-6.

[29] Temam, S., Kawaguchi, H., El-Naggar, A. K., et al. Epidermal growth factor receptor copy number alterations correlate with poor clinical outcome in patients with head and neck squamous cancer. *J. Clin. Oncol.* 2007; 25 (16): 2164-70.

[30] Sok, J. C., Coppelli, F. M., Thomas, S. M., et al. Mutant epidermal growth factor receptor (EGFRvIII) contributes to head and neck cancer growth and resistance to EGFR targeting. *Clin. Cancer Res.* 2006; 12 (17): 5064-73.

[31] Wheeler, S. E., Suzuki, S., Thomas, S. M., et al. Epidermal growth factor receptor variant III mediates head and neck cancer cell invasion via STAT3 activation. *Oncogene.* 2010; 29 (37): 5135-45.

[32] Chau, N. G., Perez-Ordonez, B., Zhang, K., et al. The association between EGFR variant III, HPV, p16, c-MET, EGFR gene copy number and response to EGFR inhibitors in patients with recurrent or metastatic squamous cell carcinoma of the head and neck. *Head Neck Oncol.* 2011; 3: 11.

[33] Gillison, M. L., Koch, W. M., Capone, R. B., et al. Evidence for a causal association between human papillomavirus and a subset of head and neck cancers. *J. Natl. Cancer Inst.* 2000; 92 (9): 709-20.

[34] Hong, A., Dobbins, T., Lee, C. S., et al. Relationships between epidermal growth factor receptor expression and human papillomavirus status as markers of prognosis in oropharyngeal cancer. *Eur. J. Cancer.* 2010; 46 (11): 2088-96.

[35] Young, R. J., Rischin, D., Fisher, R., et al. Relationship between epidermal growth factor receptor status, p16 (INK4A), and outcome in head and neck squamous cell carcinoma. *Cancer Epidemiol. Biomarkers Prev.* 2011; 20 (6): 1230-7.

[36] Kundu, S. K., Nestor, M. Targeted therapy in head and neck cancer. *Tumour Biol.* 2012; 33 (3): 707-21.

[37] Rao, S. D., Fury, M. G., Pfister, D. G. Molecular-targeted therapies in head and neck cancer. *Semin. Radiat. Oncol.* 2012; 22 (3): 207-13.

[38] Bonner, J. A., Raisch, K. P., Trummell, H. Q., et al. Enhanced apoptosis with combination C225/radiation treatment serves as the impetus for clinical investigation in head and neck cancers. *J. Clin. Oncol.* 2000; 18 (21 Suppl.): 47S-53S.

[39] Robert, F., Ezekiel, M. P., Spencer, S. A., et al. Phase I study of anti--epidermal growth factor receptor antibody cetuximab in combination with radiation therapy in patients with advanced head and neck cancer. *J. Clin. Oncol.* 2001; 19 (13): 3234-43.

[40] Bonner, J. A., Harari, P. M., Giralt, J., et al. Radiotherapy plus cetuximab for squamous-cell carcinoma of the head and neck. *N. Engl. J. Med.* 2006; 354 (6): 567-78.

[41] Bonner, J. A., Harari, P. M., Giralt, J., et al. Radiotherapy plus cetuximab for locoregionally advanced head and neck cancer: 5-year survival data from a phase 3 randomised trial, and relation between cetuximab-induced rash and survival. *Lancet Oncol.* 2010; 11 (1): 21-8.

[42] Mesia, R., Rueda, A., Vera, R., et al. Adjuvant therapy with cetuximab for locally advanced squamous cell carcinoma of the oropharynx: results from a randomized, phase II prospective trial. *Ann. Oncol.* 2013; 24 (2): 448-53.

[43] Langer, C. J., Lee, J. W., Patel, U. A., et al. Preliminary analysis of ECOG 3303: Concurrent radiation (RT), cisplatin (DDP) and cetuximab (C) in unresectable, locally advanced (LA) squamous cell carcinoma of the head and neck (SCCHN). *ASCO Meeting Abstracts.* 2008; 26 (15 suppl.): 6006.

[44] Ang, K. K., Zhang, Q. E., Rosenthal, D. I., et al. A randomized phase III trial (RTOG 0522) of concurrent accelerated radiation plus cisplatin with or without cetuximab for stage III-IV head and neck squamous cell carcinomas (HNC). *ASCO Meeting Abstracts.* 2011; 29 (15 suppl.): 5500.

[45] Ferris, R. L., Heron, D. E., Kim, S., et al. Induction docetaxel, cisplatin, and cetuximab (TPE) followed by concurrent radiotherapy, cisplatin, and cetuximab and maintenance cetuximab in patients with locoregionally advanced head and neck cancer (HNC): Mature results with HPV analysis. *ASCO Meeting Abstracts*. 2010; 28 (15 suppl.): 5515.

[46] Argiris, A., Heron, D. E., Smith, R. P., et al. Induction Docetaxel, Cisplatin, and Cetuximab Followed by Concurrent Radiotherapy, Cisplatin, and Cetuximab and Maintenance Cetuximab in Patients With Locally Advanced Head and Neck Cancer. *J. Clin. Oncol.* 2010; 28 (36): 5294-300.

[47] Lefebvre, J. L., Pointreau, Y., Rolland, F., et al. Induction chemotherapy followed by either chemoradiotherapy or bioradiotherapy for larynx preservation: the TREMPLIN randomized phase II study. *J. Clin. Oncol.* 2013; 31 (7): 853-9.

[48] Cohen, E. E. Role of epidermal growth factor receptor pathway-targeted therapy in patients with recurrent and/or metastatic squamous cell carcinoma of the head and neck. *J. Clin. Oncol.* 2006; 24 (17): 2659-65.

[49] Baselga, J., Trigo, J. M., Bourhis, J., et al. Phase II multicenter study of the antiepidermal growth factor receptor monoclonal antibody cetuximab in combination with platinum-based chemotherapy in patients with platinum-refractory metastatic and/or recurrent squamous cell carcinoma of the head and neck. *J. Clin. Oncol.* 2005; 23 (24): 5568-77.

[50] Trigo, J., Hitt, R., Koralewski, P., et al. Cetuximab monotherapy is active in patients (pts) with platinum-refractory recurrent/metastatic squamous cell carcinoma of the head and neck (SCCHN): Results of a phase II study. *ASCO Meeting Abstracts*. 2004; 22 (14 suppl.): 5502.

[51] Burtness, B., Goldwasser, M. A., Flood, W., Mattar, B., Forastiere, A. A. Phase III randomized trial of cisplatin plus placebo compared with cisplatin plus cetuximab in metastatic/recurrent head and neck cancer: an Eastern Cooperative Oncology Group study. *J. Clin. Oncol.* 2005; 23 (34): 8646-54.

[52] Hitt, R., Irigoyen, A., Cortes-Funes, H., Grau, J. J., Garcia-Saenz, J. A., Cruz-Hernandez, J. J. Phase II study of the combination of cetuximab and weekly paclitaxel in the first-line treatment of patients with recurrent and/or metastatic squamous cell carcinoma of head and neck. *Ann. Oncol.* 2012; 23 (4): 1016-22.

[53] Guigay, J., Fayette, J., Dillies, A.-F., et al. Cetuximab, docetaxel, and cisplatin (TPEx) as first-line treatment in patients with recurrent or metastatic (R/M) squamous cell carcinoma of the head and neck (SCCHN): Final results of phase II trial GORTEC 2008-03. *ASCO Meeting Abstracts*. 2012; 30 (15 suppl.): 5505.

[54] Herbst, R. S., Arquette, M., Shin, D. M., et al. Phase II multicenter study of the epidermal growth factor receptor antibody cetuximab and cisplatin for recurrent and refractory squamous cell carcinoma of the head and neck. *J. Clin. Oncol.* 2005; 23 (24): 5578-87.

[55] Vermorken, J. B., Trigo, J., Hitt, R., et al. Open-label, uncontrolled, multicenter phase II study to evaluate the efficacy and toxicity of cetuximab as a single agent in patients with recurrent and/or metastatic squamous cell carcinoma of the head and neck who failed to respond to platinum-based therapy. *J. Clin. Oncol.* 2007; 25 (16): 2171-7.

[56] Licitra, L., Storkel, S., Kerr, K. M., V et al. Predictive value of epidermal growth factor receptor expression for first-line chemotherapy plus cetuximab in patients with head

and neck and colorectal cancer: analysis of data from the EXTREME and CRYSTAL studies. *Eur. J. Cancer*. 2013; 49 (6): 1161-8.
[57] Pirker, R., Pereira, J. R., Szczesna, A., et al. Cetuximab plus chemotherapy in patients with advanced non-small-cell lung cancer (FLEX): an open-label randomised phase III trial. *The Lancet*. 2009; 373 (9674): 1525-31.
[58] Schneider-Merck, T., Lammerts van Bueren, J. J., Berger, S., et al. Human IgG2 antibodies against epidermal growth factor receptor effectively trigger antibody-dependent cellular cytotoxicity but, in contrast to IgG1, only by cells of myeloid lineage. *J. Immunol*. 2010; 184 (1): 512-20.
[59] Wirth, L. J., Allen, A. M., Posner, M. R., et al. Phase I dose-finding study of paclitaxel with panitumumab, carboplatin and intensity-modulated radiotherapy in patients with locally advanced squamous cell cancer of the head and neck. *Ann. Oncol*. 2010; 21 (2): 342-7.
[60] Kono, S. A., Haigentz, M. Jr, Yom, S. S., Saba, N. EGFR Monoclonal Antibodies in the Treatment of Squamous Cell Carcinoma of the Head and Neck: A View beyond Cetuximab. *Chemother. Res. Pract*. 2012; 2012: 901320.
[61] Bastholt, L., Specht, L., Jensen, K., et al. Phase I/II clinical and pharmacokinetic study evaluating a fully human monoclonal antibody against EGFr (HuMax-EGFr) in patients with advanced squamous cell carcinoma of the head and neck. *Radiother. Oncol*. 2007; 85 (1): 24-8.
[62] Rodriguez, M. O., Rivero, T. C., del Castillo Bahi, R., et al. Nimotuzumab plus radiotherapy for unresectable squamous-cell carcinoma of the head and neck. *Cancer Biol. Ther*. 2010; 9 (5): 343-9.
[63] Babu, K. G., Viswanath, L., Reddy, B. K., et al. An open-label, randomized, study of h-R3mAb (nimotuzumab) in patients with advanced (stage III or IVa) squamous cell carcinoma of head and neck (SCCHN): Four-year survival results from a phase IIb study. *ASCO Meeting Abstracts*. 2010; 28 (15 suppl.): 5530.
[64] Dienstmann, R., Tolcher, A. W., Papadopoulos, K. P., et al. Phase I trial of the first-in-class EGFR antibody mixture, Sym004, in patients with advanced solid tumors. *ASCO Meeting Abstracts*. 2011; 29 (15 suppl.): 3089.
[65] Machiels, J.-P. H., Specenier, P. M., Krauss, J., et al. Sym004, a novel strategy to target EGFR with an antibody mixture, in patients with advanced SCCHN progressing after anti-EGFR monoclonal antibody: A proof of concept study. *ASCO Meeting Abstracts*. 2013; 31 (15 suppl.): 6002.
[66] Stewart, J. S., Cohen, E. E., Licitra, L., et al. Phase III study of gefitinib compared with intravenous methotrexate for recurrent squamous cell carcinoma of the head and neck [corrected]. *J. Clin. Oncol*. 2009; 27 (11): 1864-71.
[67] Soulieres, D., Senzer, N. N., Vokes, E. E., Hidalgo, M., Agarwala, S. S., Siu, L. L. Multicenter phase II study of erlotinib, an oral epidermal growth factor receptor tyrosine kinase inhibitor, in patients with recurrent or metastatic squamous cell cancer of the head and neck. *J. Clin. Oncol*. 2004; 22 (1): 77-85.
[68] Yonesaka, K., Zejnullahu, K., Okamoto, I., et al. Activation of ERBB2 signaling causes resistance to the EGFR-directed therapeutic antibody cetuximab. *Sci. Transl. Med*. 2011; 3 (99): 99ra86.
[69] Harrington, K. J., Berrier, A., Robinson, M., et al. Phase II study of oral lapatinib, a dual-tyrosine kinase inhibitor, combined with chemoradiotherapy (CRT) in patients

(pts) with locally advanced, unresected squamous cell carcinoma of the head and neck (SCCHN). *ASCO Meeting Abstracts*. 2010; 28(15 suppl.): 5505.

[70] Del Campo, J. M., Hitt, R., Sebastian, P., et al. Effects of lapatinib monotherapy: results of a randomised phase II study in therapy-naive patients with locally advanced squamous cell carcinoma of the head and neck. *Br. J. Cancer*. 2011; 105 (5): 618-27.

[71] De Souza, J. A., Davis, D. W., Zhang, Y., et al. A phase II study of lapatinib in recurrent/metastatic squamous cell carcinoma of the head and neck. *Clin. Cancer Res*. 2012; 18 (8): 2336-43.

[72] Li, D., Ambrogio, L., Shimamura, T., et al. BIBW2992, an irreversible EGFR/HER2 inhibitor highly effective in preclinical lung cancer models. *Oncogene*. 2008; 27 (34): 4702-11.

[73] Yap, T. A., Vidal, L., Adam, J., et al. Phase I trial of the irreversible EGFR and HER2 kinase inhibitor BIBW 2992 in patients with advanced solid tumors. *J. Clin. Oncol*. 2010; 28 (25): 3965-72.

In: Fighting Lung Cancer through the HER Family ... ISBN: 978-1-63321-092-9
Editor: Diego Márquez-Medina

Chapter 17

Other Malignancies III. Digestive Tract

Teresa Taberner-Bonastre, M.D.
Medical Oncology Department,
Instituto Madrileño de Oncología of Madrid, Spain

Abstract

Targeted drugs against the Human Epidermal Growth Factor (HER) family of surface receptors (EGFR, HER2, HER3 and HER4) have been recently added to the anticancer pharmaceutical repertoire. The present chapter reviews the advances in the treatment of digestive malignancies that involve the anti-HER therapies. The role of monoclonal antibodies such as trastuzumab, cetuximab or panitumumab, and of tyrosine kinase inhibitors is extensively discussed.

1. Colorectal Cancer

Colorectal cancer (CRC) is the second most common malignance among European women (after breast cancer), and the third among European men (after lung and prostate cancer). However, CRC is the most common malignancy when both genders are taken together. More than 400,000 new cases are diagnosed in Europe every year, representing an annual incidence of 30-40 cases per 100,000 habitants. In 2012, over 14,000 patients died in Spain due to CRC [1].

The expression of the Epidermal Growth Factor Receptor (EGFR) in metastatic CRC widely ranges from 25% to 77%, and it has been associated with a poor prognosis [5, 6].

1.1. Cetuximab

Cetuximab, a chimeric murine/human IgG1 monoclonal antibody (mAB), promotes the EGFR internalization, and blocks the EGFR dimerization, phosphorylation, and signal transduction. The NCIC-CTG.CO.17 trial explored the efficacy of cetuximab as the third line of therapy in 572 EGFR-overexpressed metastatic CRC. Patients were previously treated (or contraindicated to be treated) with fluoropyrimidines, irinotecan, and oxaliplatin, and they were randomized to receive best supportive care with or without cetuximab. Cetuximab provided a clinical benefit in 39.4% of cases, and improved both progression-free (PFS) ($p < 0.001$) and overall survival (OS) (6.1 months versus 4.6 months; $p = 0.005$) [3].

Cunningham et al. [4] randomized 329 metastatic CRC progressing to irinotecan-based chemotherapy to receive cetuximab plus irinotecan or cetuximab alone (permitting the addition of irinotecan at disease progression). The response rate (RR) (22.9% versus 10.8%; $p = 0.007$), time to progression (4.1 months versus 1.5 months, $p < 0.001$), and median survival (8.6 months versus 6.9 months; $p = 0.48$) were significantly higher in the combination arm.

The EPIC trial [28] randomized 1,298 metastatic CRC previously treated with fluoropyrimidine, and oxaliplatin to receive second line irinotecan with or without cetuximab. Cetuximab improved the RR (16.4% versus 4.2%; $p < 0.0001$), PFS (4 months versus 2.6 months; HR 0.692, 95% CI 0.617-0.776; $p = 0.0001$), and quality of life of the patients ($p = 0.047$). However, there were no significant differences in OS (10.7 months versus 10 months; HR 0.975, 95% CI 0.854-1.114; $p = 0.71$), probably due to the administration of post-study cetuximab in 46.9% of patients from the irinotecan arm. Cetuximab related toxicity included rash, diarrhea, hypomagnesaemia, and electrolyte imbalances.

KRAS mutations are presented in 35-45% of CRC [2]. Both KRAS and NRAS proteins are involved in EGFR-triggered signaling pathways. *RAS* mutations result in constitutionally active NRAS and KRAS proteins that cannot be blocked by the EGFR inhibition. Accordingly, the benefit of cetuximab is limited to *KRAS* wild-type CRC [6]. The phase II OPUS trial [7] randomized 315 *KRAS* evaluable metastatic CRC to receive first line FOLFOX with or without cetuximab. Cetuximab significantly improved the RR ($p = 0.0027$) and PFS ($p = 0.0064$) of *KRAS* wild-type tumors only, and presented a favorable effect on survival. The CRYSTAL trial [8, 9] randomized 1,198 EGFR positive metastatic CRC to receive FOLFIRI alone or FOLFIRI plus cetuximab. The PFS was longer in the combination arm (HR 0.85, 95% CI 0.72-0.99; $p = 0.048$), and there was no significant impact in the OS (HR 0.93, 95% CI 0.81-1.07; $p = 0.31$). *KRAS* wild-type patients obtained a higher RR ($p = 0.03$), and a longer PFS (HR 0.68, 95% CI 0.5-0.94) in the combination arm. The NORDIC VII trial [10] randomized 571 metastatic CRC to receive FLOX or continuous/intermittent FLOX plus cetuximab. *KRAS* mutations were present in 39% of the tumors. Cetuximab did not obtain significant improvements in PFS (7.9 months versus 8.3 months versus 7.3 months, respectively) or OS (20.4 months versus 19.7 months versus 20.3 months, respectively).

The COIN trial [11] randomized 1,630 metastatic CRC to receive oxaliplatin and fluoropyrimidine with or without cetuximab. In *KRAS* wild-type patients (N= 729), cetuximab did not modify the PFS (8.6 months versus 8.6 months; HR 0.96, 95% CI 0.82-1.12; $p = 0.6$) or the OS (17.9 months versus 17 months; HR 1.04, 95% CI 0.87-1.23; $p = 0.67$). The RR (57% versus 64%; $p = 0.049$), skin and gastrointestinal toxic effects were increased with the addition cetuximab. Patients with *KRAS*, *BRAF* or *NRAS* mutations presented a worse prognosis than the *KRAS* wild-type ones.

The head-to-head FIRE-3 trial [12] compared the first line treatment with FOLFIRI plus cetuximab versus FOLFIRI plus bevacizumab in 336 metastatic CRC. No significant differences between cetuximab and bevacizumab were observed in the RR (44% versus 48%), the PFS (7.5 months versus 8.9 months; HR 1), or the OS (22.7 months versus 18.7 months;

HR 0.86). However, cetuximab provided a higher benefit on survival in *KRAS* wild type patients.

The benefit on RR by adding cetuximab to conventional chemotherapy has been explored in order to improve the resectability of liver metastases. The CELIM trial [13] randomized 114 metastatic CRC with non-resectable liver metastases only to receive cetuximab with either FOLFOX6 or FOLFIRI. The patients were periodically reassessed and liver surgery was offered if it was considered feasible. The objective RR was 68% versus 57%, respectively. R0 resections were performed in 38% and 30% of patients, respectively. Moreover, a retrospective analysis revealed a higher incidence of objective responses among *KRAS* wild-type patients (70% versus 41%; OR 3.42, 95% CI 1.35-8.66; p= 0.008), and an increase of resectability from 32% to 60% after induction treatment (p<0.0001).

1.2. Panitumumab

Panitumumab is a fully human IgG2 recombinant mAB with a high affinity for EGFR, whose toxic profile includes asthenia, anorexia, dermatitis and acneiform rash. In second/third line of treatment, the addition of panitumumab to chemotherapy increased both the RR and PFS. Peeters et al. [14] randomized 1,186 metastatic CRC progressing to one prior combination of chemotherapy to receive FOLFIRI with or without panitumumab. *KRAS* status was available for 91% of patients (55% *KRAS* wild-type). Panitumumab increased the RR (35% versus 10%) and PFS (5.9 months versus 3.9 months; HR 0.73; 95% CI 0.59-0.9; p= .004) in the *KRAS* wild-type patients. There was only a trend to improve the OS (14.5 months versus 12.5 months; HR 0.85, 95% CI 0.7-1.04; p= 0.12), maybe because 31% of patients in the FOLFIRI arm received subsequent anti-EGFR treatment. The efficacy of both arms of treatment was similar in *KRAS*-mutant patients. In the third line of treatment, 463 EGFR-positive metastatic CRC were randomized to receive best supportive care with or without panitumumab [15, 16]. Panitumumab improved PFS, but not OS. However, 76% of patients in the best supportive care arm received panitumumab on progression [17-19].

The phase III PRIME trial [20] randomized 1,183 metastatic CRC to receive first line FOLFOX4 with or without panitumumab. Data were prospectively analyzed on an intent-to-treat basis by *KRAS* status (93% of the patients). In the *KRAS* wild-type subgroup of patients, panitumumab increased the PFS (9.6 months versus 8 months; HR 0.8, 95% CI 0.66-0.97; p= 0.02) but not the OS (23.9 months versus 19.7 months; HR 0.83, 95% CI 0.67-1.02; p= 0.072). However, panitumumab reduced the PFS of *KRAS*-mutant patients.

In the induction setting, panitumumab was combined with XELOX in a series of 49 CRC with liver metastases [21]. The overall RR was 54%, including two complete responses, 23 partial responses, and 14 patients with stable disease. *KRAS* wild-type patients presented an overall RR of 65%.

2. Gastric Cancer

Gastric cancer (GC) is the fourth most common cancer worldwide, and the second leading cause of cancer death. The incidence and lethality of GC is decreasing in the developed countries. However, in 2012, over 5,300 and 1,720 patients died in Spain due to GC and esophageal cancer, respectively [22-24]. The standard of care for advanced GC includes fluoracil, cisplatin or oxaliplatin-based chemotherapy [25].

2.1. Anti-HER2 Therapies

The HER2 expression in gastroesophageal cancers widely varies from 2% to 45%. Malignancies from the gastro-esophageal junction (GEJC) present a higher HER2 expression than in the rest of GC (24-25% versus 9.5-12%) [26-28].

a) Trastuzumab

Trastuzumab, a humanized mAB against the HER2, was the first targeted therapy to demonstrate a survival benefit in GC and GEJC. Two Spanish phase II trials [29, 30] including 43 chemonaïve HER2-overexpressed advanced GC reported 32% RR, 64% disease control rate, and a favorable toxicity profile by combining first line cisplatin with trastuzumab.

Another phase II trial [31] reported 54.5% RR in 16 GC treated with trastuzumab, cisplatin and fluorouracil. The phase III Trastuzumab for Gastric Cancer (TOGA) trial [32] randomized 594 *HER2*-overexpressed or -amplified GC and GEJC to receive six cycles of capecitabine or fluorouracil plus cisplatin with or without trastuzumab. The OS was significantly higher in the trastuzumab arm (13.8 months versus 11.1 months; HR 0.74. 95% CI 0.60-0.91; p= 0.0046), with no significant worsening of tolerance.

b) Lapatinib

Lapatinib is a dual oral tyrosine kinase inhibitor of the HER1 and 2 receptors, with a modest first line activity in unselected and HER2-overexpressed GC [33, 34]. Lapatinib alone achieved 0-7% RR, 8-20% disease stabilization rate, and 5 months OS only. However, the combination of lapatinib and capecitabine as first line treatment for HER2-overexpressed metastatic GC, obtained 22-24% RR, and 34-45% disease stabilization rate [35, 36].

The ongoing phase III LOGIC and TYTAN trials will evaluate the combination of lapatinib and chemotherapy in advanced GC. The LOGIC trial [37] analyzing the combination of capecitabine/oxaliplatin with or without lapatinib as first-line therapy could provide survival data this year.

The TYTAN trial (N= 430) [38] compared the efficacy of paclitaxel with or without lapatinib as second-line therapy for GC. Lapatinib prolonged the OS (11 months versus 8.9 months) in the whole series, and this benefit become significant (14 months) in HER2-overexpressed patients.

c) Other Therapies

Pertuzumab, radiotherapy or DM1-conjugated trastuzumab, and pan-HER tyrosine kinase inhibitors such as dacomitinib and afatinib are being explored in GC [39].

2.2. Anti-EGFR Therapies

a) Cetuximab

The EGFR is overexpressed in 27-44% of GC and 30-60% of GEJC [40]. Several phase II trials have explored the combination of chemotherapy plus cetuximab as first line treatments for GC [41-44].

The DOCETUX trial [45] analyzed the combination of cetuximab plus cisplatin and docetaxel followed by cetuximab maintenance if clinical benefit in 72 untreated patients with advanced GC or GEJC. The overall RR was 41.2%, time to progression was 5 months, and median survival was 9 months, with a tolerable toxic profile.

A prospective Korean trial (N= 38) [46] combined cetuximab with modified FOLFOX6 regimen as first-line treatment for advanced GC. The RR was 50%, time to progression was 5.5 months, and OS was 9.9 months. The RR was significantly higher in patients with EGFR expression and low serum EGF and TGF-alpha levels (100% versus 37%; $p < 0.001$). No *EGFR* amplification or *KRAS* mutations were observed. The phase III EXPAND trial [47] randomized 904 locally advanced or metastatic GC or GEJC to receive first-line capecitabine plus cisplatin with or without cetuximab. The addition of cetuximab slightly increased the PFS (5.6 months versus 4.4 months; HR 1.09, 95% CI 0.92-1.29; p= 0.32), and worsened the toxic profile (diarrhea, hypokalemia, hypomagnesaemia, rash, and hand-foot syndrome).

b) Panitumumab

The addition of panitumumab does not improve the efficacy of chemotherapy in GC and GEJC. The phase II REAL trial reported a promising combination of epirubicin, oxaliplatin and capecitabine with panitumumab. However, in the next phase III trial [48], the addition of panitumumab decreased the OS in comparison to conventional chemotherapy. Those negative results were discussed to be due to the low dose intensity of chemotherapy in the panitumumab arm and to the recruitment of an unselected population. The REAL-3 trial [49] enrolled 553 untreated advanced GEJC to receive epirubicin, oxaliplatin and capecitabine or the same regimen with modified-doses and panitumumab. The recruitment was halted after a preplanned independent data monitoring committee review and panitumumab was withdrawn because OS decreased (11.3 months versus 8.8 months; HR 1.37, 95% CI 1.07-1.76; p= 0.013) and toxicity (diarrhea, rash, mucositis, and hypomagnesaemia) increased in the cetuximab arm.

c) Other anti-EGFR mAB

Randomized phase II trials have reported the promising activity of nimotuzumab, a humanized IgG-1 anti-EGFR mAb, in combination with irinotecan in GC progressing to fluorouracil-based chemotherapy [50], or in combination with cisplatin and S1 in the first line setting [51]. Matuzumab has been also preliminary reported to be an effective drug in phase I-II trials [52, 53].

d) EGFR Tyrosine Kinase Inhibitors

The combination of radiotherapy and erlotinib was explored in elderly patients with esophageal or GEJC (N= 17) [54], providing 35% RR, 4.5 months PFS, 7.3 months OS, and 29% estimated 1-year OS. The combination of erlotinib and FOLFOX as the first line therapy for advanced adenocarcinoma of the esophagus and GEJC (N= 33) provided 51.5% objective RR, 5.5 months PFS, and 11 months OS, with an acceptable toxicity profile [82]. The phase II SWOG-0127 trial [55] suggested that erlotinib obtained a higher RR (9% versus 0) and survival benefit (6.7 months versus 3.5 months) in GEJC than in GC.

Gefitinib alone has been explored in a phase II study [56] including 75 patients with GC or GEJC. Disease control was 18.3% only. Gefitinib in combination with cisplatin, fluorouracil, surgery, and radiation was applied to 80 locally advanced esophageal or GEJC, and compared with historical series without gefitinib. The disease control rate (40% versus 32%, p= 0.33), local control rate (76% versus 77%, p= 0.74), and 3-year OS (42% versus 28%, p= 0.06) trended to be higher in gefitinib treated patients [57].

3. Pancreatic Cancer

The incidence of pancreatic cancer (PC) in Europe and Spain is 58,000 and 6,367 new cases per year, respectively. However, PC is the fourth leading cause of cancer deaths in Europe and EEUU [58]. The EGFR expression is common in PC, and anti-EGFR therapies have been exhaustively explored in this malignancy.

3.1. EGFR Tyrosine Kinase Inhibitors

The combination of capecitabine plus erlotinib has been reported to obtain a promising RR in PC patients progressing to a first line therapy with gemcitabine [59]. The phase III Canadian PA.3 trial [60-62] randomized 569 advanced PC to receive the standard first line gemcitabine therapy with or without erlotinib. No differences in RR were observed. However, the PFS (HR 0.77, 95% CI 0.64-0.92; p= 0.004), OS (6.24 months versus 5.91 months; HR 0.82, 95% CI 0.69-0.99; p= 0.038), and 1-year OS (23% versus 17%; p= 0.023) were higher in the erlotinib arm. The Hellenic Cooperative Oncology Group analyzed the combination of gefitinib and gemcitabine as first line therapy for 53 inoperable or metastatic PC [63], reporting a 4.1 months PFS, 7.3 months OS, and 27% 1-year OS.

The EGFR tyrosine kinase inhibitors are potent radiosensitizing agents. So, erlotinib or gefitinib have been combined with radiation in order to explore an eventual role in the adjuvant setting [64-67]. They increased the ratio of local control, but resulted in very toxic combinations.

3.2. EGFR Monoclonal Antibodies

In a phase II trial [68] including 41 EGFR positive PC, the combination of cetuximab and gemcitabine obtained 12% RR, and 75% clinical benefit. The median time to progression was 3.8 months (1-year PFS 12%), OS was 7.1 months (1-year OS 31.7%), and main adverse events included rash, emesis, weight loss, and diarrhea.

The Southwest Oncology Group [69] randomized 745 unresectable locally advanced or metastatic PA to receive gemcitabine with or without cetuximab. No significant differences in the RR, PFS and OS (6.3 months versus 5.9 months, respectively; HR 1.06, 95% CI 0.91-1.23; p= 0.23) were observed. The addition of cetuximab to docetaxel and irinotecan did not achieve any benefit in a phase II trial from the Eastern Cooperative Oncology Group [70].

References

[1] Zacharakis M, Xynos ID, Lazaris A, et al. Predictors of survival in stage IV metastatic colorectal cancer. *Anticancer Res.* 2010; 30 (2): 653-60.

[2] Messa C, Russo F, Caruso MG, Di Leo A. EGF, TGF-, and EGF-R in human colorectal adenocarcinoma. *Acta Oncol.* 1998; 37: 285-9.

[3] Jonker DJ, O´Callaghan CJ, Karapetis CS, et al. Cetuximab for the treatment of colorectal cancer. *N. Engl. J. Med.* 2007; 357 (20): 2040-8.

[4] Cunningham D, Humblet Y, Siena S, et al. Cetuximab monotherapy and cetuximab plus irinotecan in irinotecan-refractory metastatic colorectal cancer. *N. Engl. J. Med.* 2004; 351 (4): 337-45.

[5] Sobrero AF, Manuel J, Fehrenbacher L, et al. EPIC: phase III trial of cetuximab plus irinotecan after fluoropyrimidine and oxaliplatin failure in patients with metastasic colorectal cancer. *J. Clin. Oncol.* 2008; 26: 2311-9.

[6] Tol J, Punt CJ. Monoclonal antibodies in the treatment of metastatic colorectal cancer: a review. *Clin. Ther.* 2010; 32 (3): 437-53.

[7] Bokemeyer C, Bondarenko I, Hartmann JT, et al. Efficacy according to biomarker status of cetuximab plus FOLFOX-4 as first-line treatment for metastatic colorectal cancer: the OPUS study. *Ann. Oncol.* 2011; 22 (7): 1535-46.

[8] Van Cutsem E, Köhne CH, Hitre E, et al. Cetuximab and chemotherapy as initial treatment for metastatic colorectal cancer. *N. Engl. J. Med.* 2009; 360: 1408-17.

[9] Van Cutsem E, Rougier P, Köhne CH, Stroch C, Schlichting M, Bokemeyer C. A meta-analysis of the CRYSTAL and OPUS studies combining cetuximab with chemotherapy (CT) as 1st- line treatment for patients with metastatic colorectal cancer: results according to KRAS and BRAF mutation status. *Eur. J. Cancer Suppl.* 2009; 7: 345.

[10] Tveit KM, Guren T, Glimelius B, et al. Randomized phase III study of 5-fluoracil/folinate/oxaliplatin given continuously or intermittently with or without cetuximab, as first-line treatment of metastatic colorectal cancer: The NORDIC VII study (NCT00145314), by the Nordic Colorectal Cancer Biomodulation Group. *Ann. Oncol.* 2009; 21 (Suppl 8): VIII9.

[11] Maughan TS, Adams RA, Smith CG, et al. Addition of cetuximab to oxaliplatin-based first-line combination chemotherapy for treatment of advanced colorectal cancer: results of the randomised phase 3 MRC COIN trial. *Lancet.* 2011; 377 (9783): 2103-14.

[12] Stintzing S, Fischer von Weikersthal L, et al. FOLFIRI plus cetuximab versus FOLFIRI plus bevacizumab as first-line treatment for patients with metastatic colorectal cancer-subgroup analysis of patients with KRAS: mutated tumours in the randomised German AIO study KRK-0306. *Ann. Oncol.* 2012; 23 (7): 1693-9.

[13] Folprecht G, Gruenberger T, Hartmann JT, et al. Tumour response and secondary resectability of colorectal liver metastases following neoadjuvant chemotherapy with cetuximab: the CELIM randomised phase 2 trial. *Lancet Oncol.* 2010; 11 (1): 38-47.

[14] Peeters M, Price TJ, Cervantes A, et al. Randomized phase III study of panitumumab with fluoracil, leucovorin and irinotecan (FOLFIRI) compared with FOLFIRI alone as second- line treatment in patients with metastatic colorectal cancer. *J. Clin. Oncol.* 2010; 28: 4706-13.

[15] Van Cutsem E, Peeters M, Siena S, et al. Open-label phase III trial of panitumumab plus best supportive care compared with best supportive care alone in patients with chemotherapy- refractory metastatic colorectal cancer. *J. Clin. Oncol.* 2007; 25: 1658-64.

[16] Van Cutsem E, Siena S, Humblet Y, et al. An open-label single-arm study assessing safety and efficacy of panitumumab in patients with metastatic colorectal cancer refractory to standard chemotherapy. *Ann. Oncol.* 2008; 19: 92-8.

[17] Siena S, Peeters M, Van Cutsem E, et al. Association of progression- free survival with patient- reported outcomes and survival: results from a randomized phase 3 trial of panitumumab. *Br. J. Cancer.* 2007; 97: 1469-74.

[18] Amado RG, Wolf M, Peeters M, et al. Wild-Type KRAS is required for panitumumab efficacy in patients with metastatic colorectal cancer. *J. Clin. Oncol.* 2008; 26: 1626-34.

[19] Peeters M, Siena S, Van Cutsem E, et al. Association of progression-free survival, overall survival, and patients-reported outcomes by skin toxicity and KRAS status in patients receiving panitumumab monotherapy. *Cancer.* 2009; 115: 1544-54.

[20] Douillard JY, Siena S, Cassidy J, et al. Randomized phase III trial of panitumumab with infusional fluoracil, leucovorin, and oxaliplatin (FOLFOX4) versus FOLFOX4 alone as first-line treatment in patients with previously untreated metastatic colorectal cancer: the PRIME study. *J. Clin. Oncol.* 2010; 28: 4697-705.

[21] Leone F, Artale S, Marino D, et al. Panitumumab in combination with infusional oxaliplatin and oral capecitabine for conversion therapy in patients with colon cancer and advanced liver metastases. The Metapan Study. *Cancer.* 2013; 119 (19): 3429-35.

[22] Luis M, Tavares A, Carvalho LS, Lara-Santos L, Araújo A, de Mello RA. Personalizing therapies for gastric cancer: molecular mechanisms and novel targeted therapies. *World J. Gastroenterol.* 2013; 19 (38): 6383- 97.

[23] Kamangar F, Dores GM, Anderson WF. Patterns of cancer incidence, mortality, and prevalence across five continents: defining priorities to reduce cancer disparities in different geographic regions of the world. *J. Clin. Oncol.* 2006; 24: 2137-50.

[24] Kelley JR, Duggan JM. Gastric cancer epidemiology and risk factors. *J. Clin. Epidemiol.* 2003; 56 (1): 1-9.

[25] Ajani JA, Moiseyenko VM, Tjulandin et al. Clinical benefit with docetaxel plus fluorouracil and cisplatin compared with cisplatin and fluorouracil in a phase III trial of advanced gastric or gastroesophageal cancer adenocarcinoma: the V-325 Study Group. *J. Clin. Oncol.* 2007; 25 (22): 3205-9.

[26] Sastre J, García-Saenz JA, Díaz-Rubio E. Chemotherapy for gastric cancer. *World J. Gastroenterol.* 2006; 12 (2): 2004-213.

[27] Field K, Michael M, Leong T. Locally advanced and metastatic gastric cancer: current management and new treatment developments. *Drugs.* 2008; 68 (3): 299-317.

[28] Sakai K, Mori S, Kawamoto T, et al. Expression of epidermal growth factor receptors on normal human gastric epithelia and gastric carcinomas. *J. Natl. Cancer Inst.* 1986; 77: 1047-52.

[29] Cortés-Funes H, Rivera F, Alés I, et al. Phase II of trastuzumab and cisplatin in patients with advanced gastric cancer with HER2/neu overexpression/ amplification. *J. Clin. Oncol.* 2007; 25: 1-2.

[30] Grávalos C, Gómez-Martín C, Rivera F, et al. Phase II study of trastuzumab and cisplatin as first-line therapy in patients with HER2-positive advanced gastric or gastroesophageal junction cancer. *Clin. Transl. Oncol.* 2011; 13: 179-84.

[31] Egamberdiev D, Djuraev M, Tuydjanova K, Nematov O. Our experience in the use of trastuzumab in patients with advanced stomach cancer. *Ann. Oncol.* 2010; 21 (Suppl 8): S839.

[32] Bang YJ, Van Cutsem E, Feyereislova A, et al. Trastuzumab in combination with chemotherapy for the treatment of HER2 positive advanced gastric or gastro-esophageal junction cancer (ToGA): a phase 3, open-label, randomised controlled trial. *Lancet.* 2010; 376: 687-97.

[33] qbal S, Goldman B, Fenoglio-Preiser CM, et al. Southwest Oncology Group study S0413: a phase II trial of lapatinib (GW572016) as first-line therapy in patients with advanced or metastatic gastric cancer. *Ann. Oncol.* 2011; 22: 2610-5.

[34] Hecht J, Urba S, Koehler M. Lapatinib monotherapy in recurrent upper gastrointestinal malignancy: phase II efficacy and biomarker analyses. ASCO Proceedings of the Gastrointestinal Cancers Symposium. 2008; 43: abstr 48.

[35] Lenz H, Zhang J, Kemner AM, Kaneko T, Yang D, Franklin N. Lapatinib capecitabine in advanced gastric cancer: An open-label phase II study of non ERBB2-targeted disease. *Ann. Oncol.* 2010; 21 (Suppl 8): S817.

[36] Pishvaian M, Sakaeva D, Hsieh R. A global, multi-center phase II trial of lapatinib plus capecitabine in gastric cancer. *J. Clin. Oncol.* 2011; 29 (Suppl 4): abstr 88.

[37] Hecht JR, Urba SG, Koehler M, Ellis C, Gagnon R, Kemner A. Lapatinib monotherapy in recurrent upper gastrointestinal malignancy: Phase II efficacy and biomarker analyses. *Proc. ASCO GI.* 2008: 43.

[38] Satoh T, Bang Y, Wang J, et al. Interim safety analysis from TYTAN: A phase III Asian study of lapatinib in combi- nation with paclitaxel as second-line therapy in gastric can- cer. *J. Clin. Oncol.* 2010; 28: 4057.

[39] Nam HJ, Ching KA, Kan J, et al. Evaluation of the antitumor effects and mechanisms of PF00299804, a pan-HER inhibitor, alone or in combination with chemotherapy or targeted agents in gastric cancer. *Mol. Cancer Ther.* 2012; 11: 439-51.

[40] Matsubara J, Nishina T, Yamada Y, et al. Impacts of excision repair cross-complementing gene 1 (ERCC1), dihydropyrimidine dehydrogenase, and epidermal growth factor receptor on the outcomes of patients with advanced gastric cancer. *Br. J. Cancer.* 2008; 98: 832-9.

[41] Han SW, Oh DY, Im SA, et al. Phase II study and biomarker analysis of cetuximab in combination with modified FOLFOX6 in advanced gastric cancer. *Br. J. Cancer.* 2009; 100: 298-304.

[42] Kim C, Lee JL, Ryu MH, et al. A prospective phase II study of cetuximab in combination with XELOX (capecitabine and oxaliplatin) in patients with metastatic and/or recurrent advanced gastric cancer. *Invest. New Drugs.* 2011; 29: 366-73.

[43] Kanzler S, Trarbach T, Seufferlein T, et al. Cetuximab with irinotecan/folinic acid/5-FU as first line treatment in advanced gastric cancer: A nonrandomized multicenter AIO phase II study. *J. Clin. Oncol.* 2009; 27: abstr 4534.

[44] Pinto C, Di Fabio, F, Siena S, et al. Phase II study of cetuximab in combination with FOLFIRI in patients with untreated advanced gastric or gastroesophageal junction adenocarcinoma (FOLCETUX study). *Ann. Oncol.* 2007; 18: 510-7.

[45] Pinto C, di Fabio F, Barone C, et al. Phase II of cetuximab in combination with cis/docetaxel as first-line treatment in patients with unresectable/metastatic gastric or gastroesophageal junction (GEJ) adenocarcinoma (DOCETUX study). *Br. J. Cancer.* 2009; 101: 1261-8.

[46] Han SW, Oh DY, Im SA, et al. Phase II study and biomarker analisis of cetuximab combined with modified FOLFOX6 in advanced gastric cancer. *Br. J. Cancer.* 2009; 100: 298-304.

[47] Lordick F, Kang YK, Chung HC, et al. Capecitabine and cisplatin with or without cetuximab for patients with previously untreated advanced gastric cancer (EXPAND): a randomised, open-label phase 3 trial. *Lancet Oncol.* 2013; 14 (6): 490-9.

[48] Chau I, Okines A, Gonzalez de Castro D, et al. REAL3: a multicenter randomized phase II/III trial of epirubicin, oxaliplatin, and capecitabine (EOC) versus modified (m) EOC plus panitumumab (P) in advanced oesophagogastric (OG) cancer – response rate (RR), toxicity, and molecular analysis from phase II. *J. Clin. Oncol.* 2011; 29 (Suppl): abstr 4131.

[49] Waddell T, Chau I, Cunningham D, et al. Epirubicin, oxaliplatin, and capecitabine with or without panitumumab for patients with previously untreated advanced oesophagogastric cancer (REAL3): a randomised, open-label phase 3 trial. *Lancet Oncol.* 2013; 14 (6): 481-9.

[50] Kim YH, Sasaki Y, Lee KH, et al. Randomized phase II study of nimotuzumab, an anti-EGFR antibody, plus iri in patients with 5-fluorouracil-based regimen-refractory advanced or recurrent gastric cancer in Korea and Japan: Preliminary results. *J. Clin. Oncol.* 2011; 29: abstr 87.

[51] Wang JW, Chi Y, Zheng Z, et al. Randomized, single-centered, phase II clinical trial of nimotuzumab plus cis and S-1 as first-line therapy in patients with advanced gastric cancer. *J. Clin. Oncol.* 2012; 30: e14668.

[52] Rao S, Starling N, Cunningham D, et al. Phase I study of epirubicin, cis and capecitabin plus matuzumab in previously untreated patients with advanced oesophagogastric cancer. *Br. J. Cancer.* 2008; 99: 868-74.

[53] Rao S, Starling N, Cunningham D, et al. Matuzumab plus epirubicin, cis and capecitabine (ECX) compared with epirubicin, cis and capecitabine alone as first-line treatment in patients with advanced oesophago-gastric cancer: A randomised, multicentre open-label phase II study. *Ann. Oncol.* 2010; 21: 2213-9.

[54] Iyer R, Chhatrala R, Shefter T, et al. Erlotinib and Radiation Therapy for Elderly Patients with Esophageal Cancer - Clinical and Correlative Results from a Prospective Multicenter Phase 2 Trial. *Oncology.* 2013; 85: 53-8.

[55] Wainberg ZA, Lin LS, DiCarlo B, et al. Phase II trial of modified FOLFOX6 and erlotinib in patients with metastatic or advanced adenocarcinoma. *Br. J. Cancer.* 2011; 105 (6): 760-5.

[56] Dragovic T, McCoy S, Fenoglio-Preiser CM, et al. Phase II trial of erlotinib in gastroesophageal junction and gastric adenocarcinomas: SWOG-0127. *J. Clin. Oncol.* 2006; 24 (30): 4922-7.

[57] Rodriguez CP, Adelstein DJ, Rice TW, et al. A phase II study of peri-operative concurrent chemotherapy, gefitinib, and hyperfractionated radiation followed by maintenance gefitinib in locoregionally advanced esophagus and gastroesophageal junction cancer. *J. Thorac. Oncol.* 2010; 5: 229-35.
[58] Oliveira-Cunha M, Newman WG, Siriwardena AK. Epidermal Growth Factor Receptor in Pancreatic Cancer. Review. *Cancers* 2011; 3:1513-26.
[59] Baselga J, Pfister D, Cooper MR, et al. Phase I studies of anti-epidermal growth factor receptor chimeric antibody C225 alone and in combination with cisplatin. *J. Clin. Oncol.* 2000; 18: 904-14.
[60] Moore MJ, Goldstein D, Hamm J, et al. Erlotinib plus gemcitabine compared with gemcitabine alone in patients with advanced pancreatic cancer. A phase III trial of the National Cancer Institute of Canada Clinical Trials Group. *J. Clin. Oncol.* 2007; 25: 1960-6.
[61] Aranda E, Manzano JL, Rivera F, et al. Phase II open- label study of erlotinib in combination with gemcitabine in unresectable and/or metastatic adenocarcinoma of the pancreas relationship between skin rash and survival (Pantar Study). *Ann. Oncol.* 2012; 23: 1919-25.
[62] Stepanski EJ, Reyes C, Walker MS, et al. The association of rash severity with overall survival: findings from patients receiving erlotinib for pancreatic cancer in the community setting. *Pancreas.* 2013; 42 (1): 32-6.
[63] Fountzilas G, Bobos M, Kalogera-Fountzila A, et al. Gemcitabine combined with gefitinib in patients with inoperable or metastatic pancreatic cancer *Cancer Invest.* 2008; 26 (8): 784-93.
[64] Loehrer PJ, Powell ME, Cardenes HR, et al. A randomized phase III study of gemcitabine in combination with radiation therapy versus gemcitabine alone in patients with localized, unresectable pancreatic cancer: E4201. *J. Clin. Oncol.* 2008; 26(15S): 4506.
[65] Iannitti D, Dipetrillo T, Akerman P, et al. Erlotinib and chemoradiation followed by maintenance erlotinib for locally advanced pancreatic cancer: a phase I study. *Am. J. Clin. Oncol.* 2005; 28 (6): 570-5.
[66] Czito BG, Willett CG, Bendell JC, et al. Increased toxicity with gefitinib, capecitabine, and radiation therapy in pancreatic and rectal cancer: phase I trial results. *J. Clin. Oncol.* 2006; 24: 656-62.
[67] Maurel J, Martin-Richard M, Conill C, et al. Phase I trial of gefitinib with concurrent radiotherapy and fixed 2-h gemcitabine infusion, in locally advanced pancreatic cancer. *Int. J. Radiat. Oncol. Biol. Phys.* 2006; 66: 1391-8.
[68] Xiong HQ, Rosenberg A, LoBuglio A, et al. Cetuximab, a monoclonal antibody targeting the epidermal growth factor receptor, in combination with gemcitabine for advanced pancreatic cancer: a multicenter phase II Trial. *J. Clin. Oncol.* 2004; 22: 2610-16.
[69] Philip PA, Benedetti J, Corless CL, et al: Phase III study comparing gemcitabine plus cetuximab versus gemcitabine in patients with advanced pancreatic adenocarcinoma: Southwest Oncology Group-Directed Intergroup Trial S0205. *J. Clin. Oncol.* 2010; 28: 3605-10.

[70] Burtness BA, Powell ME, Berlin D, et al. Phase II ECOG trial of irinotecan/docetaxel with or without cetuximab in metastatic pancreatic cancer: Updated survival and CA19–9 results. *J. Clin. Oncol.* 2008; 26 (Suppl): abstr 4642.

In: Fighting Lung Cancer through the HER Family … ISBN: 978-1-63321-092-9
Editor: Diego Márquez-Medina

Self-Correcting Test

Abbreviations

CT	computed tomography;
DFS	disease-free survival;
EGFR	epidermal growth factor receptor;
EGFR-TKI	tyrosine kinase inhibitor against the epidermal growth factor receptor;
EMT	Epithelial-to-mesenchymal transition;
HER	human epidermal growth factor receptor;
FFPE	formalin-fixed, paraffin-embedded samples;
IHC	immunochemistry;
NGS	next-generation sequencing;
NSCLC	non-small cell lung cancer;
OS	overall survival;
PFS	progression-free survival;

1. **Which of the following statements regarding lung cancer epidemiology is correct?**
    a) There are about 1.1 billion smokers worldwide and if there is no change in smoking patterns, the number will decrease to 0.6 billion by 2025.
    b) More than 80% of lung cancer patients are tobacco smokers, however, fewer than 5% of smokers develop lung carcinoma.
    c) Lung cancer is the most common cancer related to occupational exposure.
    d) Chronic obstructive pulmonary disease is not associated with an increased risk of lung cancer.
2. **Which of the following subtype of bronchogenic carcinoma is more likely associated with paraneoplastic syndromes?**
    a) Adenocarcinoma of the lung.
    b) Squamous cell carcinoma of the lung.
    c) Large cell lung cancer.
    d) Small cell lung cancer.

3. **Which of the following statements regarding lung cancer pathology is correct?**
    a) In 2011 the International Association for the Study of Lung Cancer/American Thoracic Society/European Respiratory Society introduced modifications in squamous lung cancer classification.
    b) Micropapillary invasive adenocarcinoma is recognised as a new histological subtype because of its favourable prognosis once resected.
    c) Advanced lung adenocarcinomas have predictive benefit for response rate and prognosis if *EGFR* mutation is present when EGFR-TKI therapy is applied.
    d) Small cell lung cancer is characterized by an aggressive course with metastatic disease at time of presentation but excellent response to chemotherapy.
4. **A 66-year-old man has had a chronic cough for the past year. He had an episode of hemoptysis 3 days ago. No abnormal findings are noted on physical examination. A chest x-ray demonstrates a subpleural 4 cm mass right upper lobe. A sputum sample is collected, and the sputum cytology report is negative for malignancy. Which is the initial tissue diagnostic technique modality?**
    a) CT-guided transthoracic fine needle aspiration.
    b) Endoscopic ultrasound guided fine needle aspiration.
    c) Endobronchial ultrasound guided fine needle aspiration.
    d) Videothoracoscopic lung biopsy.
5. **A 75-year-old man who has an 80 pack year history of cigarette smoking has had a chronic cough for the past 10 years. He lost weight (3 kg) during the past year. No abnormal findings are noted on physical examination. He has a chest radiograph that reveals a right hilar mass and right moderate pleural effusion. Which is the initial tissue diagnostic technique modality?**
    a) CT-guided transthoracic fine needle aspiration.
    b) Endoscopic ultrasound guided fine needle aspiration.
    c) Mediastinoscopy.
    d) Thoracentesis.
6. **What is the most appropriated treatment for a 72 years old patient diagnosed of lung adenocarcinoma with hemoptysis, liver metastases, ECOG performance status 1 and without driver mutations?**
    a) Carboplatin-paclitaxel-bevacizumab.
    b)) Cisplatin-Pemetrexed.
    c) Cisplatin-Gemcitabine.
    d) Carboplatin-paclitaxel.
7. **What of the following drugs is not approved for squamous-cell carcinoma?**
    a) Pemetrexed.
    b) Docetaxel.
    c) Bevacizumab.
    d) a and c.
8. **What treatment do you use for a patient with advanced NSCLC, squamous histology, ECOG performance status 2 and absence of mutations of *EGFR* who progressed to first line therapy?**
    a) Pemetrexed.

b) Docetaxel.
c) Erlotinib.
d) Cisplatin-gemcitabine.

9. Platinum-based doubled plus bevacizumab is an option for first line treatment in advanced NSCLC. What is false?

a) The use of bevacizumab is limited to patients with nonsquamous histology.
b) In the E4599 trial, treatment with bevacizumab showed a better progression free survival.
c) In the AVAiL trial, a significant improvement in overall survival was observed in patients treated with bevacizumab.
d) Treatment with bevacizumab of patients with squamous histology has been associated with an increased risk of pulmonary hemorrhage.

10. Regarding maintenance therapy indicates what is false:

a) In classical trial less than 33% of patients were included in the maintenance phase.
b) Immediate docetaxel after four cycles of platinum-based doublet increases PFS.
c) In the PARAMOUNT study, a statistically significant 22% reduction in the risk of death was observed.
d) In a meta-analysis, maintenance therapy did not show a statistically significant improvement in overall survival.

11. What is the sensitivity (% mutant alleles in a wild-type background) of Sanger Sequencing for detecting EGFR mutations?

a) 1%.
b) 5%.
c) 20%.
d) 50%.

12. In what state of preservation should samples be prior to performing mutational analysis profiling?

a) Snap-frozen samples.
b) Cytology.
c) FFPE samples.
d) All of the above

13. Is it possible to detect the mutational status of EGFR by IHC analysis?

a) No.
b) Yes, but only some splicing variants (EGFRvIII).
c) Yes, but only some mutations in exons 19 and 21.
d) Yes, by using some specific phospho-antibodies.

14. Which of the following technologies is based on multiplex analysis?

a) TaqMan assays
b) Sequenom OncoCarta assays.
c) Scorpion assays.
d) Bacon assays.

15. Which of the following instruments is not adapted to perform NGS technology?

a) COBAS Z480.
b) Ion Torrent.

c) MiSeq.
d) Junior^{TM}.

16. What is false?
a) Lung cancer occurs to a relatively small portion of smokers.
b) Radon has been related with lung cancer development.
c) Over the half of patients with lung cancer can be cured with conventional therapies.
d) Women are predisposed to lung cancer.

17. A higher incidence of *EGFR*-mutations have been reported in:
a) Young men.
b) Caucasian men.
c) Mine workers.
d) Elderly patients.

18. Squamous carcinomas of the lung:
a) Never harbor sensitizing *EGFR*-mutations.
b) Trend to be peripheral.
c) Could harbor sensitizing *EGFR*-mutations.
d) Are neuroendocrine tumors.

19. Human papillomavirus:
a) Affect birds, reptiles, and mammals.
b) Are small RNA viruses.
c) Produce tuberculosis.
d) Could be sexually passed on.

20. Sensitizing EGFR-mutations have not been related to:
a) Asian race.
b) Small cell histology.
c) Female gender.
d) Response to gefitinib.

21. The first molecular-targeted agent to be approved for the treatment of advanced NSCLC after failure of chemotherapy were:
a) Bevacizumab.
b) Gefitinib.
c) Erlotinib.
d) Gefitinib and Erlotinib.

22. The response rate to EGFR-TKI in *EGFR*-mutant non-small cell lung cancer exceeds:
a) 10%.
b) 50%.
c) 30%.
d) It depends on the control arm.

23. Sensitizing EGFR-mutations:
a) Increase the resistance to chemotherapy.
b) Increase the response rate to chemotherapy.
c) Increase the response rate to crizotinib.
d) None is true.

24. The IPASS and FIRST-SIGNAL trials demonstrated that:

a) Clinical criteria are as good as *EGFR* analysis to select patients to be treated with EGFR-TKI.
b) Molecular selection was better to predict response in Asian patients.
c) Molecular selection was better to predict response in Caucasian patients.
d) Clinical selection was better to predict response in Caucasian patients.

25. Benefit from EGFR-TKI is higher in:

a) First line therapy.
b) Second line therapy.
c) Maintenance therapy.
d) It is the same regardless the line of therapy.

26. Before starting therapy with EGFR-TKI:

a) Amplification of *EGFR* and *HER2* must be analyzed by FISH.
b) Amplification of *EGFR* must be analyzed by FISH.
c) Protein expression levels of EGFR must be determined by IHC.
d) Mutational analysis of the *EGFR* gene must be undertaken.

27. EGFR mutations:

a) Are always associated with sensitivity to EGFR-TKIs.
b) Are always associated with resistance to EGFR-TKIs.
c) Some are associated with resistance, but most of them are associated with sensitivity to EGFR-TKIs.
d) Are not associated with response to EGFR-TKIs.

28. *EGFR* mutations can be found:

a) Equally distributed along the 26 exons of the *EGFR* gene.
b) Only found on exon 19.
c) Only found on exon 21.
d) Mainly found on exons 19 and 21, but also on exons 18 and 20.

29. *EGFR* mutations can be detected:

a) Only by Sanger sequencing.
b) By several molecular methods with variable sensitivity.
c) Only by highly sensitive methods.
d) By FISH.

30. *EGFR* mutational status can be performed on:

a) Biopsies.
b) Cytological samples that have been paraffin-embedded.
c) Liquid cytological samples.
d) All the above are correct.

31. The following *EGFR* mutations are considered to be TKI-sensitive:

a) del19, L858R, T790M, exon 20 ins.
b) del19, L858R, ins19, G719X.
c) ins19, T790M, exon 20 ins.
d) del19, G719X, exon 20 ins.

32. A never smoker patient is admitted to the hospital with shortness of breath and found to have a right pleural effusion on chest X-ray. Thoracentesis is performed and the fluid analysis revealed a positive cytology of adenocarcinoma suggesting lung primary. After a pleural drainage, The CT-scan revealed a lung

mass in the lower right lobule with mediastinal lymph nodes. Select the correct answer:

a) The *EGFR* mutation status could be done in a sample of the pleural effusion.
b) This patient should start immediately chemotherapy.
c) Since the patient is a female, never smoker and has adenocarcinoma histology, the best approach is to start gefitinib, since the likelihood of having *EGFR* mutations is very high.
d) A lung biopsy is mandatory in order to obtain enough tissue to evaluate the *EGFR* mutations status.

33. **A 46-year-old woman, never smoker, comes to clinic to start treatment after being diagnosed of a stage IV lung adenocarcinoma. She is asymptomatic, but anxious to start treatment. Which of the following would be the best recommendation?**
    a) Take some time to perform the genotyping, which ideally should include *EGFR* and ALK.
    b) Start erlotinib immediately.
    c) Start chemotherapy immediately.
    d) Start chemotherapy and if the *EGFR* mutation turns positive, then switch to erlotinib.
34. **Which one of the following statements is true?**
    a) All the phase II trials comparing EGFR-TKI versus chemotherapy in *EGFR* mutant population have demonstrated a benefit in response rate, progression-free survival, overall survival and quality of life.
    b) All the phase II trials comparing EGFR-TKI versus chemotherapy in *EGFR* mutant population have demonstrated a benefit in response rate, progression-free survival, and quality of life.
    c) All the phase II trials comparing EGR-TKI versus chemotherapy in *EGFR* mutant population have demonstrated a benefit in response rate, overall survival and quality of life.
    d) All the phase II trials comparing EGFR-TKI versus chemotherapy in *EGFR* mutant population have demonstrated a benefit in response rate, and progression-free survival.
35. **Which one of the following statements is true when considering the *EGFR*-mutant population treatment?**
    a) As of today, no head-to-head comparison between EGFR-TKIs has been performed, but data suggest a greater benefit of gefitinib. This fact explains that gefitinib had been used in a greater number of clinical trials.
    b) Gefitinib should be used in Asian population and erlotinib should be recommended in Caucasian population.
    c) The recommendation of an specific EGFR-TKI depends mainly on the availability in every country.
    d) Afatinib should be recommended in preference to erlotinib and gefitinib since the LUX-Lung 6 results are more favorable compared to other trials and these results are applicable to both Asian and Caucasian population.

36. In reference to first-line treatment with EGFR-TKI in molecularly unselected populations, highlight the true answer:

a) In clinically selected patients such as the ones participating in the IPASS trial, mutational analysis in the available population revealed a proportion of 80% EGFR-mutant patients.

b) In the IPASS trial, Gefitinib showed non-inferiority compared to Carboplatin-Paclitaxel in clinically selected patients in the first-line setting.

c) In the First-Signal Trial, Gefitinib showed superiority compared to Cisplatin-Gemcitabine in a Korean never-smoking patients.

d) In chemotherapy-naïve Western patients unfit for platinum-based chemotherapy, vinorelbine has shown superiority when compared to Gefitinib.

37. When considering EGFR-TKI for maintenance or second-line therapy, which is the false answer?

a) The ISEL study evaluated the efficacy of Gefitinib versus placebo in the same context as the BR.21 trial.

b) In the BR.21 trial, the tumor response rate observed in the Erlotinib group was around 8%

c) In the BR.21 trial, a phase III, double blind, randomized trial in Western patients, the main benefits obtained from Erlotinib were observed in terms of Overall Survival and Disease Control Rate.

d) The TAILOR trial showed increased OS with Pemetrexed compared to Erlotinib in in the second-line setting.

38. Alterations in EGFR pathway signaling are a common finding in NSCLC. Find the false answer:

a) Expression of HER family receptors and their ligands has been linked to EGFR-TKI sensitivity in vitro.

b) Amphiregulin interacts with histone-deacetylases to promote activation of proapoptotic protein BAX, thus increasing growth inhibitory effects of EGFR-TKI in vitro.

c) Patients with Amphiregulin-positive tumors as determined by immunohistochemistry had longer OS compared to those Amphiregulin-negative in a retrospective analysis.

d) In a study conducted on tumor samples from the BR.21 trial, high circulating Amphiregulin levels were identified as an independent unfavourable prognostic factor.

39. EMT is a complex cellular program hijacked by cancer cells to invade and generate metastases. Which of the below written statements is false?

a) When undergoing EMT, a cell looses its polarity and detaches from the basal cell membrane.

b) EMT appears to be a reversible process, which may play an essential role in tumor heterogeneity and in tumor-stromal interactions.

c) Loss of tight junction proteins, such as E-cadherin and N-cadherin, precedes the acquisition of a mesenchymal phenotype.

d) Association of histone-deacetylase inhibitors and EGFR-TKI has shown benefit in preclinical models.

40. Many more discoveries will be made in the next years that will probably improve the outcomes of patients with advanced NSCLC. Until then… (One of the next is true)

a) MicroRNAs are implicated in post-transcriptional regulation of DNA polymerases and directly affect topoisomerases, modulating gene expression patterns.

b) Silibinin is a natural extract of a Mediterranean plant that has been shown to reduce miR-200c levels in NSCLC cells in vitro and in vivo.

c) VeriStrat uses mass spectrometry from a patient's tumor sample to predict outcomes with EGFR-TKI treatment.

d) Gene expression patterns (Gene signatures) have shown promising results in preclinical models, but need further prospective evaluation to show applicability in the clinical setting.

41. Choose the correct sentence:

a) The role for EGFR-targeted therapy as postoperative treatment has been clearly established.

b) Numerous phase III trials confirm the benefit of EGFR-TKI in the adjuvant setting.

c) Only retrospective cohort studies have been published with exclusively selected *EGFR* mutated tumors and adjuvant TKI therapy.

d) Currently, there are no phase II or phase III studies with surgically resected *EGFR* mutation-positive adenocarcinoma in process.

42. What reasons could explain the negative results of the SWOG 0023 and BR19 studies?

a) The population was not stratified by mutation status.

b) There was an incomplete accrual caused by a premature closure of the trial.

c) The study eligibility criteria were not based in specific clinical characteristics.

d) a, b and c are correct.

43. The analyses of retrospective cohorts series of *EGFR*-mutated patients with resected stage I-III NSCLC have shown that:

a) An improved DFS was observed in patients who received perioperative TKI therapy compared to those who did not.

b) Patients who were treated with erlotinib or gefitinib achieved a significant benefit in OS.

c) OS was improved in the mutation positive subgroup compared with patients who did not have *EGFR* mutation.

d) a and c are correct.

44. Which potential benefit of neoadjuvant treatment could be interesting to design clinical trials with EGFR-TKI?

a) It would permit to obtain quick information about sensibility of drugs using pathologic or radiologic criteria.

b) It would facilitate operation and resecability by reducing tumor size.

c) The early use of these drugs might be useful to attack micrometastatic disease.

d) All of them are correct.

45. Choose the incorrect sentence:

a) Some phase 2 and 3 trials support the use of EGFR-TKI as neoadjuvant therapy.
b) In studies with neoadjuvant EGFR-TKI, toxicity is usually mild.
c) In various phase II trials, partial responses after neoadjuvant EGFR-TKI are more common in *EGFR*-mutation positive patients.
d) Achieving a pathologic complete response after neoadjuvant treatment may predict better DFS and OS.

46. What of these mechanisms are not acquired resistant mechanisms to EGFR-TKI therapy in *EGFR* mutant tumours?

a) *MET* amplification.
b) Small-cell transformation.
c) BIM polymorphisms.
d) HGF overexpression.

47. About T790M is true that:

a) As acquired resistance mechanism confers bad prognosis in *EGFR* mutant patients.
b) Its prevalence as acquired mechanism is approximately 80%.
c) In clinic, irreversible EGFR-TKIs at conventional doses have shown higher activity against T790M mutation.
d) Any of the above is correct.

48. What is false about *MET* amplification?

a) As a mechanism of acquired resistance is a by-pass mechanism.
b) In 80% of patients with *MET* amplification as AR to EGFR-TKI coexists with T790M mutation.
c) Concomitant inhibition of EGFR and MET pathway would be required to overcome EGFR-TKI resistance in *EGFR* mutant patients.
d) a and d are correct.

49. About phenotypic transformation as acquired resistant to EGFR-TKI therapy in *EGFR* mutant patients is true that:

a) Activation of AXL tyrosine kinase receptor may mediate the acquisition of an EMT phenotype in EGFR-TKI resistant patients.
b) Phenotypic transformation is the most common mechanism of acquired resistance to EGFR-TKI therapy in *EGFR* mutant patients.
c) The histologic shift to small cell transformation does not maintain the original *EGFR* mutation and is resistant to conventional chemotherapy for small-cell carcinoma.
d) All of the above is correct.

50. Other additional genetic alterations in EGFR mutant patients with acquired resistant to EGFR-TKI are all except one:

a) PTEN mutation
b) Stem-cell properties acquisition
c) MAPK1 amplification
d) RET fusion

51. The Jackman criteria distinguish:

a) Patients with a high sensitivity to chemotherapy.

b) The sensibility to EGFR-TKI according to race.
c) The sensibility of tumor cells to combinations of chemotherapy and EGFR-TKI.
d) Primary from acquired resistance to EGFR-TKI.

52. Yang et al. reported three clinical modes of EGFR-TKI failure:
a) Dramatic, generalized, and total mode.
b) Stochastic, eventual, and chronic mode.
c) Dramatic, gradual, and local mode.
d) Initial, early, and late mode.

53. Sensitizing *EGFR*-mutations are less common in:
a) Female patients.
b) Elderly patients.
c) Former-smokers.
d) Current-smokers.

54. Combinations of chemotherapy and EGFR-TKI:
a) Have been proven safe and effective in the whole EGFR-population.
b) Only work in Asian patients.
c) Imply a continuous intake of EGFR-TKI.
d) Have been proven with short pulses of EGFR-TKI.

55. Local salvage therapies:
a) Have no application in metastatic patients.
b) Have to be applied over brain metastases only.
c) Include acupuncture followed by TKI-maintenance.
d) Are effective in selected patients and allowed TKI-maintenance.

56. Accordingly to data from a prior substudy, pemetrexed plus chemotherapy is being tested in a selected population of platinum-resistant ovarian cancer. Which subset of patients is included?
a) HER2 FISH positive ovarian cancer tumors.
b) Low-grade serous ovarian cancer tumors.
c) Mucinous ovarian cancer tumors.
d) Low HER3 mRNA serum levels in ovarian epithelial carcinoma.

57. The incidence of EGFR over-expression in squamous cell carcinoma of head and neck is:
a) 50-60%.
b) 80-90%.
c) 30-40%.
d) 60-70%.

58. Regarding to squamous cell carcinoma of head and neck, cetuximab is approved in?
a) Locally advanced disease in combination with radiotherapy.
b) Locally advanced disease in combination with radiotherapy and cisplatin.
c) Locally advanced disease in combination with radiotherapy and recurrent/metastatic disease in combination with platinum-based therapy.
d) Recurrent/metastatic disease with any chemotherapy.

59. Which EGFR-TKI has demonstrated efficacy after failure to platinum-based therapy and progression during cetuximab therapy in recurrent/metastatic disease?

a) Gefitinib.
b) Lapatinib.
c) Erlotinib.
d) Afatinib.

60. Which of the following statements is not true for trastuzumab?

a) Trastuzumab is a recombinant, monoclonal IgG-class humanized antibody.
b) Concurrent treatment with anthracycline has been associated higher rate of cardiac toxicity.
c) Trastuzumab has shown to be active in metastatic breast cancer both as single agent and in combination with chemotherapy.
d) All of the above are true.

61. The HERNATA study:

a) The study compared weekly trastuzumab and paclitaxel with vinorelbine plus trastuzumab.
b) The median time to progression in the vinorelbine arm was inferior to the control arm.
c) There was no differences in term of response rate or overall survival in both groups.
d) The toxicity profile did not favor the vinorelbine regimen.

62. In the neoadjuvant scenario, one of these statements is not true relating to pCR:

a) The addition of trastuzumab to conventional chemotherapy has shown to increase pCR rates.
b) The dual blockade with pertuzumab and trastuzumab was superior to trastuzumab plus docetaxel and superior to pertuzumab plus docetaxel in the NeoSphere study.
c) In the NeoShpere study the chemotherapy-free arm achieved a pCR of 30%.
d) In the NeoALTTO trial no significant difference in pCR rates was seen between the lapatinib and trastuzumab arms.

63. About the CLEOPATRA trial:

a) The study did not meet its primary endpoint.
b) More than 800 patients were randomized to receive as first line therapy either placebo plus trastuzumab plus docetaxel or lapatinib plus trastuzumab plus docetaxel.
c) PFS in the experimental arm was numerically superior to control arm but the differences did not achieve statistical significance.
d) The experimental arm showed to be superior in terms of PFS, response rate and OS.

64. In the last decade several anti-HER2 agents have been developed with different mechanisms of action. Which of the following is true?

a) Unlike lapatinib, neratinib is a reversible TK inhibitor of HER2 and HER1.
b) Lapatinib is a monoclonal IgG humanized antibody.

c) T-DM1 is an antibody-drug conjugate (ADC) consisting of the recombinant HER2 monoclonal antibody trastuzumab conjugated to the maytansinoid DM1 via a nonreducible thioether linkage (MCC).
d) Pertuzumab is a dual and reversible tyrosine kinase inhibitor.

65. One of these anti-HER2 drugs is approved for the treatment of gastroesophageal junction cancer.

a) Erlotinib.
b) Lapatinib.
c) Panitumumab.
d) Trastuzumab.

66. Cetuximab is indicated to treat?

a) *KRAS* mutant *NRAS* wild-type colon cancer.
b) *KRAS* mutant *NRAS* mutant colon cancer.
c) *KRAS* wild-type *NRAS* wild-type colon cancer.
d) KRAS wild-type NRAS mutant colon cancer.

67. One of these drugs is approved in combination with gemcitabine for the first-line treatment of advanced pancreatic cancer?

a) Gefitinib.
b) Cetuximab.
c) Trastuzumab.
d) Erlotinib.

68. One of these drugs is not approved for the treatment of metastatic colon cancer?

a) Panitumumab.
b) Cetuximab.
c) Bevacizumab.
d) Trastuzumab.

69. The epidermal growth factor receptor is overexpressed in?

a) Colo-rectal cancer.
b) Gastric cancer.
c) Pancreatic cancer.
d) All of them.

Answers:

1. c
2. d
3. c
4. a
5. d
6. b
7. d
8. b
9. c
10. d
11. d
12. d
13. c

14. b
15. a
16. c
17. d
18. c
19. d
20. b
21. c
22. b
23. b
24. b
25. d
26. d
27. c
28. d
29. b
30. d
31. b
32. a
33. a
34. d
35. c
36. c
37. d
38. b
39. c
40. d
41. c
42. d
43. d
44. d
45. a
46. c
47. d
48. b
49. a
50. d
51. d
52. c
53. d
54. c
55. d
56. d
57. b
58. c
59. d

60. d
61. c
62. c
63. d
64. c
65. d
66. c
67. d
68. d
69. d

Index

A

B

C

D

E

F

G

H

I

J

K

L

M

N

O

P

Q

R

S

T

U

V

W

X

Y